TOXOPLASMOSIS – RECENT ADVANCES

Edited by **Olgica Djurkovic Djakovic**

Toxoplasmosis – Recent Advances
http://dx.doi.org/10.5772/2845
Edited by Olgica Djurkovic Djakovic

Contributors

Emmanuelle Gilot-Fromont, Maud Lélu, Marie-Laure Dardé, Céline Richomme, Dominique Aubert, Eve Afonso, Aurélien Mercier, Cécile Gotteland, Isabelle Villena, Branko Bobić, Ivana Klun, Aleksandra Nikolić, Olgica Djurković-Djaković, Eva Bartova, Kamil Sedlak, Lenka Luptakova, Eva Petrovova, David Mazensky, Alexandra Valencakova, Pavol Balent, Vladimir Ivović, Marija Vujanić, Tijana Živković, Pikka Jokelainen, Jean Dupouy-Camet, Hana Talabani, Emmanuelle Delair, Florence Leslé, HélèneYera, Antoine P. Brézin, Lílian M.G. Bahia-Oliveira, Alba L.P. Rangel, Marcela S.B. Boechat, Bianca M. Mangiavacchi, Livia M. Martins, Francielle B. Ferraz, Maycon B. Almeida, Elisa M. Waked Peixoto, Flavia P. Vieira, Ricardo G. Peixe, Yoshiaki Shimada

Published by InTech

Janeza Trdine 9, 51000 Rijeka, Croatia

Publishing Process Manager Vedran Greblo
Technical Editor InTech Prepress, Novi Sad
Cover InTech Design team

Additional hard copies can be obtained from orders@intechopen.com

Toxoplasmosis – Recent Advances, Edited by Olgica Djurkovic Djakovic
p. cm.
ISBN 978-953-51-0746-0

For EU product safety concerns:
IN TECH d.o.o., Prolaz Marije Krucifikse Kozulić 3, 51000 Rijeka, Croatia,
info@intechopen.com or visit our website at intechopen.com.

Meet the editor

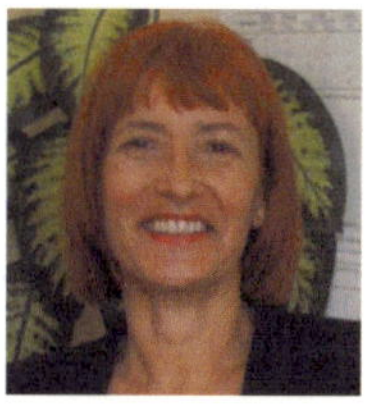

Dr Olgica Djurković-Djaković received both her medical degree and her PhD from the University of Belgrade, Serbia (then Yugoslavia), where she has pursued a scientific career ever since. Her research interest involves parasitic zoonoses, focusing on Toxoplasma gondii infection, a field in which she has published extensively. She is currently Head of the Centre of Excellence for Toxoplasmosis and Medical Entomology at the University of Belgrade Institute for Medical Research and Head of the Serbian Reference Laboratory for Toxoplasmosis. Dr Djurković-Djaković is also President of the Serbian Society of Parasitologists.

Contents

Preface

During a time span of more than a century since its recognition, the protozoan parasite *Toxoplasma gondii* has never seized to fascinate researchers. A ubiquitous organism able to infect all mammals and birds, that has been estimated to infect one third of the global human population, deserves as much. Recognized in the early days as an agent affecting the fetus, the clinical focus has moved with the advent of AIDS and increased use of treatments with immunosuppressive effect, to toxoplasmosis as an opportunistic infection, and in the recent years back again to the long known ocular disease, this time as a consequence of acquired as much as congenital disease. Developments were always associated with the use of the leading methodologies of the times, currently embodied in the penetration of molecular biology methods into medicine and microbiology, which allowed for studies of *T. gondii* and the infection it induces at the genomic level. In addition, *T. gondii* owes part of its popularity to being a very desirable model of intracellular infection quite easy to grow in the lab, offering the possibility to study various immunological, biochemical, cell biology and other aspects and providing a wealth on data on immune control, host-parasite relationship, etc. It is thus not surprising that the centenary of *T. gondii* presented an inspiration for a number of texts and books overviewing both the biology of the organism and the clinics of the disease it causes. In this regard, it is hard to find a niche for yet another book on toxoplasmosis. However, any effort on compiling a series of essays stands witness to its moment in the history of knowledge development, and offers its readers, specialist or not, a view on the current achievements and research interests.

A current approach to this zoonosis is the concept of „one health“, based on the understanding that a disease occurring between animals and man in a specific environment can only be dealt with at the interface of all „players“ involved. The structure of this book follows this concept, in that it integrates human and animal data in its respective parts. The book is opened by a formidable chapter on factors affecting the dynamics of the *T. gondii* life cycle, in which Gilot-Fromont and colleagues describe how these elements shape the spatial and temporal variability of the epidemiological dynamics, and conclude on the evolutionary and medical implications of these variations.

In line with the „one health“ concept, this part is continued by a review (Chapter 2) of both the epidemiology and the epizootiology of toxoplasmosis in South-East Europe.

Bobić and colleagues review the data published in this region in the past two decades, showing that a prevention effort requires concerted action on the animal, human and environmental side, thereby illustrating on real facts the need for a complex and unified approach advocated in Chapter 1.

The issue of epizootiology introduced by Bobić and colleagues is subject of the following two contributions, which review the current data on *T. gondii* infection in animals in the Chech Republic and Slovakia, respectively. Whereas Bartova and colleagues (Chapter 3) offer a comprehensive review of *T. gondii* infection in farm, wild and zoo animals in the Chech Republic in the last decade, in Chapter 4 Luptakova and colleagues overview their own data on toxoplasmosis in animals in Slovakia, focusing on the diagnostic methods available and discussing their advantages and pitfalls.

Part 2 is devoted to molecular epidemiology. Chapter 5 involves a text by Ivović and colleagues on the use of molecular methods for the diagnosis of toxoplasmosis, focusing on their advantages and limitations, as well as for the genotyping of strains isolated from clinical samples, providing data on the molecular epidemiology of *T. gondii* in Serbia.

The next chapter (Chapter 6) is an interesting text by P. Jokelainen, who shows that *T. gondii* strains of the most common pan-European genotype II may be, and have been, fatal for some of their animal hosts including mountain hares and foxes, in Finland but elsewhere in Europe as well. This is a good reminder that whereas insight into the parasite genotypes is expected to provide answers to many clinical questions, it is not the parasite genotype but the interplay and balance between the parasite and its host, with its different immunological responses, genetics etc., that determines the outcome of infection.

Part 3 concerns important clinical issues of toxoplasmosis. Chapter 7 is an authoritative account by Jean Dupouy-Camet and colleagues on the epidemiology of ocular toxoplasmosis as the major *T. gondii* induced clinical entity, occurring as an early or late consequence of acquired as much as of congenital disease. This relatively novel concept changes our view of acquired infection, making a strong case for the prevention of acquired infection in the general population.

Ocular toxoplasmosis in the particular setting of Brazil is further explored in Chapter 8 by Bahia-Oliveira and colleagues. As known to those familiar with the current literature, toxoplasmosis seems to be an entirely different disease in Brazil. Initially recognized after hydric epidemics, insight into strain differences at the molecular level provided explanation for the significant clinical differences observed in Brazil vs. elsewhere. Bahia-Oliveira and colleagues further explore the multifactorial nature of ocular toxoplasmosis, and based on own research on clinical, immunological and genetic parameters in a large patient series in an endemic area, propose a novel clinical classification of retinochoroidal scars in epidemiological surveys.

The book is concluded by a text on so-called pseudo-toxoplasmosis (Chapter 9), in which Shimada overviews i.e. genetic disorders causing clinical symptoms that can be initially mis-diagnosed for toxoplasmosis and in which toxoplasmosis should be ruled out in the differential diagnosis. One such case published by the author is here discussed in the light of other entities that may mimick toxoplasmosis, focusing on specific methods and examinations needed to distinguish between the two.

Dr. Olgica Djurković-Djaković
National Reference Laboratory for Toxoplasmosis
Centre of Excellence in Biomedicine
Institute for Medical Research, University of Belgrade
Serbia

Section 1

Epidemiology and Epizootiology

Chapter 1

The Life Cycle of *Toxoplasma gondii* in the Natural Environment

Emmanuelle Gilot-Fromont, Maud Lélu, Marie-Laure Dardé, Céline Richomme, Dominique Aubert, Eve Afonso, Aurélien Mercier, Cécile Gotteland and Isabelle Villena

Additional information is available at the end of the chapter

http://dx.doi.org/10.5772/48233

1. Introduction

Toxoplasma gondii (*T. gondii*) is considered as one of the most successful parasites in the world. This success is first illustrated by its worldwide distribution, from arctic to hot desert areas, including isolated islands and in cities [1]. *T. gondii* is also among the most prevalent parasites in the global human population, with around one third of the population being infected [2]. Finally, it is able to infect, or be present in, the highest number of host species: any warm-blooded animal may act as an intermediate host, and oocysts may be transported by invertebrates such as filtrating mussels and oysters [1, 3].

Beyond this ubiquitous distribution lies a fascinating transmission pattern: simply saying that *T. gondii* has a complex life cycle does not encompass all transmission routes and modes that can be used by the parasite to pass from definitive hosts (DHs), where sexual reproduction occurs, to intermediate hosts (IHs). The "classical" complex life cycle uses felids (domestic and wild-living cats) as DHs and their prey as IHs (Figure 1). Felids are infected by eating infected prey and host the sexual multiplication of the parasite. They excrete millions of oocysts that sporulate in the environment. Sporulated oocysts may survive during several years and may disperse through water movements, soil movements and microfauna. Ingesting a single sporulated oocyst may be sufficient to infect an IH and begin the asexual reproduction phase [1]. This classical life cycle thus relies on a prey-predator relationship and on environmental contamination, like other parasites, e.g., *Echinococcus multilocularis* [4].

However, beside this classical cycle, *T. gondii* shows specific abilities that allow it to use "complementary" transmission routes (Figure 1). During the phase of asexual multiplication, tachyzoites may disseminate to virtually any organ within the IH, in particular to muscles, brain, placenta, udder and gonads. Asexual forms are then infectious to new hosts, thus direct infection among IH is possible by several routes which epidemiological importance has to be discussed: vertical transmission through the placenta, pseudo-vertical transmission through the milk, and sexual transmission through the sperm [1, 5, 6]. In humans, *T. gondii* may also be transmitted during blood or organ transplant. Finally, the infectivity of asexual forms towards new IHs entails the ability for the parasite to be transmitted among IHs by carnivory. This transmission route is estimated to cause the majority of cases in humans [7], although people may also get contaminated by ingesting oocysts after a contact with contaminated soil, water, vegetables or cat litter. All the possible transmission routes among IH make the parasite able to maintain its life cycle, at least during a few generations, in the absence of DH and without environmental stage [8]. Moreover, at a high dose, oocysts from the environment may also be infectious for DHs [9], thus the parasite may bypass the IH and use a DHs-environment cycle. The infectivity of oocysts towards cats is relatively low thus the importance of this cycle may be questioned [10]. However, taken together, these observations suggest that *T. gondii* may theoretically have two distinct life cycles, one among IHs and the other one between DHs and environment.

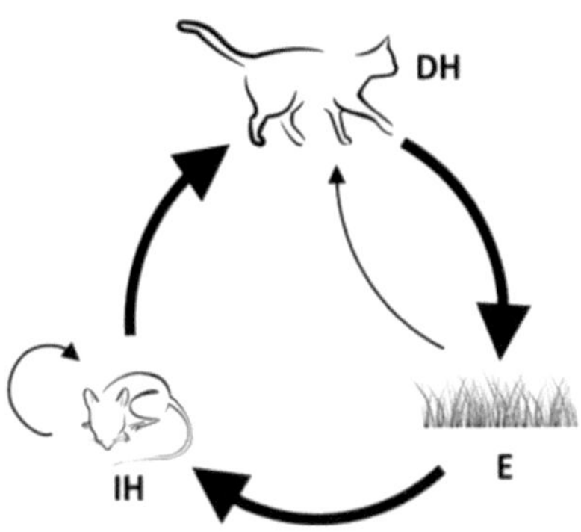

Figure 1. Life cycle of *Toxoplasma gondii*: the "classical" life cycle between intermediate hosts (IH, rodents), definitive hosts (DH, felids) and environment (E, soil) is represented with large arrows, while the "complementary" transmission routes (vertical or horizontal transmission among IHs and environment-to-cat transmission) are represented with small arrows.

Moreover, in IHs, the infection of the brain results in several specific clinical manifestations, modifications of host behaviour and life history that influence transmission. As a result of its presence in the brain of IHs, *T. gondii* manipulates host behaviour in two ways, by specifically increasing attractiveness of cat odours to rodent IHs, thus favouring transmission from IH to DH [5, 11], and by increasing the sexual attractiveness of infected males, which favours sexual transmission [6].

These numerous capacities of transmission clearly allow *T. gondii* to be distributed worldwide. However, this does not mean that the risk of toxoplasmosis is identical everywhere. On the contrary, a highly structured pattern of infection can be demonstrated, for example by comparing the level of infection of different human populations. Among countries, nationwide seroprevalences in women of childbearing age vary from less than 10% to more than 60% [12]. Within countries, a strong variability is also present: in France, the incidence of *T. gondii* varies from 1 to 68 cases per 1000 pregnancies among the 22 metropolitan regions [13]. Finally, spatial heterogeneity is also present at a more local scale, for example among districts within a region, and up to the level of families: within a village, individuals of the same family tended to have identical serological status [14]. Due to this heterogeneous distribution, the burden of toxoplasmosis and the associated socio-economic cost are unevenly distributed. Elucidating the causes of this distribution of *T. gondii* is necessary to improve prevention. However, this proves to be a difficult task, as the variability of parasite prevalence may reflect variations in many aspects of the life cycle. For example, considering the "classical" cat-environment-prey life cycle, the transmission from IH to DH likely depends on the level of predation of DHs on IHs, thus on the presence and densities of DHs and IHs, as well as on the diet of DHs. The survival of oocysts is influenced by temperature, moisture and UV radiation, thus should be determined by the meteorological conditions prevailing in the area, while dispersal depends on soil and water movements, as well as on the accumulation in invertebrates. The complementary routes of infection depend on the presence of omnivorous species (carnivory), the population dynamics of IH populations (vertical transmission) and the social structure (sexual and milk transmission).

In this chapter we aim to provide a comprehensive overview of factors that are recognized or can be expected to determine *T. gondii* dynamics in animal populations and in the environment, which constitute the reservoir of human infection, *i.e.*, a set of epidemiologically connected populations and environments in which the pathogen can be permanently maintained and from which infection is transmitted to the defined target population [15]. Although the risk for people is largely due to the quality and intensity of their contacts with this reservoir, here we only deal with variations of the cycle in the environment and in animals. We summarize which mechanisms are now established and identify areas where data are lacking. We first show that the dynamics of the life cycle varies according to the relative densities of IHs and DHs, in particular along the urban-rural-wild gradient. Then we detail the variations observed in each of these environments at different spatial scales, and the factors that have been found to influence transmission dynamics. We conclude on how the variations described here should affect human exposure and should be considered for prevention.

2. The urban- rural-wild gradient

The life cycle of *T. gondii* is dependent on populations of IHs and DHs, and on the level of predation between them. These ecological determinants are themselves dependent on their environment. Because humans exert a major influence on the structure of their environment, the first structuration of these IH-DH communities comes from the urbanization gradient. We first explicit how IHs and DHs populations vary along this gradient before detailing how these variations affect the dynamics of *T. gondii*.

2.1. Host densities and predation rates vary along a urbanization gradient

Taking advantage of a high adaptability and following human migrations, the domestic cat *Felis catus* has colonized a wide variety of habitats, ranging from urban areas to non-anthropized islands, through, agricultural areas, arid or semi-arid areas, villages or cities, from polar to equatorial climatic regions [16]. However, due to the behavioural plasticity of this species, population density and structure vary, depending on the abundance and distribution of food resources and shelters [16, 17]. In particular, cat populations are structured differently along an urban-rural-non-anthropized ("wild") gradient (Figure 2). The highest densities of cats are found in urban populations of stray cats locally more than 1000 cats/ km^2 [18, 19]. At these high densities, cats form large multimale–multifemale social groups and share their territory, as well as available resources [16]. Most resources are provided directly or not, by people (feeders, garbage) [19]. In rural areas, population density is moderate (100-300 cats/ km^2) [20, 21, 22]. Most cats have an owner who provides food and shelter but cats are generally free to roam [23]. An important part of cats diet result from predation: 15 to 90% depending on cat lifestyle [24, 16]. In rural areas, the spatial distribution of cats is based on human settlements: the social groups are based on a house or farm that provides most of the feeding and nesting resources. Around a feeding point, cats may form groups of up to 20 individuals, often constituted by related females and their kittens [16]. In fact, in such areas, a gradient can be observed between pet-owned cats mostly fed by the owner, to farm cats and feral cats mostly living on predation. Finally, feral cats occupying non-anthropized areas (sub-Antarctic, arid or forested areas), survive exclusively through predation, live at low density (1 to 10 cats/ km^2), in large and non-overlapping home ranges [25, 26].

Rodent densities also vary along the urban-rural-wild gradient (Figure 2). However, comparisons are not straightforward since many species are concerned and most of them are not present in all environments. The available estimates suggest that some species may live at very high densities in agricultural landscapes: for example, common voles *Microtus arvalis* and water voles *Arvicola terrestris* may reach 100 000 individuals/km^2 [27]. In contrast, in urban areas, the density of wood mice *Apodemus sylvaticus* was estimated to lie around 2 000 - 8 000 mice/km^2 [28, 29].

The third parameter that varies along the urban-rural-wild gradient is the rate of predation of rodents by cats, *i.e.*, how many rodents does a cat ingest per unit of time. This parameter is crucial for the transmission of *T. gondii* from IH to DH: combined with the prevalence in prey, it determines the risk for a cat to get infected. The importance of the predation rate is illustrated by the finding that cats with frequent outdoor access show higher predation rates [16] and higher prevalences than cats not allowed to roam [30, 31, 32, 33, 34]. The predation rate depends on the availability of rodents, *i.e.*, on the density of rodents relative to cats, and on the availability of other food resources provided by people. The predation rate is lowest in urban populations, ranging from 10 to 27 prey/cat/year [35, 36, 37]. For suburban and rural sites, estimated values for predation rates range from 21 to 436 prey/cat/year [10, 24, 38, 39]. Finally, the predation rate should be highest in non-anthropized areas, where cat exclusively live on predation.

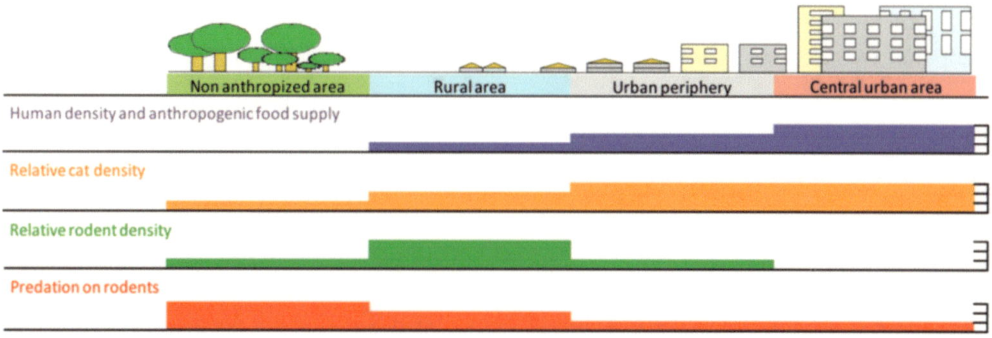

Figure 2. Variations of human density and anthropogenic food supply, cat density, rodent density and predation along an urban-rural-wild gradient. The magnitude of the bars represents the relative importance of each factor according to the degree of urbanization (modified from [4]).

Because of these variations of three key parameters of *T. gondii* cycle (densities of DHs and IHs, and predation rate), one can hypothesize that the dynamics of *T. gondii* should vary qualitatively and quantitatively along the urban-rural-wild gradient, following the specific features regarding *T. gondii* transmission in each environment. Urban areas, at least in the limited areas where cats live, support the highest densities of DHs. However, in cities, rodent densities are relatively low and predation rate is low due to the availability of anthropogenic food resources. The transmission through predation is not expected to be favoured in this case, but the DH-environment cycle should be maximized. On the contrary, in the wild environment, the level of predation of cats on rodents is maximal, but cat density is low, thus transmission should occur only by predation. Finally, rural areas combine intermediate to high values of IH and DH density, with high predation rates. Thus these may be the most favourable for the transmission of *T. gondii* [40]. This transmission should occur largely through "classical" IH-DH transmission, but transmissions among IHs and through a possible DH-environment cycle should also be possible in this case.

2.2. Variations in *T. gondii* dynamics along the urban-rural-wild gradient

The hypothesis that the dynamics of *T. gondii* transmission varies along the urban-rural gradient has been tested through a theoretical approach, using an epidemiological model [10]. The aim was to estimate the contributions of the IH-DH and DH-environment cycles in the spread of *T. gondii* according to the predation rate, with stable cat population size. The modelling approach allowed the authors to compare populations differing only by the rate of predation, all else being equal. The model first confirmed that the rural environment (here defined as having predation rates above 21 prey/cat per year [35, 36] is favourable for *T. gondii*, as transmission increases with the predation rate [10]. Seroprevalences predicted for cats ranged from 33.2 to 83.4% in the rural environment *vs.* 6.9 to 33.2% in urban areas. Moreover, in rural-type areas, the contribution of the IH-DH cycle increases with the predation rate, and may reach 70% of the transmission (Figure 3). The DH-environment cycle may theoretically be responsible for more than 50% of the transmission, but only in extremes cases with predation rates lower than 9 prey/cat/yr (Figure 3). It is noteworthy that the predicted prey seroprevalences, from 2.4 to 5 % along the gradient, was always low compared to the magnitude of cat seroprevalences.

The cat serological prevalences predicted by [10] agree with values observed along the urban rural gradient: when natural populations (as opposed to heterogeneous samples constituted from veterinary clinics or facilities) are considered, seroprevalences are clearly lower in urban (between 15 % to 26% [41, 33, 34, 42, 43]) than in rural areas (48% to 87.3% [44, 30, 45, 32, 42]). They also reach high values in non–anthropized areas: 51% in Kerguelen island [46]. In rodents, prevalence is generally low (0 – 10% [47, 46]), which renders comparisons difficult. High seroprevalences have been occasionally reported in brown rats (70% in Italy [48]) and in house mice (59% in rural and sub-urban areas in England [49]). However, these limited data do not permit to draw a clear pattern among environments in rodents. Interestingly, the usually low rodent seroprevalences are in accordance with predictions of the model [10]. The model also suggested that cat seroprevalence is less dependent on prey seroprevalence than on predation rates and prey availability. Thus obtaining accurate estimate of these two last parameters should be more important to understand *T. gondii* epidemiology than estimating rodent seroprevalence.

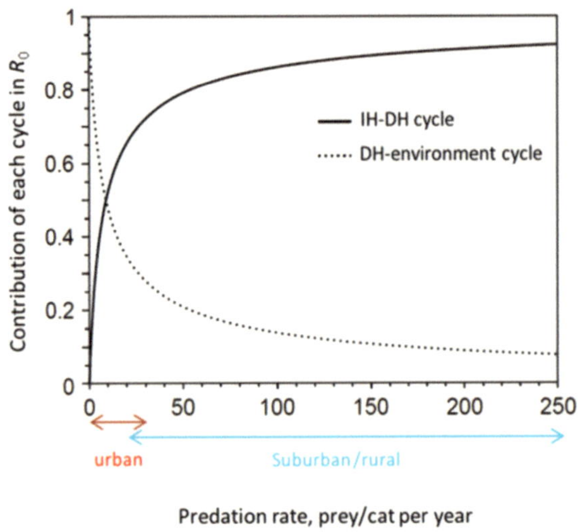

Figure 3. *Contributions of the DH-Environment and IH-DH cycles in the basic reproductive rate* R_0 *of T. gondii according to the predation rate of IHs by DHs. Predation rates below 27 prey/cat per year represent urban areas, values above 21 prey/cat per year represent rural areas. Modified with permission from* [10].

The last way to compare environments would be to compare the levels of soil contamination among environments. However, estimating the level of environmental contamination requires information on the number of new infections in cats (incidence) through longitudinal studies. Based on serological follow-up of cats, incidence was estimated to 0.26-0.39 infections/cat per year in three rural populations located in France [32]. Incidence was also estimated in one urban site (0.17 infections/cat/year [50]) and in one population living in a non-anthropized environment [46], using the age-seroprevalence relationship. Using data on oocyst shedding, Dabritz *et al.* [51, 52] estimated that 0.04 infections could occur per cat-year in cats recruited through local veterinarians in coastal cities in California (USA).

Incidences estimates may be combined to local cat densities, in order determine the number of infection that could occur each year in a given site. In urban sites, even if incidence is low, very high densities of cats lead to expect a high number of infections: 165 infections per km^2 per year could occur in the dense population studied by Afonso *et al.* [41, 50]. In rural sites where cats live in density varying between 120 and 200 cats per km^2, [32] estimated that 31 to 72 infections per km^2 per year could occur. In Kerguelen, where incidence is high but density is only 1-3 cats/km^2, the number of new cases per year would be only around 1/km^2/year. Based on the assumption that primary infected cats shed between 1 and 50 millions of potentially infectious oocysts in the environment, oocyst burden may be estimated in each case, as was proposed for rural populations [32]. The results of the cited studies are summarized in Table 1, to give a range of possible estimates for oocyst burden. This may be compared to the estimate from a recent study on owned cats living in coastal California: [51] estimated that the annual burden of oocysts in the environment ranged between 94 and 4671 oocysts/m^2.

The urban-rural-wild gradient is thus a key determinant of the *T. gondii* dynamics. The general level of transmission varies along this gradient, rural areas being particularly favourable for *T. gondii* transmission. Moreover, the relative importance of different transmission routes is not equivalent along this gradient. In particular, the DH-environment cycle may become significant at very low levels of predation rate, especially in urban areas. These variations are expected to influence the risk for other target species, and especially for people, to get infected. In particular, generally speaking, the level of soil contamination is expected to be highest in the areas where urban feral cats are concentrated, and lowest in the wild environment. However, with each environment, spatial and temporal heterogeneities are present. They will be detailed in the following paragraphs.

Population	Kerguelen (Non-anthropized)	Aimargues, Saint-Just Chaleyssin, Barisey (Rural)	Lyon Croix-Rousse (Urban)
Seroprevalence in cats (%)	36.2 – 55.0	47.4 – 55.1	18.6
Incidence in cats (number of new infections/cat/year)	0.28 – 0.65	0.26 – 0.39	0.17
Number of new cat infections/km^2	0.66 – 1.3	31 - 72	165
Oocyst burden (number deposited /year/m2)	17 - 33	775 - 1800	4125

Table 1. Estimated levels of contamination by oocysts in five populations located in different environments. The table summarizes the studies of one population in a non-anthropized island (2 study sites) [46], three rural populations [32] and one urban population [41]. Oocyst burdens are estimated considering that an infected cat produces 25 millions oocysts.

3. Urban toxoplasmosis

Urban landscapes are characterized by highly fragmented natural or semi-natural habitats resulting in a mosaic of patches varying in size and quality. Dispersal abilities of animal species between patches are generally affected by roads or by distance to the nearest patches [53, 54]. Many animal species are thus restricted to parks, artificial forest fragments or recreation areas [55]. This results in local extinctions, increased local population density, or social disturbance. Natural populations of domestic cats are present in urban areas in various sites including hospital gardens [56], parks [57, 58], cemeteries or squares [59], taking advantage of the abundance of shelters, food wastes linked to human activity or food provided by cat lovers [59, 17, 54]. Densities regularly exceed 250 cats per km^2 [16], and can reach up to 2000 cats per km^2 like in urban parks in Italy [58].

In urban areas, rodent densities are heterogeneous and generally strongly related to vegetation cover, predation pressure [29], and/or on how the presence of rodents is controlled by trapping or poisoning. For example, the density of field mouse *Apodemus sp.* can range from no individual in areas occupied by dense populations of predators, to 20,000 individuals per km^2 in isolated patches [28, 29]. Communities of small mammals can persist at high density in small habitat patches sparsely settled by predators [28]. It is therefore unlikely that cat and IHs populations coexist at high densities in the same habitat patches. In addition, urban cats are attracted by food provided by humans, easily accessible all over the year, and that requires no effort of predation. The presence of such a resource can reduce the motivation to hunt in cats [16, 59]. Observations made on urban cats in hunting activity are thus rare in such areas [41]. The altered predator-prey dynamics limits IH-HD *T. gondii* transmission, however toxoplasmosis does occur in urban hosts. Most surveys conducted in stray cats show low prevalences ranging from 5 to 20% [60, 61, 62, 41]. However, high values have occasionally been found: 35.4% in Sao Paolo [62], 51.9 Barcelona [63], 70.2 in Ghent, Belgium [64]. These cases may correspond to areas where cats have access to predation.

The high local densities of cats also entail a high local level of environmental contamination by *T. gondii* oocysts. Beside density, in such areas, cats often use the same place to defecate where they burry or expose their faeces as scent marks [16, 65], and a single location may be used by several cats when cat density is high [66]. Moreover, this behaviour is expected to favour the direct contamination of cats by oocysts while defecating, since oocyst load in defecating areas is extremely high, and cats are exposed through scratching the soil, before cleaning their paws and fur. These defecation sites spread over cat territory cumulate a high concentration of oocysts in areas closed to humans. A study of a cat population living in the Croix-Rousse hospital (Lyon, France) showed that defecation sites were the areas most often found to be positive for *T. gondii* DNA, and may be viewed as hot spots of environmental risk to humans [50]. Similarly, in Poland and in China, contaminated soil samples have been found in public parks and sand pits [67, 68]. Contact with soil, and particularly gardening and consumption of raw vegetables have been demonstrated to be significant risk factors for toxoplasmosis in humans [69, 7, 70]. Contact with defecation sites is thus expected to result in a high risk of infection, but, because contaminated sites represent a low proportion of the area, only a few humans are likely to be directly exposed. These persons include children playing in sand pits, persons feeding the cats, gardeners, maintenance workers in these sites and also dog owners who allow pets to roam in these sites and become indirectly exposed through contact with dogs [71, 67, 68].

Overall, toxoplasmosis in urban areas should be characterized by heterogeneous dynamics, with usually low levels of prevalence in cats, but locally high levels of soil contamination, which may favour the environment-DH cycle.

4. Heterogeneity in the rural environment

Rural areas, and in particular agricultural landscapes, are suitable for *T. gondii* transmission, due to the high densities of both DHs and IHs [72], and to the high level of predation. However, this does not mean that rural areas are evenly infected. Spatial and temporal variations have been detected at several scales. We first present the temporal dynamics to identify mechanisms of heterogeneity that may also explain spatial variations.

4.1. Temporal dynamics

A temporal variability in the dynamics of *T. gondii* life cycle has been detected, both at the year-to-year level and between seasons. It is first important to notice that temporal variability is uneasy to study using serological data, because of the lifelong persistence of antibodies. In long-lived species, temporal variations in the rate of appearance of new cases (incidence) may be masked by the persistence of antibodies. The easiest ways to study temporal dynamics of *T. gondii* should be to consider short-lived species, species where antibody response does not persist lifelong, individual serological follow-up, or to consider indicators of acute infection, *i.e.*, type M immunoglobulins or oocyst excretion in cats.

Due to the difficulty to organize long-term surveys, year-to-year variations have been found in a few populations only: in roe deer *Capreolus capreolus* in Spain [73] and in Sweden [74], in red deer *Cervus elaphus* in Scotland [75], as well as in Canadian seals [76]. Tizard *et al.* [77] performed the largest survey to our knowledge, with nearly 12,000 persons studied over 14 years. This survey revealed inter-annual 6-year cycles and showed that year-to-year variations follow rainfall levels with a correlation coefficient as strong as 0.71. Accordingly, a longitudinal survey of rural populations of domestic cats in France showed important interannual variations in incidence among years, related to variations in the level of rainfall [32]. In an urban site, seroprevalence in cats was highest during years with a hot and moist weather or with a moderate and less moist weather [41]. The same trend was observed during a long-term follow-up of two populations of roe deer, with maximal seroprevalence under cold/dry, or cool/moist years [78].

The first explanation that has been proposed for the correlation between meteorological conditions and *T. gondii* dynamics involves the survival of oocysts. The free stage of *T. gondii* is subject to hard environmental conditions: in the terrestrial environment, its survival in soil depends on temperature and moisture. Oocyst survival is maximal (> 200 days) for temperatures comprised between -6°C and +20 °C [79]. Above +20°C, dessication of oocysts may occur [41, 80, 81], but moisture should prevent it [82, 83]. Under-6°C, the survival of oocysts is reduced and their capacity to sporulate is lost [79], although one may hypothesize that snow cover may protect them from cold. Meteorological variations are thus expected to determine the survival of oocysts. Oocyst survival has also been demonstrated as one of the parameters that most influence predictions given by a mathematical model [10]. However, other factors may also vary with meteorological conditions and influence *T. gondii* life cycle. In particular, the population dynamics of rodents is affected by climate-driven vegetation growth [84]. Specifically, when winter is mild, survival is high and rodent populations comprise many adult or old individuals, which are the age groups most often infected. Thus the risk of encountering an infected prey is expected to increase after mild winters [32]. This mechanism would contribute to the high transmission of *T. gondii* after mild winters, in combination with high oocyst survival.

Meteorological conditions are also expected to act at the seasonal level. Oocyst survival should be lowest during dry, hot summer periods, and during very cold winters. Moreover, the population dynamics of hosts follows seasonal cycles: most births of rodents and cats occur in spring and summer. However, since many kittens carry maternal derived antibodies [41], the susceptible populations may increase in summer for rodents and in fall for cats. We thus propose the following pattern (Figure 4): in summer, the low survival of oocysts would lead to a low level of environmental contamination. However, the renewal of the pool of susceptible rodents at the same period may boost *T. gondii* transmission. The proportion of infected rodents would increase during summer and fall, thus increasing the risk for cats to get infected. During fall and winter, kittens would have a maximal risk to get infected and excrete oocysts. Finally, in spring, most cats born during the previous year and highly exposed through hunting would have terminated their oocyst excretion thus the rate of soil contamination would decrease. However, due to the survival of oocysts, the prevalence in rodents would continue to rise, and would reach its maximal value at the beginning of spring when reproduction starts again, giving birth to naïve rodents. Following this scenario, the infection of domestic herbivores would increase at the end of fall and in winter, when cats excrete oocysts, specifically within farm buildings [85], but could continue up to the following spring, due to the high survival of oocysts. The risk for infection of people would thus be maximal in winter when oocyst contamination and herbivore infections are frequent, and may persist up to the following spring.

Because of the methodological difficulties presented above, many studies do not find any seasonal pattern [47], and few data come in support of this hypothesis. Tizard *et al.*, considering only high titres, found a clear decrease of human infections in fall [77]. This decrease was interpreted as a consequence of the dry summer period, corresponding to low oocyst survival. In Serbia, new infections occurred more often between October and April than the rest of the year [86]. A seasonal pattern was also found in the proportion of cat faeces presenting oocysts in Germany. Faeces collected between January and June (0.09%) were significantly less often infected than those collected during the second part of the year, between July and December (0.31%) [87]. These observations are concordant with the above

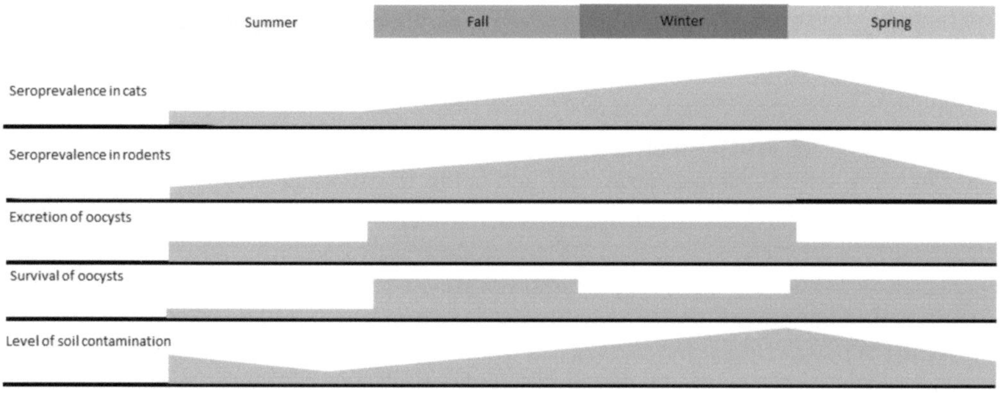

Figure 4. Possible seasonal pattern of the transmission of *T. gondii.*

scenario, however, more detailed data and/or a theoretical approach are needed to fully confirm the proposed pattern. Should this pattern be confirmed, the variability of risk with time should be taken into account for management and prevention recommendations.

4.2. Spatial heterogeneity

Spatial heterogeneity of the infection in the rural environment has been demonstrated both between regions and between areas within and around villages. Farm animals, being restrained to agricultural areas, are particularly relevant to analyse spatial heterogeneities of the circulation of *T. gondii*. However, studies concerning other species or humans may provide useful information when the studied processes concern farms as well as surrounding areas.

At the between-region scale, heterogeneity has essentially been shown to correlate with climatic variations. The hypothesis of relationships between humidity, temperature and *T. gondii* prevalence has been suggested in cattle in Serbia [88] and in sheep in Spain [89]: regions with high humidity and moderate temperatures are considered as most favourable for the sporulation and survival of oocysts. However, few data allowed authors to formally analyse these relationships in farm animals. When comparing the incidence of toxoplasmosis in rural cats living in three villages from distinct regions in France, Afonso *et al.* found that the difference between the villages was explained by their level of rainfall [32]. Other surveys, considering wild-living species and humans, are in accordance with the hypothesis of a climate-driven dynamics. Regional seroprevalences in woman in France vary with temperature: they increase when mean temperature increases, but decrease when the mean number of days below -5°C increases in the region [13]. In a national survey on the wild boar *Sus scrofa*, the number of 10-day periods below -6°C was also found as a determinant of *T. gondii* seroprevalence [90]. Still in the wild boar, in Corsica, prevalence was highest at high altitude, where rainfalls are abundant and temperatures are low [91]. Overall, these and previous results (4.1) underline the importance of climate and meteorological conditions in driving the temporal and spatial dynamics of *T. gondii*. These environmental conditions probably also act at a very local scale, for example to affect soil contamination in South-oriented versus North-oriented slopes, however this has not been studied.

Within villages, the spatial organization of host populations leads to heterogeneities of *T. gondii* between central villages, farm areas and fields. In particular, farm buildings and their surroundings, which shelter both cats and IHs, constitute an important source of infection for the surrounding areas. The spatial distribution of cases around a pig farm [72], and a mathematical modelling approach [92] both confirmed that farms represent a source for the whole rural environment. Farms also represent a source of infection for the surrounding wild areas: in Corsica, the seroprevalence in wild boar increased with the density of farms in the county [91].

Finally, the dynamics of *T. gondii* is also variable among farms. As expected, the presence of cats often determines the risk of a farm being infected [93, 94], thus cat control is a key to the control of toxoplasmosis in farms [95], as well as rodent control [96]. Other factors reported to influence *T. gondii* prevalence are related to herd management: size and isolation of herd, presence of a water point, type of feeding [97, 93]. These factors represent interesting control points [96].

Overall, the rural environment, and in particular farms and their surroundings, are a major source of infection, including for other areas. In particular, rural areas and farms are the gate for *T. gondii* to circulate between the wild and domestic environments, thus their spatial distribution, management and level of biosecurity are determinant in the possibility for *T. gondii* to mix domestic and sylvatic cycles.

5. A sylvatic cycle for *T. gondii*?

Being able to infect many species, *T. gondii* is common in wildlife, both in DHs and IHs [2, 98, 46, 1]. The question of a sylvatic cycle, and of whether such a cycle would be separated from the transmission in the domestic area, has been raised. A possible interpenetration between domestic and wild cycles would have important consequences for the management of *T. gondii,* since limiting the propagation of the parasite among domestic animals is only feasible if there is no major wild source. The main tools available to investigate this question are the analysis of genotypes that are present in both areas, and the understanding of transmission pathways through epidemiological surveys.

However, the situation differs between temperate and tropical areas. Section 5.1 reviews the factors associated with *T. gondii* infection in wild animals in temperate areas, and assesses the risk of inter-transmission between domestic and wild cycles with its consequences in terms of zoonotic hazard, animal health and population dynamics of highly susceptible wild species. Section 5.2 shows that in Europe, and to a lesser extent in North America, strains found in wildlife are similar to local strains found in domestic animals and the environment. Finally, section 5.3 deals with the specific situation of tropical areas, where the separation between domestic and wild cycles is clearer than in the temperate areas.

5.1. The dynamics of *T. gondii* in wildlife in temperate climates

T. gondii infection in wildlife does not occur with the same probability in any species or place. Wild-living species first have variable levels of susceptibility and exposure. Exposure is largely determined by life history traits, especially feeding behaviour. In birds, where *T. gondii* infection can be present at a high level in many wild birds without any clinical impact, exposure to *T. gondii* is highest in carnivorous species [99]. High *T. gondii* seroprevalence is also reported in large predator species as Lynx and the European wildcat [100, 101] which is of epidemiological significance because infected felids shed oocysts in the wild environment.

Among non-carnivorous species, the risk of infection is related to the risk of encountering oocysts, thus to the level of contact with potentially contaminated soil. In rodents and lagomorphs, home-range size, energy requirements and life expectancy are all expected to be related to the probability to encounter *T. gondii* oocysts. As these traits are correlated to body size [102, 103, 104, 46], large rodents species are more often found positive than small ones [46]. Body size is thus a relevant indicator of prevalence in a given species, and also an indicator of the risk for predators to get infected by preying on that species. Finally, omnivores such as wild boar can acquire toxoplasmosis by incidentally ingesting infected rodents and mainly by rooting and feeding from soil contaminated with oocysts excreted by cats, as shown for other species with similar behaviour, *e.g.*, poultry [105]. On the same way, nutria *Myocastor coypus* is a terrestrial herbivorous but can also eat small insects that can disseminate oocysts and mussels, which can accumulate oocysts [106, 107, 108]. Nutria and wild boar are thus particularly exposed to infection by *T. gondii* [109, 110]. Besides being potential source of *T. gondii* for scavengers, they constitute relevant species to monitor the burden of oocysts in the wild environment and to study factors associated with the dynamic of *T. gondii* infection.

The relationship between feeding behaviour and *T. gondii* infection may also act within species: in a predator species for example, differences of feeding behaviour between genders can lead to a *T. gondii* infection higher in one group compared to others. In an insular population, male cats were more often infected than females, which may be related to the fact that males are heavier and may feed on lagomorphs more often than females, which prey mainly on small mammals [46].

Beside species feeding ecology, wild-living populations also have a spatially and temporally structured risk. Like for rural populations (see 4), climatic and meteorological conditions are significant factors explaining the spatio-temporal variations of *T. gondii* in wild populations [111, 91, 90, 78, 112]. Another determinant factor is the proximity of agricultural activity: in Corsican wild boar, seroprevalence was highest in counties with high farm densities [91]. The presence of domestic cats, including farm cats or feral cats essentially living on predation, and wildcats and hybrid that may live close to rural areas [113], is probably an important factor explaining the connection between the wild and domestic life-cycles of *T. gondii*. Cats roaming into forest or rural landscape searching for preys may shed oocysts and contaminate the soil grazed by herbivorous or omnivorous IHs. The domestic-wild interconnection is thus expected to increase with the proportion of predatory cats in populations and their densities. This connection is also expected to increase with landscape fragmentation, which increases the surfaces where wild animals may come in contact with cats habitat. Generally, the level of anthropization is a relevant proxy for the presence of domestic cats and risk of toxoplasmosis in wild-living populations: in Sweden and Finland, the north-South gradient found in ungulates and hares, respectively, has been interpreted as the result of a declining presence of human settlements and cats in the North [74, 114, 115]. In Chile, the prevalence in American minks *Neovison vison* was highest at proximity of human settlements [116]. Finally, when wild-living cats are present, they constitute a strong determinant of *T. gondii* in wildlife: at the national level, *T. gondii* prevalence in French wild boar is high in the area of presence of the European wildcat *Felis silvestris* [90]; in Alaska, the prevalence of infection in herbivorous species reflects the distribution of lynx *Felis canadensis* in the area [117]. Here it is important to underline that, in order to find relevant explanatory spatial factors, these have to be measured at the appropriate scale. For example, farm density may not be an appropriate estimator of the domestic cat population when considered at the country level [90]. Similarly, as stated earlier (4.2.), oocyst survival depends on the conditions experienced by oocysts in their microenvironment, whose range can be lower than the home range of the studied host population, and also lower than the scale at which meteorological data are usually obtained [90]. The difficulty to obtain data at the right spatial scale may explain that some spatial patterns were not elucidated [118, 119].

On the other hand, the presence of cats or anthropized area is not the single way remote areas may be contaminated. Within the natural environment, long-distance dispersal of *T. gondii* is possible either as oocysts or cysts within IHs. An example of the first process is the contamination of marine mammals along the Northern Pacific American coast. Genetic as well as epidemiological studies suggest that southern sea otters *Enhydra lutris nereis* may be contaminated following fecal contamination of soil by domestic and wild felids flowing from land to sea through surface runoff, followed by the accumulation of oocysts in filter-feeding marine invertebrates [120]. The dispersal of oocysts within the marine environment is poorly known, but Massie and al. [121] recently proposed that migratory filter-feeding fish, like northern anchovies *Engraulis mordax* and Pacific sardines *Sardinops sagax*, may spread *T. gondii* throughout the ocean. On the other hand, the long-distance dispersal of *T. gondii* within IHs may be illustrated in the case of the isolated archipelago of Svalbard, where cats are absent. In this area, arctic foxes were found to carry *T. gondii*, whereas 751 grazing herbivores tested were all seronegative, indicating that contamination by oocysts is uncommon in the area. Prestrud *et al.* [122, 123] proposed that *T. gondii* may have been transported to arctic area by migratory birds.

All these processes act to spread *T. gondii* from domestic to wild, and within the wild environment. A possible consequence of this large transmission is the threat on conservation efforts of highly susceptible species [124]. In most species, *T. gondii* infection is generally unapparent, provoking only mild symptoms. However, a limited number of highly susceptible species have been discovered, in which *T gondii* infection leads to frequent clinical disease and mortality. Marsupials and New World monkeys, which have evolved largely separately from cats, are among the most vulnerable species [2, 125]. Fatal toxoplasmosis is also well-documented in hares (*Lepus sp.*), in northern Europe [114] and Japan [126]. Hares that die of toxoplasmosis are in general in a normal nutritional state and the disease is acute. The explanations for the failure to achieve equilibrium between the host and parasite mainly focus on the host characteristics: a possible lack of cellular immune response [127, 128], the negative impact of stress (food and diet disturbances, exposure to cold, concurrent infections) on the immune response of this species, or even the cumulative effect of immunosuppression induced by toxoplasmosis and stress [129] have been proposed. A clinical expression of toxoplasmosis is also observed in a felid, the Pallas' cats *Otocolobus manul* when raised in captivity [130, 131]. In fact, wild Pallas' cats have minimal opportunity for exposure to *T. gondii* in their isolated natural habitat in Central Asia and, typically, do not become infected with this parasite until being brought into captivity. This could explain their extreme susceptibility to toxoplasmosis [132], which could threaten conservation programs devoted to this species [133]. Although no specific case has been documented in the wild, *T. gondii* may threaten local wild-living populations, for example when new human settlements come in contact with isolated endangered populations.

5.2. *T. gondii* strains in wildlife at temperate latitudes

Despite the presence of a sexual cycle, *T.gondii* maintains a highly clonal population structure. The majority of isolates found belong to one of the three clonal lineages referred to as type I, II and III [134]. Recently, a fourth clonal lineage, called haplogroup 12, has been identified based on isolates from wildlife in the United States [135].

In Europe, the majority of isolates from wildlife contain type II strains, with a few type III strains. From 26 *T. gondii* positive extracts from red fox *Vulpes vulpes* from Belgium submitted to a genotyping analysis with 15 microsatellite markers [136], 25 were type II and only one type III [137]. Similarly, using six loci microsatellite analysis, only type II strains were observed in 46 French isolates including 21 from wild boar [138], 12 from roe deer, 9 from foxes, one from mouflon *Ovis aries*, red deer and mallard *Anas platyrhynchos* [139] and one from tawny owl *Strix aluco* [140]. Using the same molecular technique, Jokelainen *et al.* [141] also identified the clonal type II in 15 DNA extracts from hare (*Lepus sp.*) in Finland. In a recent study in Central and in Eastern Germany, Hermann *et al.* [87] determined the complete genotype has been determined for twelve samples tissues from red foxes, using nine PCR-RFLP markers. In addition to *T. gondii* clonal type II apico II and apico I, type III and *T. gondii* showing non-canonial allele pattern were observed. Interestingly, this study showed evidence of a mixed infection, as well as infection with a *T. gondii* genotype that may represent a recombination of *T. gondii* types II and III.

Su *et al.* [142] developed a standardized restriction fragment length polymorphism (RFLP) typing scheme based on nine mostly unlinked nuclear genomic loci and one apicoplast marker. These markers enable one to distinguish the archetypal from atypical types. In addition, mixed strains in samples can be easily detected by these markers. Mixed infection of *T. gondii* strains in IHs has been previously reported [134, 143]. Detection of mixed infection is of particular interest in epidemiological studies. For genetic exchange, the DH must ingest different types of parasites from their prey at nearly the same time. The frequency of mixed infections in IHs is a relevant indicator of the likelihood of the genetic exchange to occur in the field. In Svalbard, a Norvegian arctic archipelago, 55 artic foxes *Vulpes lagopus* were found infected with *T. gondii*: 27 (49.1%) harboured clonal type II (17/27 were apico I and 10/27 apico II) and four (7.3%) had clonal type III [123]. Strains from 22 foxes (40%) could not be fully genotyped, but two (3.6%) shared more than one allele at a given locus. Again, the most prevalent genotype in this study was clonal type II (with apico alleles I and II) with a few types III genotypes.

It is noteworthy that type II is also the dominant type in domestic mammals in Europe. For instance, Dumètre *et al.* [144] showed by multilocus microsatellite analysis the predominance of type II in sheep, which has also been previously described in humans. In the same way, Halos *et al.* [145] analysed 433 hearts of sheep by using PCR-restriction fragment length polymorphism and microsatellite markers on parasites isolated after bioassay in mice. All 46 genotypes belonged to type II, except for one strain from the Pyrenees mountains area, which belonged to genotype III, which is the first non-type II genotype found in sheep in Europe [146], Denmark [147] and France [144]. This similarity between strains found in wildlife and domestic species in Europe suggests that no clear separation exists between the two cycles.

In North America, strains of *T. gondii* are more diverse. A recent study [148] analysed 169 *T. gondii* isolates from various wildlife species including DHs and IHs, and revealed the large dominance of a recently designated fourth clonal type, called type 12, followed by the type II and III lineages. These three major lineages accounted for 85% of strains from wildlife in North America [148]. The strains isolated from wildlife in North America are thus more diverse, but may also be more different from strains found in the domestic environment than in Europe. Although type 12 has been identified from pigs and sheep in the USA, it may be more specifically found in wildlife [135]. The relative high diversity in *T. gondii* genotypes isolated from wildlife samples compared to those from domestic animals raised the question as to whether distinct gene pools exist for domestic and sylvatic hosts [149].

5.3. The wild environment in tropical areas

The wild environment in tropical areas is still characterized by high fauna diversity, and large areas preserved from influence of humans and of domesticated animals, including cats. Studies on *T. gondii* seroprevalence conducted on tropical wild animals, mainly in South America, show the wide circulation of *T. gondii* in the wild environment of these countries. As in temperate climate [150], the prevalence of *T. gondii* infection was higher in carnivorous or carrion-eaters, or those that accidentally consume oocysts while foraging for food on the ground than in arboreal animals [151]. It was also remarkably high in aquatic mammals such as free-living Amazon River dolphins *Inia geoffrensis* [152]. Remote human population living in wild environment may also exhibit high seroprevalence level for *T. gondii* infection, for example 60.4% in Amerindian tribes [153] or 38.9% in Pygmies from Central Africa [154]. As domestic cats are generally absent from this environment, wild felids are the main source of water and soil contamination. Thirty-nine species of felids have been described, of which 20 live in humid tropical areas [155, 156]. The capacity of oocyst excretion has been demonstrated in captivity, and high seroprevalences were found on free-living felids [157]. In captive Neotropical felids from Southern Brazil, wild-caught felids were three-times more likely to be infected when compared to zoo-born animals [158]. The different species of wild felids varied in home range and resource requirements, but they generally have larger hunting areas and dietary intake than domestic cats, especially the largest ones [159]. This could result in a high opportunity to ingest *T. gondii* infected preys. So, despite the fact that the ecology of *T. gondii* in the wild tropical environment has been poorly studied, the different behaviour of wild felids compared to that of domestic cats and the number of possible IHs suggest a complex ecology of this parasite in this environment leading to a high genetic diversity [160].

This high genetic diversity in tropical wild-life in connection with a sylvatic life cycle has been firstly evoked in French Guiana where severe cases of human toxoplasmosis were detected after eating Amazonian undercooked game or drinking untreated river water [161, 162, 163]. These cases were due to highly atypical strains, all with unique genotype, as determined by microsatellite analysis [164]. The difference between these strains acquired from the Amazonian environment and strains from the anthropized environment of French Guiana was further documented by strain sampling in animals from the different compartments [165].

Compared to the strains of the anthropized environment, the "wild" strains from the Amazonian rainforest in the Guianas exhibited a remarkably high genetic diversity [162, 164, 165]. Whereas the majority of strains from the adjacent anthropized environment are clustered into a few widespread lineages, the "wild" population of strains does not exhibit any clear genetic clustering/structure nor any linkage disequilibrium, supporting the hypothesis of an important circulation and mixing in this environment. This could be connected to the high level of biodiversity in Amazonian neotropical rainforest. This biodiversity concerns the different protagonists of *T. gondii* life cycle (DH, IH and environment). This part of the world may be considered as one of the most important hotspot of diversity with at least 183 mammal species, including 8 of thirty nine known wild felid species, and 718 bird species in French Guiana [165]. The corresponding high level of diversity among *T. gondii* strains may reflect the "natural" population structure of this parasite (before the time of domestication of cats and development of farming) within the true complexity of less disturbed ecosystems. The relative richness of potential hosts that exists within the tropics may have resulted in a correspondingly more diverse range of genotypes of the parasite that can co-exist in such an environment. Under this hypothesis, *T. gondii* would have developed a plurality of alleles to increase its colonization potential [160, 162]. In addition, the larger home ranges of wild felids compared to domestic cats can also strongly influence hybridization patterns and gene flow of the parasite and thus the genetic structure of pathogen populations. The high prevalence in IHs, added to wild felid ecology (diet and home range), could suggest that DHs are more frequently infected by multiple *T. gondii* genotypes, which then cross and recombine before transmission to a new IH. The possibility of reinfection by different strains is known for humans [166]. It has never been explored for felids, but may be hypothesized as another source of increasing diversity.

Most tropical countries are also characterized by an ongoing anthropization with development of farming and settlement in deforested areas. At the confluence between the two environments, wild animals may penetrate in anthropized areas and domestic animals come in contact with the wild through wild game, soil or running water. The increasing pressure of anthropization reduces the hunting area of wild carnivores, including felids and favours their penetration in domestic area. The predatory activity of wild felines or stray cats around these disturbed environments (consumption of chickens, dogs, cats…) would ensure gene flow between the two populations of strains. The consequences of this interpenetration in terms of *T. gondii* genotypes are diverse: (i) detection of *T. gondii* strains with "hybrid" genotypes between the "wild" population and the anthropized population reflecting genetic exchanges, (ii) strains from the wild environment found in domestic animals, such as stray dogs, or (iii), on the opposite, strains from the anthropized environment found in wild animals [165]. In parallel, the influence of human activities with urbanization, fragmentation of landscape, deforested areas, farming, domestication of cats and other animals, modifies *T. gondii* ecology reducing the number of ecological niches. This process favours an impoverishment of *T. gondii* genetic diversity with the selection of a few strains well adapted to a small number of domestic species [167, 168]. Transportation of these strains through large distances by human trade exchange and transportation of animals lead to introduction of domestic strains in the wild environment and occasionally to expansion of clonal lineages. In tropical countries, this is evidenced by the so-called *Caribbean* genotypes found in the anthropized areas of French Guiana and in several Caribbean Islands, or in Africa, where the same African lineages were found in different countries [169, 170, 171].

Finally, the dynamics of *T. gondii* in wildlife and its interaction with domestic areas show a contrasted pattern. In most European countries, due to the large anthropization, any wild-living individual lives relatively close to domestic areas. Farming and cat domestication occurred long time ago. Farms constitute the reservoir of infection, from which a few genotypes adapted to farm species irradiate in the surrounding environment [72]. This could explain the widespread occurrence of only a few well adapted clonal lineages (types II and III) even in wild animals. In other temperate or cold countries, such as the U.S.A. or Canada where large territories are non-anthropized, the genotypic diversity of *T. gondii* in the wild animals is present [148, 149, 172]. The diversity is maximal in tropical areas, due to high host diversity and large non-anthropized areas. Thus the risk of transmission of toxoplasmosis from wildlife has not the same consequences everywhere. In tropical areas, specific "wild" strains may be transmitted, thus the transmission risk is relatively easy to characterize through strain genotyping, while in Europe, a case of infection acquired from wildlife would pass unnoticed due to the similarity of strains. The risk of infection from wildlife may be analyzed through genotyping strains in tropical areas, but through epidemiological surveys in Europe.

6. Conclusion: consequences for the management of zoonotic transmission

Like other IHs, humans can be infected either by cysts containing bradyzoits, or by oocysts of *T. gondii*. Tissue cysts are responsible for meat-borne infection (pork, lamb, beef or poultry are possible source of contamination), while sporulated oocysts lead to infection by ingesting particles of soil (after gardening for example) or by consuming unwashed raw fruits or vegetables, or untreated water [2, 145, 173, 174, 175]. However, the crucial question of the relative part of risk related to bradyzoits versus oocysts remains open. Different approaches have been used to estimate the relative importance of sources of contamination, using risk-factor analyses or estimation of the fraction of attributable risk, either in the general population (chronic infection) or in cases of seroconversion in pregnant women. These studies clearly identified the ingestion of undercooked meat as a risk factor [7, 13, 173, 176]. However, this result is probably partly due to this risk being easier to characterize than the risk due to oocysts. Another way to get an idea of the relative part of risk related to cysts or oocysts is to undertake a quantitative assessment of the risk of toxoplasmosis [177]. Recently, in the Netherlands, Opsteegh *et al.* performed a quantitative microbial risk assessment (QMRA) for meat-borne toxoplasmosis, which predicted high numbers of infections per year. The study also demonstrated that, even with a low prevalence of infection in cattle, consumption of beef constitutes an important source of infection [178]. However, the risk assessment remains limited by the lack of detailed information on which fraction of meat is more contaminated in carcass: although seroprevalences are available for farm animals from many countries [2], the correlation between seropositivity and detection of parasites in meat is weak. In terms of veterinary medicine, there is no surveillance system for animal toxoplasmosis and only cases of abortions (due to *T. gondii* or other causes) have to be declared. The meat-borne risk analysis is also limited by the low level of information on the food cooking practices, and on the contamination of species consumed less often, such as game [90, 91, 78].

Up to now, the risk analyses essentially used information on, and produced estimates about, meat-borne toxoplasmosis. These studies permitted to identify control points for the management of meat-producing animals. For example, in intensively managed swine farms, modern biosecure management practices have resulted in reduced levels of infection in swine raised in confinement [96, 179, 180]. In organic livestock production systems, farm-management factors including feeding are thought to play an important role in the on-farm prevalence of *T. gondii* [181]. To limit *T. gondii* infection in such farms, recommended practices include exclusion of cats or other wildlife, strict rodent control and restriction of human entry in pig barns [182]. These measures could be effective in other species to reduce the level of contamination of meat. On the contrary, organic pork meat may pose a specific risk of transmitting T. *gondii* to humans [183]. However, due to the capacity of dissemination of *T. gondii*, the objective of a completely *T. gondii*-free meat seems difficult, but feasible using pre-harvest measures for prevention of T. gondii infection [184].

On the other hand, working to reduce the level of infection in meat does not act on the risk of toxoplasmosis due to direct contact with oocysts, which stays largely unknown and unmanaged. Limiting the level of contamination in meat may even result in the increase of the relative risk due to oocysts. The importance of oocysts in the overall contamination rate remains difficult to assess, due to the lack of information on the level of environmental contamination and to the difficulty to characterize the level of contact of people with contaminated areas. In this framework, a better knowledge of the life cycle of *T. gondii* in its natural environment should help to characterize the risk due to oocysts. For example, the estimates provided in Table 1 give an order of magnitude of the expected differences between environments. Moreover, two recent methodological advances should improve our knowledge of environmental contamination. First, new methods to detect oocysts in soil [185] and water [186, 187, 188] have been proposed, based on molecular detection or immunocapture. Being highly sensitive, these methods should allow researchers to better characterize areas and periods at risk of contamination. A few studies have already measured the level of soil and water contamination [50, 68, 189]. These studies confirmed that the risk in urban areas is spatially structured at the very local scale, and they should help to identify areas most contaminated in other environments. The second useful tool that should bring relevant information is the development of methods to detect antibodies specifically linked to infection by oocysts [190]. This test, based on western blot assay detecting for IgG positive serums antibodies to sporozoites, allowed the authors to determine the proportion of cases that had contacts with oocysts in Chile, both in humans [191] and in swine [192]. In North America, a survey using this method shows that a high proportion of mothers of congenitally infected infants had primary infection with oocysts [193].

These new analytical tools should help to identify the origin of contamination, and thus solve several fundamental and practical questions regarding *T. gondii* life cycle. For example, estimating the frequency of infection from oocysts in cats of urban and rural area should help to estimate the part of the DH-environment life cycle in different environments. In people, these tools should help to assess if the relative role of oocyst and meat-born infection varies according to the area (urban versus rural populations for example). In such case, prevention measures should focus on specific aspects depending on the exposure of people. These elements should help to reduce the burden of toxoplasmosis in human and animal populations.

Author details

Emmanuelle Gilot-Fromont[1,2,*], Maud Lélu[3], Marie-Laure Dardé[4], Céline Richomme[5], Dominique Aubert[6], Eve Afonso[7], Aurélien Mercier[4], Cécile Gotteland[1,6], Isabelle Villena[6]
[1]*UMR CNRS 5558 Laboratoire de Biométrie et Biologie Evolutive, Université Lyon 1, Villeurbanne, France.*
[2]*VetAgro-Sup Campus Vétérinaire, Université de Lyon, Marcy l'Etoile, France,*
[3]*NIMBioS, University of Tennessee, Knoxville, Tennessee, USA,*
[4]*INSERM UMR1094, Tropical Neuroepidemiology, School of Medicine, Institute of Neuroepidemiology and Tropical Neurology, CNRS FR 3503 GEIST, University of Limoges, Limoges, France,*
[5]*ANSES, Nancy laboratory for rabies and wildlife, Technopole agricole et vétérinaire, Malzéville, France,*
[6]*Laboratoire de Parasitologie-Mycologie, EA 3800, UFR de Médecine, SFR Cap Santé, FED 4231, University of Reims Champagne-Ardenne, Reims, France,*
[7]*Department Chrono-environnement, UMR CNRS 6249 USC INRA, University of Franche-Comté, Besançon, France*

Acknowledgement

The authors thank Aurélien Dumètre, René Ecochard, Michel Langlais, Dominique Pontier, Philippe Thulliez and Stéphane Romand for their help in elaborating the 10-year research period that produced part of the results presented here. This project has been supported by the Agence Française de Sécurité Sanitaire de L'Environnement et du Travail (AFSSET) and by the Agence De l'Environnement et de la Maitrise de l'Energie (ADEME), with additional grants from Grünenthal France Laboratory (EA), Institut National de la Recherche Agronomique (INRA, CR), Région Champagne-Ardenne (EA, ML and CG), Département des Ardennes (ML), Communauté de Communes de l'Argonne Ardennaise (ML) and the National Institute for Mathematical and Biological Synthesis (NIMBioS, sponsored by the National Science Foundation, the U.S. Department of Homeland Security, and the U.S. Department of Agriculture, ML).

7. References

[1] Dubey JP (2010) Toxoplasmosis of animals and humans, second edition. Boca Raton: CRC Press. 313 p.

* Corresponding Author

[2] Tenter AM, Heckeroth AR, Weiss LM (2000) *Toxoplasma gondii*: from animals to humans. Int. j. parasitol. 30: 1217-1258.

[3] Miller MA, Miller WA, Conrad PA, James ER, Melli AC, Leutenegger CM, Dabritz HA, Packham AE, Paradies D, Harris M, Ames J, Jessup DA, Worcester K, Grigg ME (2008) Type X *Toxoplasma gondii* in a wild mussel and terrestrial carnivores from coastal California: new linkages between terrestrial mammals, runoff and toxoplamosis of sea otters. Int. j. parasitol 58: 928-937.

[4] Deplazes P, Hegglin D, Gloor S, Romig T (2004) Wilderness in the city: the urbanization of *Echinococcus multilocularis*. Trends parasitol 20 : 77-84.

[5] House PK, Vyas A, Sapolsky R (2011) Predator cat odors activate sexual arousal pathways in brains of *Toxoplasma gondii* infected rats. PLoS ONE 6: e23277.

[6] Dass SAH, Vasudevan A, Dutta D, Soh LJT, Salposky RM, Vyas A (2011) Protozoan parasite *Toxoplasma gondii* manipulates mate choice in rats by enhancing attractiveness of males. PLoS ONE 6: e27229.

[7] Cook AJC, Gilbert RE, Buffolano W, Zufferey J, Petersen E, Jenum PA, Foulon W, Semprini AE, Dunn DT (2000) Sources of *Toxoplasma* infection in pregnant women: European multicentre case-control study. Br. med. j. 321: 142-147.

[8] Beverly JKA (1959) Congenital transmission of toxoplasmosis through successive generations of mice. Nature 183: 1348-1349.

[9] Dubey JP (2006) Comparative infectivity of oocysts and bradyzoites of *Toxoplasma gondii* for intermediate (mice) and definitive (cats) hosts. Vet. parasitol. 140: 69-75.

[10] Lélu M, Langlais M, Poulle ML, Gilot-Fromont E (2010) Transmission dynamics of *Toxoplasma gondii* along an urban-rural gradient. Theor. popul. biol. 78: 139–147.

[11] Berenreiterova M, Flegr J, Kubena AA, Nemec P (2011) The Distribution of *Toxoplasma gondii* Cysts in the Brain of a Mouse with Latent Toxoplasmosis: Implications for the Behavioral Manipulation Hypothesis. PLoS One 6: e28925.

[12] Pappas G, Roussos N, Falagas ME (2009) Toxoplasmosis snapshots: Global status of *Toxoplasma gondii* seroprevalence and implications for pregnancy and congenital toxoplasmosis. Int. j. parasitol. 39: 1385-1394.

[13] Berger F, Goulet V, Le Strat Y, Desenclos JC (2008) Toxoplasmose chez les femmes enceintes en France : évolution de la séroprévalence et de l'incidence et facteurs associés, 1995-2003. Bulletin Epidemiologique Hebdomadaire 14-15: 117-121.

[14] Gilot-Fromont E, Riche B, Rabilloud M (2009) Seroprevalence of *Toxoplasma gondii* in a rural population in France: detection of a household effect. BMC infect. dis. 9: 76.

[15] Haydon DT, Cleaveland S, Taylor LH, Laurenson K (2002) Identifying Reservoirs of Infection: A Conceptual and Practical Challenge. Emerg. infect. dis. 8: 1468-1473.

[16] Turner DC, Bateson PB (2000) The Domestic cat: the biology of its behaviour. Cambridge University Press.

[17] Macdonald DW (1983) The ecology of carnivore social behaviour. Nature 301: 379-384.

[18] Page RJC, Ross J, Bennett DH (1993) Home ranges of feral cats at Avonmouth Docks (United Kingdom). Rev. sci. tech. OIE 12: 23-26.

[19] Calhoon RE, Haspel C (1989) Urban cat populations compared by season, subhabitat and supplemental feeding. J. anim. ecol. 58: 321-328.

[20] Liberg O (1980) Spacing pattern in a population of rural free-roaming domestic cats. Oikos 35: 336-349.

[21] Pontier D, Rioux N, Heizmann A (1995) Evidence of selection on the orange allele in the domestic cat *Felis catus*: the role of social structure. Oikos 73: 299-308.

[22] Fromont E, Artois M, Pontier D (1998) Epidemiology of feline leukemia virus (FeLV) and structure of domestic cat populations. J. wildl. manage. 62: 978-988.

[23] Liberg O (1981) Predation and social behaviour in a population of domestic cats. An evolutionary perspective. Ph. D. Thesis, Univ. Lund (Sweden), 135 p.

[24] Liberg O (1984) Food habits and prey impact by feral and house-based domestic cats in a rural area in southern Sweden. J. mammal. 65: 424-432.

[25] Say L, Gaillard JM, Pontier D. (2002) Spatiotemporal variation in cat population density in a sub-Antarctic environment. Polar biol. 25: 90–95.

[26] Say L, Devillard S, Natoli E, Pontier D (2002) The mating system of feral cats (*Felis catus* L.) in a sub-Antarctic environment. Polar biol. 25: 838–842.

[27] Le Louarn H, Quéré JP (2003) Les Rongeurs de France. Faunistique et biologie. INRA éditions, Paris, 256pp.

[28] Dickman CR, Doncaster CP (1987) The Ecology of Small Mammals in Urban Habitats. I. Populations in a Patchy Environment. J. anim. ecol. 56: 629-640.

[29] Baker PJ, Ansell RJ, Dodds PAA, Webber CE, Harris S (2003) Factors affecting the distribution of small mammals in an urban area. Mammal rev. 33: 95-100.

[30] Dubey JP, Saville WJA, Stanek J, Reed SM (2002) Prevalence of *Toxoplasma gondii* antibodies in domestic cats From rural Ohio. J. parasitol. 88: 802-803.

[31] Miró G, Montoya A, Jimenez S, Frisuelos C, Mateo M, Fuentes I (2004) Prevalence of antibodies to *Toxoplasma gondii* and intestinal parasites in stray, farm and household cats in Spain. Vet. parasitol. 126: 249-255.

[32] Afonso E, Thulliez P, Gilot-Fromont E (2010) Local meteorological conditions, dynamics of seroconversion to *Toxoplasma gondii* in cats (*Felis catus*) and oocyst burden in a rural environment. Epidemiol. infect. 138: 1105–1113.

[33] Wu SM, Zhu XQ, Zhou DH, Fu BQ, Chen J, Yang JF, Song HQ, Weng YB, Ye DH (2011) Seroprevalence of *Toxoplasma gondii* infection in household and stray cats in Lanzhou, northwest China. Parasites & Vectors 4: 214-218.

[34] Zhang H, Zhou DH, Zhou P, Lun ZR, Chen XG, Lin RQ, Yuan ZG, Zhu XQ (2009) Seroprevalence of *Toxoplasma gondii* infection in stray and household cats in Guangzhou, China. Zoonoses public health 56: 502-505.

[35] Barratt DG (1998) Predation by house cats, *Felis catus* (L.), in Canberra, Australia. II. Factors affecting the amount of prey caught and estimates of the impact on wildlife. Wildlife res. 25: 475-487.

[36] Baker PJ, Bentley AJ, Ansell RJ, Harris S (2005) Impact of predation by domestic cats *Felis catus* in an urban area. Mammal rev. 35: 302-312.

[37] Woods M, McDonald RA, Harris S (2003) Predation of wildlife by domestic cats *Felis catus* in Great Britain. Mammal rev. 33: 174–188.

[38] Gillies C, Clout M (2003) The prey of domestic cats (*Felis catus*) in two suburbs of Auckland City, New Zealand J. zool. 259: 309-315.

[39] Kays RW, DeWan AA (2004) Ecological impact of inside/outside house cats around a suburban nature reserve. Anim. conserv. 7: 273-283.

[40] Rosenthal BM (2009) How has agriculture influenced the geography and genetics of animal parasites? Trends parasitol. 25: 67-70.

[41] Afonso E, Thulliez P, Gilot-Fromont E (2006) Transmission of *Toxoplasma gondii* in an urban population of domestic cats (*Felis catus*). Int. j. parasitol. 36: 1373-1382.

[42] Hornok S, Edelhofer R, Joachim A, Farkas R, Berta K, Repasi A, Lakatos B (2008) Seroprevalence of *Toxoplasma gondii* and *Neospora caninum* infection of cats in Hungary. Acta vet. hung. 56: 81-88.

[43] Lee SE, Kim NH, Chae HS, Cho SH, Nam HW, Lee WJ, Kim SH, Lee JH (2011) Prevalence of *Toxoplasma gondii* infection in feral cats in Seoul, Korea. J. parasitol. 97, 153-155.

[44] Dubey JP, Weigel RM, Siegel AM, Thuilliez P, Kitron UD, Mitchell MA, Mannelli A, Mateus-Pinilla NE, Shen SK, Kwok OCH, Todd KS (1995) Sources and reservoirs of *Toxoplasma gondii* infection on 47 swine farms in Illinois. J. parasitol. 81: 723-729.

[45] Cavalcante GT, Aguiar DM, Chiebao D, Dubey JP, Ruiz VLA, Dias RA, Camargo LMA, Labruna MB, Gennari SM (2006) Seroprevalence of *Toxoplasma gondii* antibodies in cats and pigs from rural Western Amazon, Brazil. J. parasitol. 92: 863-864.

[46] Afonso E, Thulliez P, Pontier D, Gilot-Fromont E (2007) Toxoplasmosis in prey species and consequences for prevalence in feral cats: not all prey species are equal. Parasitology 134: 1963-1971.

[47] Dabritz HA, Miller MA, Gadner IA, Packham AE, Atwill ER, Conrad PA (2008) Risk factors for *Toxoplasma gondii* infection in wild rodents from central coastal California and a review of *T. gondii* prevalence in rodents. J. parasitol. 94: 675–683.

[48] Genchi G, Polidori GA, Zaghini L, Lanfranchi P (1991) Aspetti epidemiologici della toxoplasmosi nell'allevamento intensivo del suino. Arch. vet. ital. 42, 105–111.

[49] Marshall PA, Hughes JM, Williams RH, Smith JE, Murphy RG, Hide G (2004) Detection of high levels of congenital transmission of *Toxoplasma gondii* in natural urban populations of *Mus domesticus*. Parasitology 128: 39-42.

[50] Afonso E, Lemoine M, Poulle ML, Ravat MC, Romand S, Thulliez P, Villena I, Aubert D, Riche B, Rabilloud M, Gilot-Fromont E (2008) Spatial distribution of soil contamination by *Toxoplasma gondii* in relation to cat defecation behaviour in an urban area. Int. j. parasitol. 38: 1017-1023.

[51] Dabritz HA, Miller, Atwill ER, Gardner IA, Leutenegger CM, Melli AC, Conrad PA (2007) Detection of *Toxoplasma gondii*-like oocysts in cat feces and estimates of the environmental oocyst burden. J. am. vet. med. assoc. 231: 1676–1684.

[52] Dabritz HA, Atwill ER, Gardner IA, Miller MA, Conrad PA (2006) Outdoor fecal deposition by free-roaming cats and attitudes of cat owners and nonowners toward stray pets, wildlife, and water pollution. J. am. vet. med. assoc. 229: 74-81.

[53] Forman RTT, Godron M (1986) Landscape ecology. Wiley and Sons, New York, USA.

[54] McKinney ML (2002) Urbanization, biodiversity, and conservation. BioScience 52: 883-890.

[55] Bradley CA, Altizer S (2007) Urbanization and the ecology of wildlife diseases. Trends ecol. evol. 22: 95-102.
[56] Zaunbrecher KI, Smith RE (1993) Neutering of feral cats as an alternative to eradication programs. J. am. vet. med. assoc. 203: 449-452.
[57] Neville PF, Remfry J (1984) Effect of neutering on two groups of feral cats. Vet. rec. 114: 447-450.
[58] Natoli E (1985) Spacing pattern in a colony of urban stray cats (*Felis catus* L.) in the historic centre of Rome. Appl. anim. behav. sci. 14: 289-304.
[59] Haspel C, Calhoon RE (1989) Home ranges of free ranging cats (*Felis catus*) in Brooklyn, New York. Can. j. zool. 67: 178-181.
[60] Salant H, Spira DT (2004) A cross-sectional survey of anti-*Toxoplasma gondii* antibodies in Jerusalem cats. Vet. parasitol. 124: 167-177.
[61] Jittapalapong S, Nimsupan B, Pinyopanuwat N., Chimnoi W, Kabeya H, Maruyama S (2006) Seroprevalence of *Toxoplasma gondii* antibodies in stray cats and dogs in the Bangkok metropolitan area, Thailand. Vet. parasitol. 145: 138-141.
[62] Pena HJF, Soares RM, Amaku M, Dubey JP, Gennari SM (2006) *Toxoplasma gondii* infection in cats from Saõ Paulo state, Brazil: seroprevalence, oocyst shedding, isolation in mice, and biologic and molecular characterization. Res. vet. sci. 81: 58-67.
[63] Gauss CBL, Almeria S, Ortuno A, Garcia F, Dubey JP (2003) Seroprevalence of *Toxoplasma gondii* Antibodies in Domestic Cats from Barcelona, Spain. J. parasitol. 89: 1067-1068.
[64] Dorny P, Speybroeck N, Verstraete S, Baeke M, De Becker A, Berkvens D, Vercruysse J (2002) Serological survey of *Toxoplasma gondii*, feline immunodeficiency virus and feline leukaemia virus in urban stray cats in Belgium. Vet. rec. 151: 626-629.
[65] Corbett LK (1979) Feeding ecology and social organization of wildcats (*Felis silvetris*) and domestic cats (*Felis catus*) in Scotland. Scotland: University of Aberdeen.
[66] Uga S, Minami T, Nagata K (1996) Defecation habits of cats and dogs and contamination by *Toxocara* eggs in public park sandpits. Am. j. trop. med. hyg. 54: 122-126.
[67] Lass A, Pietkiewicz H, Modzelewska E, Dumètre A, Szostakowska B, Myjak P (2009) Detection of *Toxoplasma gondii* oocysts in environmental soil samples using molecular methods. Eur. j. clin. microbiol. Infect. dis. 28: 599-605.
[68] Du F, Feng HL, Nie H, Tu P, Zhang QL, Hu M, Zhou YQ, Zhao JL (2012) Survey on the contamination of *Toxoplasma gondii* oocysts in the soil of public parks of Wuhan, China. Vet. parasitol. 184: 141-146.
[69] Bobić B, Jevremović I, Marinković J, Šibalić D, Djurković-Djaković O (1998) Risk factors for *Toxoplasma* infection in a reproductive age female population in the area of Belgrade, Yugoslavia. Eur. j. epidemiol. 14: 605-610.
[70] Kortbeek LM, De Melker HE, Veldhuijzen IK, Conyn-Van Spaendonck MAE (2004) Population-based *Toxoplasma* seroprevalence study in the Netherlands. Epidemiol. infect. 132: 839-845.
[71] Frenkel JK, Hassanein KL, Hassanein RS, Brown E, Thulliez P, Quintero-Nunez R (1995) Transmission of *Toxoplasma gondii* in Panama city, Panama: A five-year prospective

cohort study of children, cats, rodents, birds, and soil. Am. j. trop. med. hyg. 53: 458-468.

[72] Lehmann T, Graham DH, Dahl E, Sreekumar C, Launer F, Corn JL, Gamble HR, Dubey JP (2003) Transmission dynamics of *Toxoplasma gondii* on a pig farm. Infect. genet. evol. 3: 135–141.

[73] Gauss CB, Dubey JP, Vidal D, Cabezon O, Ruiz-Fons F, Vicente J, Marco I, Lavin S, Gortazar C, Almería S (2006) Prevalence of *Toxoplasma gondii* antibodies in red deer (*Cervus elaphus*) and other wild ruminants from Spain. Vet. parasitol. 136: 193-200.

[74] Malmsten J, Jakubek EB, Bjorkman C (2011) Prevalence of antibodies against *Toxoplasma gondii* and *Neospora caninum* in moose (*Alces alces*) and roe deer (*Capreolus capreolus*) in Sweden. Vet. parasitol. 177: 275-280.

[75] Williamson JMW, Williams H (1980) Toxoplasmosis in farmed red deer (*Cervus elaphus*) in Scotland. Res. vet. sci. 29: 36–40.

[76] Simon A, Chambellant M, Ward BJ, Simard M, Proulx JF, Levesque B, Bigras-Poulin M, Rousseau AN, Ogden NH (2011) Spatio-temporal variations and age effect on *Toxoplasma gondii* seroprevalence in seals from the Canadian Arctic. Parasitology 138: 1-7.

[77] Tizard IR, Fish NA, Quinn JP (1976) Some observations on the epidemiology of toxoplasmosis in Canada. J. hyg. Camb. 77: 11–21.

[78] Gotteland C, Aubert A, Gilbert P, Moinet M, Klein F, Villena I, Game Y, Gilot-Fromont E (submitted) *Toxoplasma gondii* in natural populations of Ungulates in France : prevalence and spatio-temporal variations.

[79] Dumètre A, Dardé ML (2003) How to detect *Toxoplasma gondii* oocysts in environmental samples? FEMS microbiol. rev. 27: 651-661.

[80] Davies, CM, Altavilla N, Krogh M, Ferguson CM, Deere DA, Ashbolt NJ (2005) Environmental inactivation of *Cryptosporidium* oocysts in catchment soils. J. appl. microbiol. 98: 308-317.

[81] Langkjær M, Roepstorff A (2008) Survival of *Isospora suis* oocysts under controlled environmental conditions. Vet. parasitol. 152: 186-193.

[82] Frenkel JK, Ruiz A, Chinchilla M (1975) Soil survival of *Toxoplasma* oocysts in Kansas and Costa Rica. Am. j. trop. med. hyg. 24: 439–443.

[83] Lélu M, Villena I, Dardé ML, Aubert D, Geers R, Dupuis E, Marnef F, Poulle ML, Gotteland C, Dumètre A, Gilot-Fromont E (2012) Quantitative assessment of the survival of *Toxoplasma gondii* oocysts in soil. Appl. env. microbiol. doi: 10.1128/AEM.00246-12.

[84] Stenseth NC,Viljugrein H, Jedrejewski W, Mysterud A, Pucek Z (2002) Population dynamics of *Clethrionomys glareolus* and *Apodemus flavicollis* : seasonal components of density dependence and density independence. Acta theriol. 47 (Suppl. 1): 39–67.

[85] Tizard R, Harmeson J, Lai CH (1978) The Prevalence of Serum Antibodies to *Toxoplasma gondii* in Ontario Mammals. Can. j. comp. med. 42: 177-183.

[86] Bobić B, Klun I, Nikolić A, Nikolić A, Vujanić M, Zivković T, Ivović V, Djurković-Djakovic O (2010) Seasonal variations in human *Toxoplasma* infection in Serbia. Vector borne zoonotic dis. 10: 465–469.

[87] Herrmann DC, Pantchev N, Vrhovec MG, Barutzki D, Wilking H, Fröhlich A, Lüder CG, Conraths FJ, Schares G (2010) Atypical *Toxoplasma gondii* genotypes identified in oocysts shed by cats in Germany. Int. j. parasitol. 40: 285-292.

[88] Klun I, Djurkovic-Djakovic O, Katic-Radivojevic S, Nikolic A (2006) Cross-sectional survey on *Toxoplasma gondii* infection in cattle, sheep and pigs in Serbia: seroprevalence and risk factors. Vet. parasitol. 135: 121–131.

[89] Panadero R, Painceira A, López C, Vázquez L, Paz A, Díaz P, Dacal V, Cienfuegos S, Fernández G, Lago N, Díez-Baños P, Morrondo P (2010) Seroprevalence of *Toxoplasma gondii* and *Neospora caninum* in wild and domestic ruminants sharing pastures in Galicia (Northwest Spain). Res. vet. sci 88: 111–115.

[90] Beral M, Rossi S, Aubert D, Gasqui P, Terrier ME, Klein F, Geers R, Abrial D, Gilot-Fromont E, Richomme C, Hars J, Jourdain E (submitted) Environmental factors associated with the seroprevalence of *Toxoplasma gondii* in wild boar (*Sus scrofa*), France.

[91] Richomme C, Afonso E, Tolon V, Ducrot C, Halos L, Alliot A, Perret C, Thomas M, Boireau P, Gilot-Fromont E (2010) Risk factors for *Toxoplasma gondii* infection in wild boar from the Mediterranean island of Corsica. Epidemiol. infect. 138: 1257–1266.

[92] Langlais M, Lélu M, Avenet C, Gilot-Fromont E (2012) A simplified model system for *Toxoplasma gondii* spread within a heterogeneous environment. Nonlinear Dynamics, doi: 10.1007/s11071-011-0255-4.

[93] Lopes WDZ, dos Santos TR, dos Santos da Silva R, Rossanese WM, de Souza FA, D'Ark de Faria Rodrigues J, Paranhos de Mendonça R, Soares VE, da Costa AJ (2010) Seroprevalence of and risk factors for *Toxoplasma gondii* in sheep raised in the Jaboticabal, microregion, São Paulo State, Brazil. Res. vet. sci 161: 324-326.

[94] Mainar RC, de la Cruz C, Asencio A, Dominguez L, Vazquez-Boland IA (1996) Prevalence of agglutination antibodies to *Toxolasma gondii* in small ruminants of the Madrid region, Spain, and identification of factors influencing seropositivity by multivariate analysis. Vet. res. com. 20: 153-159.

[95] Mateus-Pinilla NE, Hannon B, Weigel M (2002) A computer simulation of the prevention of the transmission of *Toxoplasma gondii* on swine farms using a feline *T-gondii* vaccine. Prev. vet. med. 55: 17–36.

[96] Kijlstra A, Jongert E (2008) Control of the risk of human toxoplasmosis transmitted by meat. Int. j. parasitol. 38: 1359–1370.

[97] Gilot-Fromont E, Aubert D, Belkilani S, Hermitte P, Gibout O, Geers R, Villena I (2009) Landscape, herd management and within-herd seroprevalence of *Toxoplasma gondii* in beef cattle herds from Champagne-Ardenne, France. Vet. parasitol. 161: 36-40.

[98] Hill DE, Chirukandoth S, Dubey JP (2005) Biology and epidemiology of *Toxoplasma gondii* in man and animals. Anim. health res. rev. 6: 41-61.

[99] Cabezón O, García-Bocanegra I, Molina-López R, Marco I, Blanco JM, Höfle U, Margalida A, Bach-Raich E, Darwich L, Echeverría I, Obón E, Hernández M, Lavín S, Dubey JP, Almería S (2011) Seropositivity and risk factors associated with *Toxoplasma gondii* infection in wild birds from Spain. PloS ONE 6: 1–7.

[100] Sobrino R, Cabezón O, Millán J, Pabón M, Arnal MC, Luco DF, Gortázar C, Dubey JP, Almería S (2007) Seroprevalence of *Toxoplasma gondii* antibodies in wild carnivores from Spain. Vet. parasitol. 148: 187-192.

[101] García-Bocanegra I, Dubey JP, Martínez F, Vargas A, Cabezón O, Zorrilla I, Arenas A, Almería S (2010). Factors affecting seroprevalence of *Toxoplasma gondii* in the endangered Iberian lynx (*Lynx pardinus*). Vet. parasitol. 167: 36-42.

[102] Degen AA, Kam M, Khokhlova IS, Krasnov BR, Barraclough TG (1998) Average daily metabolic rate of rodents: habitat and dietary comparisons. Funct. ecol. 12: 63–73.

[103] Speakman JR (2005) Body size, energy metabolism and lifespan. J. exp. biol. 208: 1717–1730.

[104] Ottaviani D, Cairns SC, Oliverio M, Boitani L (2006) Body mass as a predictive variable of homerange size among Italian mammals and birds. J. zool. 269: 317–330.

[105] Ruiz A, Frenkel JK (1980) Intermediate and transport hosts of *Toxoplasma gondii* in Costa Rica. Am. J. trop. med. hyg. 29: 1161–1166.

[106] Lindsay DS, Phelps KK, Smith SA, Flick G, Sumner SS, Dubey JP (2001) Removal of *Toxoplasma gondii* oocysts from seawater by Eastern oysters (*Crassostrea virginica*). J eukariot. microbiol. 48: S197-S198.

[107] Putignani L, Mancinelli L, Del Chierico F, Menichella D, Adlerstein D, Angelici MC, Marangi N, Berrilli F, Caffara M, di Regalbono A (2011) Investigation of *Toxoplasma gondii* presence in farmed shellfish by nested PCR and real-time PCR fluorescent amplicon generation assay (FLAG). Exp. parasitol 127: 409-417.

[108] Dubey JP (2004) Toxoplasmosis - a waterborne zoonosis. Vet. parasitol. 126: 57-72.

[109] Bollo E, Pregel P, Gennero S, Pizzoni E, Rosati S, Nebbia P, Biolatti B (2003) Health status of a population of nutria (*Myocastor coypus*) living in a protected area in Italy. Res. vet. sci. 75: 21-25.

[110] Nardoni S, Angelici MC, Mugnaini L, Mancianti F (2011). Prevalence of *Toxoplasma gondii* infection in *Myocastor coypus* in a protected Italian wetland. Parasite and Vectors 23: 240-243.

[111] Almeria S, Calvete C, Pages A, Gauss CBL, Dubey, JP (2004). Factors affecting the seroprevalence of *Toxoplasma gondii* infection in wild rabbits (*Oryctolagus cuniculus*) from Spain. Vet. parasitol. 123: 265–270.

[112] Gamarra JA, Cabezón O, Pabón M, Arnal MC, Luco DF, Dubey JP, Gortázar C, Almería S (2008) Prevalence of antibodies against *Toxoplasma gondii* in roe deer from Spain. Vet. parasitol. 153: 152–156.

[113] Germain E, Benhamou S, Poulle ML (2008) Spatio-temporal sharing between the European wildcat, the domestic cat and their hybrids. J. zool. 276: 195–203.

[114] Jokelainen P, Isomursu M, Näreaho A, Oksanen A (2011) Natural *Toxoplasma gondii* infections in European brown hares and mountain hares in Finland: proportional mortality rate, antibody prevalence, and genetic characterization. J. wildl. dis. 47: 154–163.

[115] Jokelainen P, Näreaho A, Knaapi S, Oksanen A, Rikula U, Sukura A (2010) *Toxoplasma gondii* in wild cervids and sheep in Finland: north-south gradient in seroprevalence. Vet. parasitol. 171: 331-336.

[116] Sepúlveda MA, Muñoz-Zanzi C, Rosenfeld C, Jara R, Pelican KM, Hill D (2011) *Toxoplasma gondii* in feral American minks at the Maullín river, Chile. Vet. parasitol. 175: 60–65.

[117] Stieve E, Beckmen K, Kania SA, Widner A, Patton S (2010) *Neospora caninum* and *Toxoplasma gondii* antibody prevalence in Alaska wildlife. J. wildl. dis. 46: 348-355.

[118] Vikoren T, Tharaldsen J, Fredriksen B, Handeland K (2004) Prevalence of *Toxoplasma gondii* antibodies in wild red deer, roe deer, moose, and reindeer from Norway. Vet. parasitol. 120: 159-169.

[119] Zarnke RL, Dubey JP, Kwok OC, Ver Hoef JM (2000) Serologic survey for *Toxoplasma gondii* in selected wildlife species from Alaska. J. wildl. dis. 36: 219-224.

[120] Miller MA, Miller WA, Conrad PA, James ER, Melli AC, Leutenegger CM, Dabritz HA, Packham AE, Paradies D, Harris M, Ames J, Jessup DA, Worcester K, Grigg ME (2008) Type X *Toxoplasma gondii* in a wild mussel and terrestrial carnivores from coastal California: New linkages between terrestrial mammals, runoff and toxoplasmosis of sea otters. Int. j. parasitol. 38: 1319–1328.

[121] Massie GN, Ware MW, Villegas EN, Black MW (2010) Uptake and transmission of *Toxoplasma gondii* oocysts by migratory, filter-feeding fish. Vet. parasitol. 169: 296-303.

[122] Prestrud KW, Asbakk K, Fuglei E, Mørk T, Stien A, Ropstad E, Tryland M, Gabrielsen GW, Lydersen C, Kovacs KM, Loonen MJ, Sagerup K, Oksanen A (2007) Serosurvey for *Toxoplasma gondii* in arctic foxes and possible sources of infection in the high Arctic of Svalbard. Vet parasitol. 150: 6-12.

[123] Prestrud KW, Asbakk K, Mørk T, Fuglei E, Tryland M, Su C (2008) Direct high-resolution genotyping of *Toxoplasma gondii* in arctic foxes (*Vulpes lagopus*) in the remote arctic Svalbard archipelago reveals widespread clonal Type II lineage. Vet parasitol. 158: 121-128.

[124] Maubon D, Ajzenberg D, Brenier-Pinchart MP, Dardé ML, Pelloux H (2008) What are the respective host and parasite contributions to toxoplasmosis? Trends parasitol. 24: 299–303.

[125] Innes EA (1997) Toxoplasmosis: comparative species susceptibility and host immune response. Comp. immunol. microbiol. infect. dis. 20: 131-138.

[126] Shimizu K (1958) Studies on toxoplasmosis I: An outbreak of toxoplasmosis among hares (*Lepus timidus ainu*) in Sapporo. Jap. j. vet. res. 6: 157–166.

[127] Gustafsson K, Järplid B (1997) *Toxoplasma gondii* infection in the mountain hare (*Lepus timidus*) and domestic rabbit (*Oryctolagus cuniculus*). I. Pathology. J. comp. pathol. 117: 351–360.

[128] Gustafsson K, Wattrang E, Fossum C, Heegaard PMH, Lind P, Uggla A (1997) *Toxoplasma gondii* infection in the mountain hare (*Lepus timidus*) and domestic rabbit (*Oryctolagus cuniculus*). II. Early immune reactions. J. comp. pathol. 117: 361–369.

[129] Sedlak K, Literak I, Faldyna M, Toman M, Benak J (2000) Fatal toxoplasmosis in brown hares (*Lepus europaeus*): Possible reasons of their high susceptibility to the infection. Vet. parasitol. 93: 13–28.

[130] Kenny DE, Lappin MR, Knightly F, Baler J, Brewer M, Getzy DM (2002) Toxoplasmosis in Pallas' cats (*Otocolobus felis manul*) at the Denver Zoological Gardens. J. zoo wildl. med. 33: 131-138.

[131] Basso W, Edelhofer R, Zenker W, Möstl K, Kübber-Heiss A, Prosl H (2005) Toxoplasmosis in Pallas' cats (*Otocolobus manul*) raised in captivity. Parasitology 130: 293-299. Erratum in: Parasitology 130: 586.

[132] Brown M, Lappin MR, Brown JL, Munkhtsog B, Swanson WF (2005) Exploring the ecologic basis for extreme susceptibility of Pallas' cats (*Otocolobus manul*) to fatal toxoplasmosis. J wildl dis. 41: 691-700.

[133] Convention on international trade in threatened species (2001) Checklist of CITES species Convention on International Trade in Threatened Species, Geneva, Switzerland, http://www.felineconservation.org/feline_species/pallas__cat.htm.

[134] Ajzenberg D, Bañuls AL, Tibayrenc M, Dardé ML (2002) Microsatellite analysis of *Toxoplasma gondii* shows considerable polymorphism structured into two main clonal groups. Int j. parasitol. 32:27-38.

[135] Su C, Khan A, Zhou P, Majumdar D, Ajzenberg D, Dardé ML, Xing-Quan Zhu XQ, Ajioka JW, Rosenthal BM, Dubey JP, Sibley LD (2012) Globally diverse *Toxoplasma gondii* isolates comprise six major clades originating from a small number of distinct ancestral lineages. Proc. nat. acad. sci. doi: 10.1073/pnas.1203190109.

[136] Ajzenberg D, Collinet F, Mercier A, Vignoles P, Dardé ML (2010) Genotyping of *Toxoplasma gondii* isolates with 15 microsatellite markers in a single multiplex PCR assay. J. clin. microbiol. 48: 4641-4645.

[137] De Craeye S, Speybroeck N, Ajzenberg D, Dardé ML, Collinet F, Tavernier P, Van Gucht S, Dorny P, Dierick K (2010) *Toxoplasma gondii* and *Neospora caninum* in wildlife: common parasites in Belgian foxes and Cervidae? Vet. parasitol. 178: 64-69.

[138] Richomme C, Aubert D, Gilot-Fromont E, Ajzenberg D, Mercier A, Ducrot C, Ferté H, Delorme D, Villena I (2009) Genetic characterization of *Toxoplasma gondii* from wild boar (*Sus scrofa*) in France. Vet. parasitol. 164: 296–300.

[139] Aubert D, Ajzenberg D, Richomme C, Gilot-Fromont E, Terrier ME, de Gevigney C, Game Y, Maillard D, Gibert P, Dardé ML, Villena I (2010) Molecular and biological characteristics of *Toxoplasma gondii* isolates from wildlife in France. Vet. parasitol. 171: 346-349.

[140] Aubert D, Terrier ME, Dumètre A, Barrat J, Villena I (2008) Prevalence of *Toxoplasma gondii* in raptors from France. J. wildl. dis. 44: 172-173.

[141] Jokelainen P, Isomursu M, Nareaho A, Oksanen A (2010) *Toxoplasma gondii* killing European brown hares and mountain hares in Finland: Proportional mortality rate, seroprevalence, and genetic characterization. 9th Biennial Conference of the European Wildlife, Association, Vlieland, The Netherlands, 13 to 16 September 2010.

[142] Su C, Zhang X, Dubey JP (2006) Genotyping of *Toxoplasma gondii* by multilocus PCR-RFLP markers: a high resolution and simple method for identification of parasites. Int. j. parasitol. 36: 841-848.

[143] Aspinall TV, Marlee D, Hyde JE, Sims PF (2002) Prevalence of *Toxoplasma gondii* in commercial meat products as monitored by polymerase chain reaction - food for thought? Int. j. parasitol. 32: 1193-1199.

[144] Dumètre A, Ajzenberg D, Rozette L, Mercier A, Dardé ML (2006) *Toxoplasma gondii* infection in sheep from Haute-Vienne, France: seroprevalence and isolate genotyping by microsatellite analysis. Vet. parasitol. 142: 376-379.

[145] Halos L, Thébault A, Aubert D, Thomas M, Perret C, Geers R, Alliot A, Escotte-Binet S, Ajzenberg D, Dardé ML, Durand B, Boireau P, Villena I (2010) An innovative survey underlining the significant level of contamination by *Toxoplasma gondii* of ovine meat consumed in France. Int. j. parasitol. 40: 193-200.

[146] Owen MR, Trees AJ (1999) Genotyping of *Toxoplasma gondii* associated with abortion in sheep. J parasitol. 85: 382-384.

[147] Jungersen G, Jensen L, Rask MR, Lind P (2002) Non-lethal infection parameters in mice separate sheep Type II *Toxoplasma gondii* isolates by virulence. Comp. immunol. microbiol. infect. dis. 25: 187-195.

[148] Dubey JP, Velmurugan GV, Rajendran C, Yabsley MJ, Thomas NJ, Beckmen KB, Sinnett D, Ruid D, Hart J, Fair PA, McFee WE, Shearn-Bochsler V, Kwok OC, Ferreira LR, Choudhary S, Faria EB, Zhou H, Felix TA, Su C (2011) Genetic characterisation of *Toxoplasma gondii* in wildlife from North America revealed widespread and high prevalence of the fourth clonal type. Int. j. parasitol. 41: 1139-1147.

[149] Wendte JM, Gibson AK, Grigg ME (2011) Population genetics of *Toxoplasma gondii*: new perspectives from parasite genotypes in wildlife. Vet. parasitol. 182: 96-111.

[150] Smith DD, Frenkel JK (1995) Prevalence of antibodies to *Toxoplasma gondii* in wild mammals of Missouri and east central Kansas: biologic and ecologic considerations of transmission. J. wildl. dis. 31: 15-21.

[151] de Thoisy B, Demar M, Aznar C, Carme B (2003) Ecologic correlates of *Toxoplasma gondii* exposure in free-ranging neotropical mammals. J. wildl. dis. 39: 456-459.

[152] Santos PS, Albuquerque GR, da Silva VM, Martin AR, Marvulo MF, Souza SL, Ragozo AM, Nascimento CC, Gennari SM, Dubey JP, Silva JC. (2011) Seroprevalence of *Toxoplasma gondii* in free-living Amazon River dolphins (*Inia geoffrensis*) from central Amazon, Brazil. Vet. parasitol. 29: 171-173.

[153] Sobral CA, Amendoeira MR, Teva A, Patel BN, Klein CH (2005) Seroprevalence of infection with *Toxoplasma gondii* in indigenous Brazilian populations. Am. j. trop. med. hyg. 72: 37-41.

[154] Berengo A, Pampiglione S, De Lalla F (1974) Serological studies on toxoplasmosis in some groups of Babiga Pygmies in Central Africa. Riv. parassitol. 35: 81-86.

[155] Johnson WE, Eizirik E, Pecon-Slattery J, Murphy WJ, Antunes A, Teeling E, O'Brien SJ (2006) The late Miocene radiation of modern Felidae: a genetic assessment. Science 311: 73-77.

[156] IUCN SSC Group CS (1996) Cat Website. Available: http://lynx.uio.no/lynx/catsgportal/cat-website/20_cat-website/home/index_en.htm. 02.04.2012.

[157] Elmore SA, Jones JL, Conrad PA, Patton S, Lindsay DS, Dubey JP (2010) *Toxoplasma gondii*: epidemiology, feline clinical aspects, and prevention. Trends parasitol. 26: 190-196.

[158] Ullmann LS, da Silva RC, de Moraes W, Cubas ZS, dos Santos LC, Hoffmann JL, Moreira N, Guimaraes AM, Montaño P, Langoni H, Biondo AW (2010) Serological survey of *Toxoplasma gondii* in captive Neotropical felids from Southern Brazil. Vet. parasitol. 172: 144-146.

[159] Bevins SN, Carver S, Boydston EE, Lyren LM, Alldredge M, Logan KA, Riley SP, Fisher RN, Vickers TW, Boyce W, Salman M, Lappin MR, Crooks KR, VandeWoude S (2012) Three pathogens in sympatric populations of pumas, bobcats, and domestic cats: implications for infectious disease transmission. PLoS ONE 7: e31403.

[160] Boothroyd JC (2009) Expansion of host range as a driving force in the evolution of *Toxoplasma*. Mem. inst. Oswaldo Cruz 104: 179-184.

[161] Carme B, Demar-Pierre M (2006) [Toxoplasmosis in French Guiana. Atypical neo-tropical features of a cosmopolitan parasitosis]. Med. trop. (Mars) 66: 495-503.

[162] Carme B, Demar M, Ajzenberg D, Dardé ML (2009) Severe acquired toxoplasmosis caused by wild cycle of *Toxoplasma gondii*, French Guiana. Emerg. infect. dis. 15: 656-658.

[163] Dardé ML, Villena I, Pinon JM, Beguinot I (1998) Severe toxoplasmosis caused by a *Toxoplasma gondii* strain with a new isoenzyme type acquired in French Guyana. J. clin. microbiol. 36: 324.

[164] Ajzenberg D, Banuls AL, Su C, Dumetre A, Demar M, Carme B, Dardé ML (2004) Genetic diversity, clonality and sexuality in *Toxoplasma gondii*. Int. j. parasitol. 34: 1185-1196.

[165] Mercier A, Ajzenberg D, Devillard S, Demar MP, de Thoisy B, Bonnabau H, Collinet F, Boukhari R, Blanchet D, Simon S, Carme B, Dardé ML (2011) Human impact on genetic diversity of *Toxoplasma gondii*: Example of the anthropized environment from French Guiana. Infect. genet. evol. 11: 1378-1387.

[166] Elbez-Rubinstein A, Ajzenberg D, Dardé ML, Cohen R, Dumètre A, Yera H, Gondon E, Janaud JC, Thulliez P (2009) Congenital toxoplasmosis and reinfection during pregnancy: case report, strain characterization, experimental model of reinfection, and review. J. infect. dis. 199: 280-285.

[167] Grigg ME, Bonnefoy S, Hehl AB, Suzuki Y, Boothroyd JC (2001) Success and virulence in *Toxoplasma* as the result of sexual recombination between two distinct ancestries. Science 294: 161-165.

[168] Su C, Evans D, Cole RH, Kissinger JC, Ajioka JW, Sibley LD (2003) Recent expansion of *Toxoplasma* through enhanced oral transmission. Science 299: 414-416.

[169] Mercier A, Devillard S, Ngoubangoye B, Bonnabau H, Bañuls AL, Durand P, Salle B, Ajzenberg D, Dardé ML (2010) Additional Haplogroups of *Toxoplasma gondii* out of Africa: Population structure and mouse-virulence of strains from Gabon. PLoS negl. trop. dis 4: e876.

[170] Ajzenberg D, Yera H, Marty P, Paris L, Dalle F, Menotti J, Aubert D, Franck J, Bessieres MH, Quinio D, Pelloux H, Delhaes L, Desbois N, Thulliez P, Robert-Gangneux F,

Kauffmann-Lacroix C, Pujol S, Rabodonirina M, Bougnoux ME, Cuisenier B, Duhamel C, Duong TH, Filisetti D, Flori P, Gay-Andrieu F, Pratlong F, Nevez G, Totet A, Carme B, Bonnabau H, Dardé ML, Villena I (2009) Genotype of 88 *Toxoplasma gondii* isolates associated with toxoplasmosis in immunocompromised patients and correlation with clinical findings. J. infect. dis. 199: 1155-1167.

[171] Lehmann T, Marcet PL, Graham DH, Dahl ER, Dubey JP (2006) Globalization and the population structure of *Toxoplasma gondii*. Proc. natl. acad. sci. U S A 103: 11423-11428.

[172] Dubey JP, Quirk T, Pitt JA, Sundar N, Velmurugan GV, Kwok OC, Leclair D, Hill R, Su C (2008) Isolation and genetic characterization of *Toxoplasma gondii* from raccoons (*Procyon lotor*), cats (*Felis domesticus*), striped skunk (*Mephitis mephitis*), black bear (*Ursus americanus*), and cougar (*Puma concolor*). J. parasitol. 94: 42-45.

[173] Kapperud G, Jenum PA, Stray-Pedersen B, Melby KK, Eskild A, Eng J (1996) Risk factors for *Toxoplasma gondii* infection in pregnancy. Results of a prospective case-control study in Norway. Am. j. epidemiol. 144: 405-412.

[174] Bowie WR, King AS, Werker DH, IsaacRenton JL, Bell A, Eng SB, Marion SA (1997) Outbreak of toxoplasmosis associated with municipal drinking water. Lancet 350: 173-177.

[175] Aubert D, Villena I (2009) Detection of *Toxoplasma gondii* oocysts in water: proposition of a strategy and evaluation in Champagne-Ardenne Region, France. Memorias Do Instituto Oswaldo Cruz 104: 290-295.

[176] Baril L, Ancelle T, Goulet V, Thulliez P, Tirard-Fleury V, Carme B (1999) Risk factors for *Toxoplasma* infection in pregnancy: A case-control study in France. Scand. j. infect. dis. 31: 305-309.

[177] AFSSA (2005) Toxoplasmose : état des connaissances et évaluation du risque lié à l'alimentation Rapport du groupe de travail « *Toxoplasma gondii* » de l'Afssa. http://www.anses.fr/cgi-bin/countdocs.cgi?Documents/MIC-Ra-Toxoplasmose.pdf.

[178] Opsteegh M, Prickaerts S, Frankena K, Evers EG (2011) A quantitative microbial risk assessment for meatborne *Toxoplasma gondii* infection in The Netherlands. Int. j. food microbiol. 150: 103-114.

[179] Kijlstra A, Meerburg BG, Mul MF (2004) Animal-friendly production systems may cause re-emergence of *Toxoplasma gondii*. Njas-Wageningen Journal of Life Sciences 52: 119-132.

[180] van der Giessen J, Fonville M, Bouwknegt M, Langelaar M, Vollema A (2007) Seroprevalence of *Trichinella spiralis* and *Toxoplasma gondii* in pigs from different housing systems in The Netherlands. Vet. parasitol. 148: 371-374.

[181] Meerburg BG, Van Riel JW, Cornelissen JB, Kijlstra A, Mul MF (2006) Cats and goat whey associated with *Toxoplasma gondii* infection in pigs. Vector-Borne and Zoonotic Diseases 6: 266-274.

[182] Kijlstra A, Meerburg B, Cornelissen J, De Craeye S, Vereijken P, Jongert E (2008) The role of rodents and shrews in the transmission of *Toxoplasma gondii* to pigs. Vet. parasitol. 156: 183-190.

[183] Dubey JP, Hill DE, Rozeboom DW, Rajendran C, Choudhary S, Ferreira LR, Kwok OC, Su C (2012) High prevalence and genotypes of *Toxoplasma gondii* isolated from organic pigs in northern USA. Vet parasitol. in press.

[184] Kijlstra A, Jongert E (2009) Toxoplasma-safe meat: close to reality? Trends parasitol. 25: 18-22.

[185] Lélu M, Gilot-Fromont E, Aubert D, Afonso E, Dupuis E, Gotteland C, Dardé ML, Marnef F, Poulle ML, Richaume-Jolion A, Villena I (2011) Development of a sensitive method for *Toxoplasma gondii* oocysts extraction in soil samples. Vet. parasitol. 183: 59-67.

[186] Villena I, Aubert D, Gomis P, Ferté H, Inglard JC, Denis-Bisiaux H, Dondon JM, Pisano E, Ortis N, Pinon JM (2004) Evaluation of a strategy for *Toxoplasma gondii* oocyst detection in water. Appl. environ. microbiol. 70: 4035–4039.

[187] Kourenti C, Karanis P (2006) Evaluation and applicability of a purification method coupled with nested PCR for the detection of *Toxoplasma* oocysts in water. Lett. appl. microbiol. 43: 475-481.

[188] Borchardt MA, Spencer SK, Bertz PD, Ware MW, Dubey JP, Alan Lindquist HD (2009) Concentrating *Toxoplasma gondii* and *Cyclospora cayetanensis* from surface water and drinking water by continuous separation channel centrifugation. J. appl. microbiol. 107: 1089-1097.

[189] Du F, Zhanga Q, Yu Q, Hu M, Zhou Y, Zhao J (2012) Soil contamination of Toxoplasma gondii oocysts in pig farms in central China. Vet. parasitol. doi:10.1016/j.vetpar.2011.12.036.

[190] Hill D, Coss C, Dubey JP, Wroblewski K, Sautter M, Hosten T, Muñoz-Zanzi C, Mui E, Withers S, Boyer K, Hermes G, Coyne J, Jagdis F, Burnett A, McLeod P, Morton H, Robinson D, McLeod R (2011) Identification of a sporozoite-specific antigen from *Toxoplasma gondii*. J. parasitol. 97: 328-37.

[191] Muñoz-Zanzi CA, Fry, P Lesina B, Hill D (2010) *Toxoplasma gondii* Oocyst–specific Antibodies and Source of Infection. Emerg. infect. dis 16: 1591-1596.

[192] Muñoz-Zanzi C, Tamayo R, Balboa J, Hill D (2012) Detection of oocyst-associated toxoplasmosis in swine from Southern Chile. Zoonoses pub. health. doi: 10.1111/j.1863-2378.2012.01471.x.

[193] Boyer K, Hill D, Mui E, Wroblewski K, Karrison T, Dubey JP, Sautter M, Noble AG, Withers S, Swisher C, Heydemann P, Hosten T, Babiarz J, Lee D, Meier P, McLeod R (2011) Toxoplasmosis Study Group. Unrecognized ingestion of *Toxoplasma gondii* oocysts leads to congenital toxoplasmosis and causes epidemics in North America. Clin. infect. dis. 53: 1081-1089.

Chapter 2

Toxoplasma gondii Infection in South-East Europe: Epidemiology and Epizootiology

Branko Bobić, Ivana Klun, Aleksandra Nikolić and Olgica Djurković-Djaković

Additional information is available at the end of the chapter

http://dx.doi.org/10.5772/50831

1. Introduction

Toxoplasmosis is a globally distributed parasitic zoonosis. Cats and other *Felidae* are the definitive host of the *Toxoplasma gondii* parasite, in whose intestines the sexual cycle takes place, and they are the primary source of infection to all animals including humans, by way of contaminating the environment with oocysts excreted in the feces (Dubey, 2010). Herbivores are infected by ingestion of food and water contaminated by oocysts, and carnivores by eating tissue cysts present in the flesh of infected animals. Omnivores including humans are infected by both routes – by oocysts via improperly washed vegetables or fruits, contaminated water or hands, and by tissue cysts via improperly processed or raw meat. Vertical transmission, from mother to offspring, may occur, and is the cause of congenital toxoplasmosis (CT). CT is actually the major *T. gondii*-induced clinical entity, which, along with opportunistic infection in immunocompromised patients, defines the clinical significance of toxoplasmosis. The gravity of the potential consequences of CT on the one hand, and the preventability of the disease on the other, call for implementation of prevention programs. A prerequisite for an adequate choice of prevention strategy is continuous monitoring of the local epidemiological situation.

This chapter reviews the epidemiology and epizootiology of *T. gondii* infection in South-East Europe (SEE). SEE is here considered as the territory comprising the Balkan Peninsula (35° – 46°53' N latitude, 13°23' – 30° E longitude), bordered by the Adriatic Sea to the west, the Mediterranean Sea to the south, the Black Sea to the east and the rivers Sava and Danube to the north, encompassing the countries descending from ex-Yugoslavia including Slovenia, Croatia, Bosnia & Herzegovina, Serbia, Montenegro and FYR of Macedonia (FYRoM), as well as Albania, Bulgaria and mainland Greece. Most of the area is mountainous, while the climate varies from Mediterranean to moderate. The whole region has a combined area of 550,000 km^2 and a population of 55 million.

2. Epidemiology of toxoplasmosis in SEE

We analysed epidemiological data published in the last 20 years for all SEE countries except Bulgaria and Bosnia & Herzegovina for which none were available. Data in the published reports were obtained using a wide array of immunodiagnostic assays which may somewhat limit comparisons. Indeed, the tests in use have varied over time both among and within individual countries, and included the Sabin-Feldman test (SFT), complement fixation test (CFT), indirect fluorescence (IFAT) to direct agglutination (DA) and ELISA, whether in-house or commercial; the latter ones were obtained from various manufacturers. However, this limitation applies to any such review (Gilbert & Peckham, 2002), and moreover, the pattern of infection observed in the region despite the variety of tests with their different specificities, sensitivities, cut-offs etc., rather emphasizes the described trends.

The vast majority of epidemiological data on toxoplasmosis in SEE comes from studies in women of generative age, and a few from studies in immunocompromised patients.

2.1. Toxoplasmosis in generative age women

Data on the prevalence of *T. gondii* infection in SEE countries are presented in Figure 1. In the last ten years, the prevalence has not surpassed 50% anywhere in the region, ranging from 20% in Greece (Diza et al., 2005) to 49% in Albania (Maggi et al., 2009). Wide differences in the prevalence of infection are generally characteristic of Europe, since the infection prevalence is currently ranging from 8.2% in Switzerland (Lausanne and Geneva) (Zufferey et al., 2007) to 57.6% in Timisoara-Romania (Olariu et al., 2008). Differences in the prevalence of *T. gondii* infection are commonly explained by differences in life-style habits pertaining to risk factors for transmission in particular milieus. Not many studies on infection risk factors have been published in SEE countries, but those available identified consumption of undercooked meat as the leading risk factor for transmission in Serbia and, more recently, in Albania (Bobić et al., 1998; 2003; 2007; Maggi et al., 2009), and contact with soil in northern Greece and FYRoM (Decavalas et al., 1990; Diza et al., 2005; Cvetković et al., 2010). Exposure to soil was also considered to account for the higher prevalence of infection in rural *vs.* urban women in Croatia.

Continuous monitoring of the prevalence of *T. gondii* infection in women of childbearing age in Slovenia, Serbia and Greece has showed a significant decrease in the infection prevalence since the eighties onwards. The largest decrease, from 86% in 1988 to 31% in 2007 (Bobić et al., 2003; 2007), was noted in Serbia. Furthermore, a trend of decreasing prevalence has been shown during the last decade in FYRoM, from 25% in 2002 to 20% in 2005 (Cvetković et al., 2003; 2010) and in Montenegro, a rather dramatic one, from 41% in 2001 to 27% in 2007 (Mišković et al., 2003; Rajković & Vratnica, 2008). These data suggest that a decrease in the prevalence is a region-wide feature (Fig. 1).

A decreasing trend of *T. gondii* infection prevalence noted in the SEE region is obviously part of a Europe-wide changing pattern of *T. gondii* infection over the last 30 years (Aspöck & Pollak, 1992; Nowakowska et al., 2006; Berger et al., 2009). Many factors have contributed

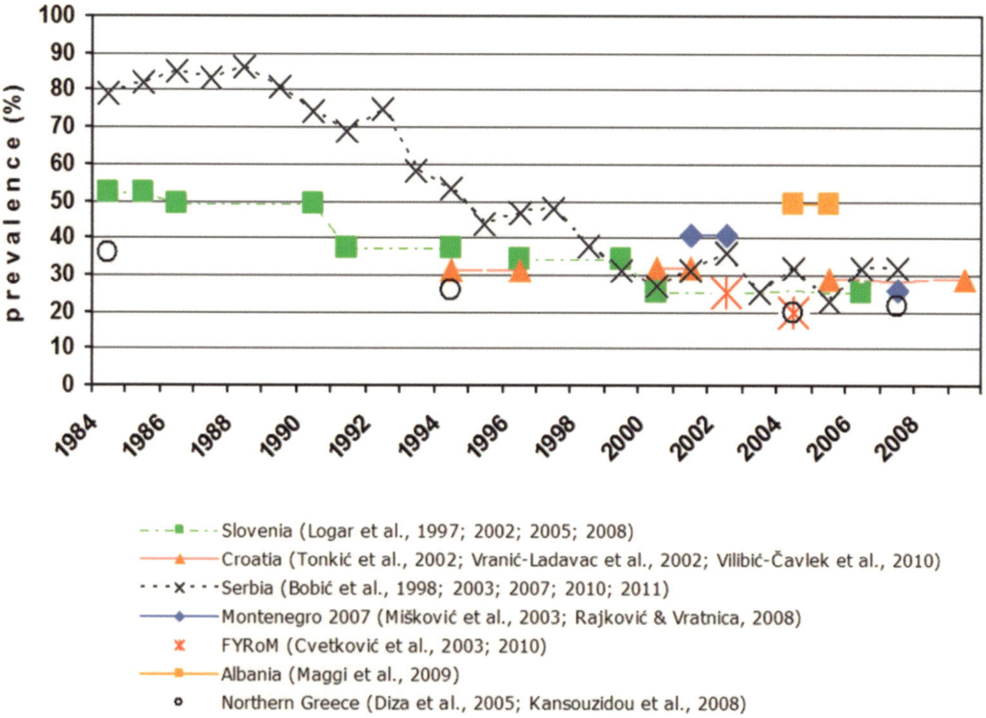

Figure 1. Prevalence of *Toxoplasma gondii* infection in generative age women in South-East Europe countries (1984-2009)

to such a change, including increased public awareness as a result of health education, better hygiene on livestock farms, and more frequent use of frozen meat. However, according to the SEE data, the listed factors seem not to be exhaustive; although better farming conditions along with the increased consumption of frozen meat (freezers now present in most households) may have contributed to a decrease in the infection prevalence in Serbia and Albania, a decreasing trend was also noted in FYRoM and Greece where consumption of undercooked meat was not found to be a risk factor.

It appears that, according to reports from the eastern part of the region, there is a north-to-south decrease in the infection prevalence (Table 1). For instance, in 1994, the prevalence ranged from 69% in southern Hungary (as a region neighbouring the SEE to the north) (Szénási et al., 1997), over 53% in Serbia (Bobić et al., 2003) to 26% in northern Greece (Diza et al., 2005). This trend was also evident within SEE in all years for which comparative data were available (2002: Serbia 36%, FYRoM 25%; 2004: Serbia 32%, Northern Greece 20%; 2007: Serbia 31%, Northern Greece 21%) (Cvetković et al., 2003; Diza et al., 2005; Bobić et al., 2007; Kansouzidou et al., 2008; Bobić et al., 2011). Moreover, a significant north-to-south decrease in the infection prevalence was also shown within Serbia itself (Bobić et al., 2003). The north-to-south decrease in the prevalence of infection within SEE suggests a possible influence of climatic conditions, which vary across the region from continental to Mediterranean, and over time as well.

Year	South Hungary	Serbia	FYR Macedonia	Northern Greece
1991	73% (1)	69% (2)		
1992	70% (1)	75% (2)		
1993	64% (1)	58% (2)		
1994	69% (1)	53% (2)		26% (6)
2002		36% (3)	25% (4)	
2004		32% (3)	20% (5)	20% (6)
2007		31% (8)		21% (7)

1) Szénási et al., 1997; 2) Bobić et al., 1997; 3) Bobić et al., 2007; 4) Cvetković et al., 2003; 5) Cvetković et al., 2010; 6) Diza et al., 2005; 7) Kansouzidou et al., 2008; 8) Bobić et al., 2011

Table 1. Decrease of prevalence of *Toxoplasma gondii* infection from North to South in three SEE countries

Seasonality of infection was examined in Slovenia (Logar et al., 2005) in the west and Serbia (Bobić et al., 2010) in the east. Both studies showed a strong seasonality, with significantly more cases of acute infection in the winter than in the summer months (Fig. 2). In Slovenia, seasonality of infection was attributed to "more frequent and closer contacts with potentially *T. gondii* infected cats, which prefer to stay indoors during this period" (Logar et al., 2005). In contrast, more cases of acute infection in the winter in Serbia were explained by a higher influence of undercooked meat consumption in the winter period (Bobić et al., 2010).

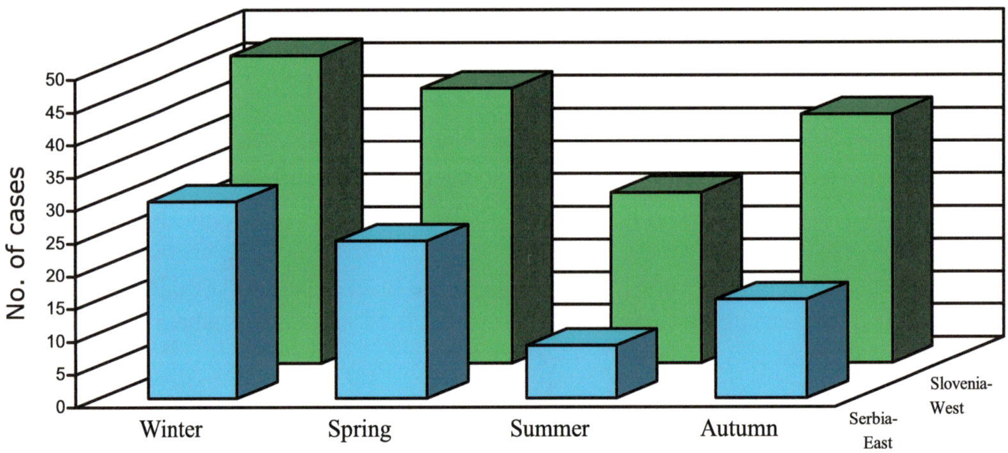

Figure 2. Seasonality of *Toxoplasma gondii* infection in Slovenia (1999-2004) and Serbia (2004-2008) (Logar et al., 2005; Bobić et al., 2010)

Accordingly, the decrease in the prevalence of *T. gondii* infection in the SEE seems independent of the varying influence of risk factors for infection transmission throughout the region. However, this may prove not to be entirely true, as the above analysis was based on the limited data reported, which were often not acquired through systematic nation-wide research, and which were mainly derived from epidemiological questionnaires of variable precision level. For an accurate insight into the risk factors of major significance for human *T. gondii* infection, more research, based on larger patient series and carried out in different SEE areas, including case-control studies, would be preferable.

2.2. Toxoplasmosis in immunocompromised patients

Toxoplasmosis is a major opportunistic infection causing life-threatening disease in immunocompromised individuals, which is considered to be a consequence of reactivation of previously latent infection. Although opportunistic infection due to *T. gondii* has long been known in organ/tissue transplantations and patients with malign or systemic diseases on treatment with immunosuppressive effect, data on toxoplasmosis in the immunocompromised population in SEE are available only from groups of HIV-infected individuals and even these are scarce. In Serbia, out of a cohort of 339 patients diagnosed with AIDS during a five year period (1991-95), 288 were tested for *T. gondii* infection and the prevalence was 44.1% (Djurković-Djaković et al., 1997). A more recent Croatian study of 219 blood donors and 166 HIV-infected patients referred to the Zagreb University Hospital for Infectious Diseases "Dr. Fran Mihaljević" in 2000-2001, the seroprevalence of toxoplasmosis was 52.5% and 51.8%, respectively (Đaković-Rode et al., 2010), confirming that the prevalence of *T. gondii* infection among HIV-positive individuals is similar to that in the general population. Interestingly, whereas the risk for developing TE was not associated with age, sex or HIV transmission risk factor in Serbia (Djurković-Djaković et al., 1997), the Croatian study established a higher risk of *T. gondii* infection (OR 2.37) for men who have sex with men (Đaković-Rode et al., 2010). In the Serbian study, of the 288 examined HIV-infected patients, 31 developed toxoplasmic encephalitis, indicating an overall attack rate of 7.8%. At the time, the cumulative incidence of toxoplasmic encephalitis in *T. gondii*-seropositive patients was estimated at 32.7% for 60 months. However, the subsequent wide use of highly active antiretroviral treatment has allowed for good control of formerly AIDS-defining opportunistic infections including toxoplasmosis, significantly decreasing their significance.

2.3. Molecular epidemiology

Although the population structure of *T. gondii* isolates throughout the world is currently a major research interest in the field of toxoplasmosis (Ajzenberg et al. 2002; Sibley et al., 2009), such studies are at its beginning in SEE. As concerns the data on *T. gondii* genotypes present in the SEE region, there is a single published report of a type II strain genotype isolated from a case of congenital toxoplasmosis in Serbia (Djurković-Djaković et al. 2006). Current data on this issue in Serbia are reported elsewhere in this book (Ivović et al.). It is to be hoped that with the increased use of molecular methodologies in the region, work will be performed which will contribute to the pan-European map of *T. gondii* genotypes.

2.4. Prevention of human toxoplasmosis

Strategies for the prevention of CT include general screening-in-pregnancy programs and health education, and countries with a low prevalence of infection generally opt for health education (Kravetz et Federman, 2005; Gilbert and Peckham, 2002), while those with a high prevalence adopt screening-in-pregnancy programs (Aspöck & Pollak, 1992; Thulliez, 1992). In the SEE, a systematic program for the prevention of CT based on serological screening of pregnant women and health education has been implemented in Slovenia, while no other country has a systematic prevention program (Logar et al, 2002). The changing pattern of infection across the region currently complicates the choice of prevention strategy. A decrease in the prevalence of infection in women of childbearing age implies a rising proportion of women susceptible to infection in pregnancy, which, in turn, may lead to an increase in the incidence of congenital infections. Indeed, an increase in the incidence of primary infections in pregnancy has been shown through systematic screening-in-pregnancy programs; in Austria, which has been screening all pregnant women ever since 1975, the decrease in *T. gondii* prevalence from 50% to 37% during the 1980s was followed by an increase in the incidence of primary infections in pregnancy from 0.4% to 0.8% (Aspöck & Pollak, 1992). Similarly, in Slovenia, the decrease in the prevalence of infection from the early 1980s onwards, therefore before the introduction of the systematic prevention program in 1995, has been associated with an increased incidence of infections in pregnancy from 0.33% in the early 1980s to 0.75% in the early 1990s and to 0.94% in the late 1990s (Logar et al., 1995; 2002).

The decreasing prevalence of *T. gondii* infection and a possible subsequent increase in the incidence of primary infections in pregnancy warrants introduction of CT prevention programs in the SEE countries. A prerequisite for such programs to be cost-effective, however, is an accurate assessment of the proportion of women of childbearing age susceptible to infection in pregnancy and the subsequent incidence of CT. These data are not yet available for most of the SEE, and are further complicated by the changing pattern of infection across the region. Thus, a sound and financially sustainable alternative that may be recommended for all of the SEE, similar to what has been recommended for Serbia (Bobić et al., 2003), includes health education of all women of childbearing age focusing on the locally significant risk factors for infection transmission in particular countries.

Health education is an adequate preventive measure for uninfected immunocompromised patients too.

3. Epizootiology of toxoplasmosis in SEE

Epizootiological surveillance of *T. gondii* infection in meat animals is important both as a measure essential for animal health and economics of livestock production, and for assessment of the risk for human health, as infected meat animals represent an important reservoir for human infection.

Throughout SEE, few data are available on *T. gondii* infection in animals and most are not the result of systematic research. Early reports, in particular from Serbia/Yu, dealt with isolation of viable *T. gondii* from various species. By bioassay of brains and/or hearts in ground squirrels (*Spermophilus citellus*) *T. gondii* was isolated from 0.25% chickens (Simitch et al., 1961); and 0.7% pigs, 0% sheep and cattle, 6.2% guinea fowl, 3.8% turkeys, 3.6% ducks, 1% geese and 0% pigeons (Simić et al., 1967). By mouse bioassay, *T. gondii* has been isolated from pork, and from pig and sheep diaphragms in Croatia/Yu (Wikerhauser et al., 1983; 1988). In Bosnia/Yu, Živković and Arežina (1991) reported apparent *T. gondii* in smears from muscle tissues of farmed layers.

The data on strain isolation in animals are scarce; researchers in Bulgaria have reported isolation of both virulent and avirulent strains of *T. gondii* from domestic and wild animals, but did not perform genetic typing (Arnaudov, 1978; Arnaudov et al., 2003; Arnaudov & Arnaudov, 2005). In Serbia, genotyping of *T. gondii* strains isolated from animals (sheep, pigs, pigeons) is in progress, and the first results confirm the dominance of type II strains (unpublished data).

Earlier serological investigations of various animal species in SEE countries showed a prevalence of 37% for cattle, 30% for sheep, 26% for pigs, 17% for horses, 41% for dogs, 25% for cats, 52% for house mice and 20% for rats in Serbia, but except for pigs, they were carried out on samples of limited size (Šibalić, 1977). In Bulgaria, Nankov (1968) has shown a 15.7% prevalence in hares, and Arnaudov (1971, 1973) reported a prevalence of 32.6% for sheep and 27.2% for goats.

An overview of studies of *T. gondii* infection in animals in SEE countries in the last 20 years is presented in Table 2. Evidently, data are not available for a half of the SEE countries.

As in humans, and similar to the rest of Europe and elsewhere (Tenter et al., 2000; Hall et al., 2001), data on the prevalence in animals vary quite widely in SEE. The highest prevalence has been reported for cattle, sheep and goats (Table 2). While farming practices are similar throughout the SEE region, differences within the region mostly occur in the climatic conditions and terrain characteristics.

The single nation-wide survey on *T. gondii* infection in meat animals in SEE, performed recently in Serbia, showed high seroprevalence rates of 76.3% in cattle and 84.5% in sheep and a lower one, of 28.9%, in pigs (Klun et al., 2006). This study showed that cattle from Western Serbia were at an increased risk of infection compared to all other regions (Table 3), possibly associated with a comparably increased humidity in this region (Klun et al., 2006). The levels of specific antibody determined in the cattle were relatively low (not above 1:400),

Country	Species	No. examined	% Positive	Test (cut-off)	Origin of animals	Ref.
Croatia	Goats	79	13.9	MAT (1:20)	Farms	Rajković-Janje et al., 1993
	Goats	100	4	MAT (1:20)	Farms	
	Σ Goats	179	8.4	MAT (1:20)	Σ	
	Sheep	unknown	11.6 (sheep) 9.4 (lambs)	DAT	Farms	Rajković-Janje et al., 1994
	Sheep	unknown	0.5	DAT	Nomadic	
	Σ Sheep	334	4.8	DAT	Σ	
	Sheep	unknown	48.4	ELISA	10 farms	Marinculić et al., 1997
	Chickens	716	0.4	Bioassay	Abattoir	Kutičić & Wikerhauser, 2000
	Rats	142	1.4	Bioassay	Pig farms	Kutičić et al., 2005
	Mice	86	0	Bioassay	Pig farms + households	

Serbia	Cattle	611	76.3	MAT (1:25)	Farms + abattoir	Klun et al., 2006
	Sheep	511	84.5	MAT (1:25)	Farms	
	Pigs	605	28.9	MAT (1:25)	Farms + abattoir	
	Horses	250	30.8	MAT (1:25)	Farms	Klun, 2005
	Sheep	367	7.1	unknown	Aborting sheep	Vidić et al., 2007
	Sheep	30	36.7	IFAT (1:20)	Farm	Laloševič et al., 2008
	Pigs	488	9.2	MAT (1:25)	Abattoir	Klun et al., 2011
	Goats	356	74.7	MAT (1:25)	Farms	Djokić et al., 2011
	Rats	80	27.5	MAT (1:25)	Urban	Vujanić et al., 2011
	Rats	144	7.6	Microscopy		
	Mice	12	3	Microscopy		
	Rats	144	10.4	Real-time PCR		
	Mice	12	83.3	Real-time PCR		
	Pigeons	30	13.3	MAT (1:25)	Urban (wild)	Personal observations
Bulgaria	Wild animals (7 species)	643	0 – 16.7	Agar gel micro precipitation	Wild	Arnaudov et al., 2003
	Sheep	380	48.2	IHAT (1:10)	Farms	Prelezov et al., 2008
	Goats	364	59.8	IHAT (1:10)		
Greece (mainland)	Sheep	840	53.4	IFAT	Farms	Kontos et al., 2001
	Sheep	450	58.5	ELISA		
	Cattle	105	20	ELISA	Dairy farms	Diakou et al., 2005a
	Sheep	350	52.6	ELISA	Mixed stock farms	Diakou et al., 2005b
	Goats	280	62.9			
	Sheep	184/182	52.2/50.5	ELISA (a)	Organic farms	Ntafis et al., 2007
	Goats	229/167	22.3/18	ELISA (a)		
	Horses/ equids	753/773	1.7/1.8	ELISA (a)	Farms	Kouam et al., 2010
	Dogs	2512	31.8	ELISA	unknown	Haralabidis & Diakou, 1999
	Pigeons	379	5.8	ELISA	Domestic flocks	Diakou et al., 2011
	Pigeons	50	0	ELISA	Urban (wild)	
	Σ Pigeons	429	5.1	ELISA	Σ	

(a) Mean $OD_{negative\ controls}$ + 3SD

Table 2. *Toxoplasma gondii* infection in animals in SEE countries in the last 20 years

which is consistent with reports on the rapid decrease of *T. gondii* antibody in cattle (Dubey et al., 1985). Cattle are relatively resistant to *T. gondii* infection (Dubey and Thulliez, 1993), but it is unclear whether this is associated with fast elimination of cysts from cattle tissues (Dubey, 1983), or there is inconsistent cyst formation following infection. In addition to farm location in the western region, the only other risk factor determined for cattle infection was small herd size. According to the type of housing, the results showed that access to outside pens was protective as compared to total confinement. This apparently paradoxical finding may represent a further argument for the importance of the way in which feed is kept, or possibly indicates involvement of other farm factors not identified in this type of study.

The same study showed a prevalence of 85% in sheep in Serbia, of which 10% had high antibody levels of ≥1:1600, suggestive of acute infection. Although arbitrary, the cut-off of 1:1600 is even conservative since Dubey and Welcome (1988) had considered a titre of 1:1024 high. However, correlation with ovine abortions could not be established, since etiological laboratory diagnosis of ovine abortions in Serbia does not include diagnosis of *T. gondii*. Regionwise, similarly as with cattle, sheep from Western Serbia were at an increased risk of infection as compared to all other regions (Table 3). An increased risk of infection was also found in state-owned vs. private large flocks. Compared to other SEE countries, the prevalence of 85% is quite high; in Croatia and Bulgaria the highest recorded prevalence in sheep is 48%, and in Greece 58.5% (Table 2). This is also evident in goats; compared with the prevalence of 74.7% established in Serbia (Djokić et al., 2011), it was lower in Greece (62.9%) (Diakou et al., 2005b) and Bulgaria (59.8%) (Prelezov et al., 2008), and very markedly so in Croatia – 8.4% (Rajković-Janje et al., 1993).

An outbreak of toxoplasmosis in sheep has recently been reported; massive abortions (60%) occurred in a flock of 500 dairy sheep in Northern Greece at 110-130 days of pregnancy, diagnosed upon observation of tissue cysts in brain smears of aborted fetuses, and by serological (ELISA) examinations of mother and fetal serum samples. The abortion rate declined immediately upon instituting sulfadimidine therapy (Giadinis et al., 2011).

In horses, who generally have lower seroprevalence values than small ruminants (van Knapen et al., 1982), a prevalence of 30.8% has been determined in a study in Serbia (Klun, 2005), *vs.* only 1.7% in Greece (Kouam et al., 2010).

In pigs, an overall seroprevalence of 29% was established in Serbia (Klun et al., 2006). Of those seropositive, 4% were likely to be in the acute stage of infection, indicating continuous presence of infection reservoirs in the environment. Risk factors included age and farm type (Table 3). Since pigs are continuously exposed to infection, the increase in the risk of infection with age, ranging from 15% in market weight age pigs to 41% in adults, was expected, and repeated previous findings (Dubey et al., 1991; Dubey et al., 1995; Weigel et al., 1995; Damriyasa et al., 2004). Pigs on finishing type farms were four-fold more likely to be infected than those from farrow-to-finish farms. According to these results, it was proposed that a national strategy to reduce the level of *T. gondii* infection in pigs should include a shift towards the development of more farrow-to-finish farms, as well as vigilance in farm management and implementation of zoo-hygienic measures at finishing farms. Damriyasa et al. (2004) stated that *T. gondii* seropositivity is an indicator of the hygienic status of the pig farm.

Species	Factor	Adjusted OR	95% CI	*P*-value
Cattle	Herd size			
	Large (n>100)	1.00		
	Small (n<10)	2.19	1.28–3.75	0.004
	Type of housing			
	Stable only	1.00		
	Access to outside pens	0.37	0.21–0.67	0.001
	Access to pasture	0.72	0.25–2.07	0.548
	Region			
	Northern Serbia	1.00		
	Western Serbia	2.04	1.10–3.79	0.024
	Central/Eastern Serbia	0.97	0.32–2.90	0.951
	Belgrade District	0.60	0.30–1.20	0.148
Sheep	Farm type			
	Private large (n>100)	1.00		
	State-owned (n>100)	4.18	2.18–8.00	<0.001
	Private small (n<10)	1.79	0.55–5.81	0.332
	Region			
	Northern Serbia	1.00		
	Western Serbia	4.66	1.18–18.32	0.028
	Central/Eastern Serbia	0.82	0.25–2.73	0.748
Pigs	Age group			
	Market weight (<8 months)	1.00		
	Adult (≥8 months)	3.87	2.60–5.76	<0.001
	Farm type			
	Farrow-to-finish	1.00		
	Finishing	3.96	1.97–7.94	<0.001

Table 3. Risk factors for *T. gondii* infection in meat animals in Serbia in 2003. Final logistic regression models. Results presented as adjusted odds ratio (OR) and 95% confidence intervals (CI) (modified from Klun et al., 2006)

A recent study on *T. gondii* infection in slaughter pigs in Serbia (Klun et al., 2011) showed, however, a three-fold lower prevalence of 9.2% in a total of 488 swine from abattoirs in the vicinity of Belgrade. This difference was largely attributed to the difference in the studied samples since the latter one consisted of a large majority (96%) of market-weight pigs, who generally have a much lower prevalence than adult pigs. Similarly to the 2006 study, risk factors for infection in slaughter pigs included age and farm type with a 41-fold higher likelihood of infection in adult *vs.* market-weight pigs ($p<0.001$), and a 15-fold higher likelihood of infection in pigs of all ages from smallholders' finishing type farms ($p<0.001$) *vs.* those from farrow-to-finish intensive farms.

On the other hand, the modern approach in farm management to provide for the welfare of the animals as well as organic food for human consumption is to develop animal-friendly (organic) farms. According to experiences from the Netherlands (Kijlstra et al., 2004), development of such farms may result in an increase in *T. gondii* infection. Nevertheless, a single report from organic sheep and goat farms in Greece (Ntafis et al., 2007) showed similar prevalence rates to those in animals from conventionally managed farms (Kontos et al., 2001; Diakou et al., 2005b).

A major reason for the control of *T. gondii* infection in meat animals is the reduction of the reservoir of human infection. Cattle are generally thought not to be significant in this context (Dubey and Thulliez, 1993). However, beef is often consumed undercooked ('rare' beef steaks, roast beef, steak tartar), and at least one outbreak of toxoplasmosis whose source was raw beef has been documented (Smith, 1993). In addition, one out of four beef samples randomly chosen from UK retail outlets tested positive for *T. gondii* by PCR (Aspinall et al., 2002). These facts, along with the circumstantial evidence provided by the data on the high prevalence of cattle infection of 92% in Italy and 69% in France (see Tenter et al., 2000), and now in Serbia, countries in which human infection is highly prevalent as well, all suggest a role for cattle as a *T. gondii* reservoir for human infection. In addition, Bobić et al. (2007) have demonstrated that among all the meat consumed, undercooked beef presents the highest risk for human infection in Serbia. Similarly, although Opsteegh et al. (2011a) did not establish a correlation between seropositivity and the detection of parasites in cattle, a study in which the relative contribution of sheep, beef and pork products to human *T. gondii* infection in the Netherlands was quantified (by Quantitative Microbial Risk Assessment), showed that beef is indeed an important source even if the seroprevalence in cattle is low (Opsteegh et al., 2011b).

On the other hand, according to official statistical reports (RZS, 2006–2010), pork represents approximately 50% of all meat consumed in Serbia. Thus, although pigs were the least infected of the examined species, given the findings that the prevalence increases with age and reaches 41% in sows (Klun et al., 2006), pork consumption may significantly contribute to human infection. When used for cooking, pork is generally properly thermally processed, but in most of the SEE countries' tradition mature pork is also highly valued for making delicatessen meat products. Raw or improperly cured sausages and ham are the source of small (family) epidemics of trichinellosis which, in spite of mandatory meat examination for

Trichinella spiralis, occasionally occur in Serbia (Djordjević 1989, Čuperlović et al., 2005), and thus, are a quite plausible source of human *T. gondii* infection as well.

For most meat animals, although a trend is generally (worldwide) difficult to establish due to the scarcity of studies in most countries (no two time points), there is no visible reduction in the prevalence of *T. gondii* infection, as opposed to the decreasing trend in humans, discussed in detail earlier in this chapter (and explained by reasons including increased frozen meat use, better farm management etc.). For the most part, farming practices and environmental contamination have not changed, and except for the intensive pig farms in which a major reduction in *T. gondii* prevalence has occurred, a decline in the prevalence of *T. gondii* infection in meat animals is yet to be achieved. Moreover, for strictly herbivorous species that require outdoor access, this is probably impossible (Kijlstra & Jongert, 2009).

Ubiquitous contamination of the environment is also evident from the presence of *T. gondii* in both farm and urban rodents (Kutičić et al., 2005; Vujanić et al., 2011), wild animals, and pigeons (Arnaudov et al., 2003; Arnaudov & Arnaudov, 2005; Diakou et al., 2011) (Table 2). In dogs, studies performed in Greece have shown a prevalence ranging from 21.2% to 30.8% (Chambouris et al., 1989), and of 31.8%, in a large series of 2512 dogs from the regions of Macedonia and Thrace (Haralabidis & Diakou, 1999). As long as there is evidence of such widespread environmental contamination in SEE, a change for the better and a decrease of *T. gondii* infection in meat animals may hardly be expected in the absence of energetic and systematic prevention measures throughout the region.

4. Conclusion

Existing strategies for the prevention of toxoplasmosis in countries which have been implementing them for years have led to a decrease in its incidence, but have not solved the problem of congenital infection. This clearly shows that new comprehensive strategies for the prevention of toxoplasmosis are needed. These should be based on accurate and validated data on (1) the routes and risk factors for human infection on local level, which will allow for a more efficient health education; (2) routes and risk factors for meat animal infection to diminish infection reservoirs; (3) environmental contamination. Epidemiological and epizootiological data presented in this chapter show how far along this road we have come, and more importantly, how far we still have to go to achieve successful prevention of *T. gondii* infection in the SEE region.

Author details

Branko Bobić, Ivana Klun, Aleksandra Nikolić and Olgica Djurković-Djaković*
National Reference Laboratory for Toxoplasmosis, Centre for Parasitic Zoonoses (Centre of Excellence in Biomedicine), Institute for Medical Research, University of Belgrade, Serbia

* Corresponding Author

Acknowledgement

This work has been supported by project grant No. III 41019 from the Ministry of Education and Science of Serbia.

5. References

[1] Ajzenberg D, Cogné N, Paris L, Bessieres MH, Thulliez P, Fillisetti D, Pelloux H, Marty P, Dardé ML (2002): Genotype of 86 *Toxoplasma gondii* isolates associated with human congenital toxoplasmosis and correlation with clinical findings. J Infect Dis 186: 684–689.

[2] Arnaudov D (1971): [Study on the prevalence of toxoplasmosis in farm animals]. Vet Sci (Sofia) 8: 61-67.

[3] Arnaudov D (1973): [Comparative studies on complement binding test, indirect haemagglutination reaction and agar gel microprecipitation for diagnostics of toxoplasmosis in farm animals]. Vet Sci (Sofia) 10: 43-53.

[4] Arnaudov D (1978): [Comparative studies of the virulent and immunogenic properties of the *Toxoplasma* strains isolated from domestic animals]. Vet Med Nauki 15: 38-46.

[5] Arnaudov D, Arnaudov A (2005): Isolation *of Toxoplasma gondii* from domestic and wild animals. Balkan Scientific Conference on Biology, Plovdiv, Bulgaria, May 19-21. Proceedings (ed. by Gruev B, Nikolova M, Donev A): pp. 41-47.

[6] Arnaudov D, Kozojed V, Jíra J, Stourac L (1976): [Immunoepizootological study of ovine toxoplasmosis]. Vet Med (Praha) 21: 375-384.

[7] Arnaudov D, Arnaudov A, Kirin D (2003): Study on the Toxoplasmosis among wild animals, J Exp Path Parasitol *BAS* (Sofia) 6: 51-54.

[8] Aspinall TV, Marlee D, Hyde JE, Sims PF (2002); Prevalence of *Toxoplasma gondii* in commercial meat products as monitored by polymerase chain reaction – food for thought? Int J Parasitol 32: 1193-1199.

[9] Aspöck H, Pollak A (1992): Prevention of prenatal toxoplasmosis by serological screening of pregnant women in Austria. Scand J Infect Dis 84 (Suppl): 32-37.

[10] Berger F, Goulet V, Le Strat Y, Desenclos JR (2009): Toxoplasmosis among pregnant women in France: risk factors and change of prevalence between 1995 and 2003. Rev Epidemiol Sante Publique 57: 241-248.

[11] Bobić B, Djurković-Djaković O, Šibalić D, Jevremović I, Marinković J, Nikolić A, Vuković D (1996): Epidemiological relationship of the cat and human toxoplasma infection in Belgrade. Acta Vet (Belgrade) 45: 155-160.

[12] Bobić B, Jevremović I, Marinković J, Šibalić D, Djurković-Djaković O (1998): Risk factors for *Toxoplasma* infection in a reproductive age female population in the area of Belgrade, Yugoslavia. Eur J Epidemiol 14: 605-610.

[13] Bobić B, Nikolić A, Djurković-Djaković O (2003): Identification of risk factors for infection with *Toxoplasma gondii* in Serbia as a basis of a programme for prevention of congenital toxoplasmosis. Srp Arh Celok Lek 131: 162-167.

[14] Bobić B, Nikolić A, Klun I, Vujanić M, Djurković–Djaković O (2007): Undercooked meat consumption remains the major risk factor for *Toxoplasma* infection in Serbia. Parassitologia 49: 227-230.

[15] Bobić B, Klun I, Nikolić A, Vujanić M, Živković T, Ivović V, Djurković-Djaković O (2010): Seasonal variations in human *Toxoplasma* infection in Serbia. Vector Borne Zoonotic Dis 10: 465-469.

[16] Bobić B, Nikolić A, Klun I, Djurković-Djaković O (2011): Kinetics of Toxoplasma infection in the Balkans. Wien Klin Wochenschr 123 (Suppl 1): 2-6.

[17] Chambouris R, Stünzner D, Sebek Z, Sixl W, Köck M (1989): [Toxoplasmosis in dogs in Greece]. Geogr Med (Suppl 3): 19-22.

[18] Čuperlović K, Djordjević M, Pavlovic S (2005): Re-emergence of trichinellosis in southeastern Europe due to political and economic changes. Vet Parasitol 132: 159-166.

[19] Cvetković D, Grdanoska T, Panovski N, Petrovska M (2003) *Toxoplasma gondii* antibodies in women during reproductive period - our experiences. 1st FEMS Congress of European microbiologists, Ljubljana, Slovenia, June 29 – July 3. Abstract book: p. 271.

[20] Cvetković D, Bobić B, Jankovska G, Klun I, Panovski N, Djurković-Djaković O (2010): Risk factors for *Toxoplasma gondii* infection in pregnant women in FYR of Macedonia. Parasite 17: 183-186.

[21] Đaković-Rode O, Židovec-Lepej S, Vodnica Martucci M, Lasica Polanda J, Begovac V (2010): [Prevalence of antibodies against *Toxoplasma gondii* in patients infected with human immunodeficiency virus in Croatia]. Croatian J Infect 30: 5-10.

[22] Damriyasa IM, Bauer C, Edelhofer R, Failing K, Lind P, Petersen E, Schares G, Tenter AM, Volmer R, Zahner H (2004): Cross-sectional survey in pig breeding farms in Hesse, Germany: seroprevalence and risk factors of infections with *Toxoplasma gondii*, *Sarcocystis spp.* and *Neospora caninum* in sows. Vet Parasitol 126: 271-286.

[23] Decavalas G, Papapetropoulou M, Giannoulaki E, Tzigounis V, Kondakis XG (1990): Prevalence of *Toxoplasma gondii* antibodies in gravidas and recently aborted women and study of risk factors. Eur J Epidemiol 6: 223-226.

[24] Diakou A, Papadopoulos E, Haralabidis S, Papachristou F, Karatzias H, Panousis N (2005a): Prevalence of Parasites in Intensively Managed Dairy Cattle in Thessaloniki Region, Greece. Cattle practice 13: 51-54.

[25] Diakou A, Papadopoulos E, Panousis N, Giadinis N, Karatzias C (2005b): *Toxoplasma gondii* and *Neospora* spp. infection in sheep and goats mixed stock farming. Proceedings of the 6th International Sheep Veterinary Congress, Hersonissos, Crete, Greece, June 17-21: p. 170.

[26] Diakou A, Papadopoulos E, Antalis V, Gewehr S (2011): *Toxoplasma gondii* infection in wild and domestic pigeons (*Columba livia*). In: Hahn C, Fromm B (eds.). Parasites and infectious diseases in a changing world. Programme and Proceedings from the 4th Conference of the Scandinavian-Baltic Society for Parasitology, Oslo, Norway, June 19-22: p. 79.

[27] Diza E, Frantzidou F, Souliou E, Arvanitiduu M, Gioula G, Antoniadis A (2005): Prevalence of *Toxoplasma gondii* in northern Greece during the last 20 years. Clin Microbiol Infect 11: 719-723.

[28] Djokić V, Klun I, Musella V, Ivović V, Rinaldi L, Djurković-Djaković O (2011): *Toxoplasma gondii* infection in goats in Serbia: shades of grey. 3rd CAPARA WGs Workshop & MC Meeting, Limassol, Cyprus, November 10-12. Programme & Abstract book: p. 22.

[29] Djordjević M (1989): Raširenost trihineloze svinja u nekim enzootskim područjima SR Srbije i poređenje pouzdanosti nekih direktnih metoda, PhD Thesis, Belgrade University School of Veterinary Medicine.

[30] Djurković-Djaković O, Bobić B, Vuković D, Marinković J, Jeftović Dj (1997): Risk for toxoplasmic encephalitis in AIDS patients in Yugoslavia. Int J Infect Dis 2: 74-78.

[31] Djurković-Djaković O, Klun I, Khan A, Nikolić A, I Knezević-Ušaj S, Bobić B, Sibley LD (2006): A human origin type II strain of *Toxoplasma gondii* causing severe encephalitis in mice. Microbes Inf 8: 2206-2212.

[32] Dubey JP (1983): Distribution of cysts and tachyzoites in calves and pregnant cows inoculated with *Toxoplasma gondii* oocysts. Vet Parasitol 13: 199-211.

[33] Dubey JP (2010): Epidemiology. In: Dubey JP: Toxoplasmosis of animals and humans. 2nd ed., CRC Press, Boca Raton, USA. pp: 46-47.

[34] Dubey JP, Thulliez P (1993): Persistence of tissue cysts in edible tissues of cattle fed *Toxoplasma gondii* oocysts. Am J Vet Res 54: 270-273.

[35] Dubey JP, Welcome FL (1988): *Toxoplasma gondii*-induced abortion in sheep. J Am Vet Med Assoc 193: 697-700.

[36] Dubey JP, Desmonts G, McDonald C, Walls KW (1985): Serologic evaluation of cattle inoculated with *Toxoplasma gondii*: comparison of Sabin-Feldman dye test and other agglutination tests. Am J Vet Res 46: 1085-1088.

[37] Dubey JP, Leighty JC, Beal VC, Anderson WR, Andrews CD, Thulliez P (1991): National seroprevalence of *Toxoplasma gondii* in pigs. J Parasitol 77: 270-274.

[38] Dubey JP, Weigel RM, Siegel AM, Thulliez P, Kitron UD, Mitchell MA, Mannelli A, Mateus-Pinilla NE, Shen SK, Kwok OCH, Todd KS (1995): Sources and reservoirs of *Toxoplasma gondii* infection on 47 swine farms in Illinois. J Parasitol 81: 723-729.

[39] Giadinis ND, Terpsidis K, Diakou A, Siarkou V, Loukopoulos P, Osman R, Karatzias H, Papazahariadou M (2011): Massive toxoplasma abortions in a dairy sheep flock and therapeutic approach with different doses of sulfadimidine. Turk J Vet Anim Sci 35: 207-211.

[40] Gilbert RE, Peckham CS (2002): Congenital toxoplasmosis in the United Kingdom: to screen or not to screen? J Med Screen 9: 135-141.

[41] Hall S, Ryan M, Buxton M (2001): The epidemiology of *Toxoplasma* infection. In: Joynson DHM, Wreghitt TG (Eds.). Toxoplasmosis: a Comprehensive Clinical Guide. Cambridge University Press, Cambridge, pp. 58-124.

[42] Haralabidis ST, Diakou AN (1999): Toxoplasmosis, leishmaniosis, toxacariosis and filariosis of the dog in Macedonia and Thrace. Proceedings of the 5th Hellenic Congress in Small Animal Veterinary Medicine, Athens, Greece, March 27-29: pp. 168-170.

[43] Kansouzidou A, Kaftantzi A, Vamvaka E, Koltsida M, Karambaxoglou D (2008): Laboratory diagnosis of *Toxoplasma gondii* infection in population in northern Greece. 18th European Congress of Clinical Microbiology and Infectious Diseases, Barcelona, Spain, April 19-22. Abstract book: R2418.

[44] Kijlstra A, Jongert E (2009): Toxoplasma-safe meat: close to reality? Trends Parasitol 25: 18-22.

[45] Kijlstra A, Eissen OA, Cornelissen J, Munniksma K, Eijck I, Kortbeek T (2004): *Toxoplasma gondii* infection in animal-friendly pig production systems. Invest Ophthalmol Vis Sci 45: 3165-3169.

[46] Klun I (2005): Seroepizootiological study of *Toxoplasma gondii* infection in ungulates in Serbia. MSc Thesis, Belgrade University School of Veterinary Medicine

[47] Klun I, Djurković-Djaković O, Katić-Radivojević S, Nikolić A (2006): Cross-sectional survey on *Toxoplasma gondii* infection in cattle, sheep and pigs in Serbia: seroprevalence and risk factors. Vet Parasitol 135: 121-131.

[48] Klun I, Vujanić M, Yera H, Nikolić A, Ivović V, Bobić B, Bradonjić S, Dupouy-Camet J, Djurković-Djaković O (2011): *Toxoplasma gondii* infection in slaughter pigs in Serbia: seroprevalence and demonstration of parasites in blood. Vet Res 42(1): 17.

[49] van Knapen F, Franchimont JH, van der Lugt G (1982): Prevalence of antibodies to toxoplasma in farm animals in the Netherlands and its implication for meat inspection. Vet Q 4: 101-105.

[50] Kontos V, Boutsini S, Haralabidis S, Diakou A, Athanasiou L, Magana O, Nomikou K (2001): Ovine Toxoplasmosis. An Epizootiological Research. Proceedings of the 3rd Hellenic Symposium in Farm Animals Veterinary Medicine, Thessaloniki, Greece, November 9-11: p. 81.

[51] Kouam MK, Diakou A, Kanzoura V, Papadopoulos E, Gajadhar AA, Theodoropoulos G (2010): A seroepidemiological study of exposure to Toxoplasma, Leishmania, Echinococcus and Trichinella in equids in Greece and analysis of risk factors. Vet Parasitol 170: 170-175.

[52] Kravetz JD, Federman DG (2005): Toxoplasmosis in pregnancy. Am J Med 118: 212-216.

[53] Kutičić V, Wikerhauser T (2000): A survey of chickens for viable toxoplasms in Croatia. Acta Vet Hung 48: 183-185.

[54] Kutičić V, Wikerhauser T, Gracner D (2005): A survey of rats and mice for latent toxoplasmosis in Croatia: a case report. Vet Med – Czech, 50: 513-514.

[55] Lalošević V, Lalošević D, Boboš S, Simin S (2008): (Seroprevalence of *Toxoplasma gondii* infection in Srbobran region]. Savr Poljoprivr 57: 38–43.

[56] Logar J, Novak-Antolič Ž, Zore A (1995): Serological screening for toxoplasmosis in pregnancy in Slovenia. Scand J Infect Dis 27: 163-164.

[57] Logar J, Petrovec M, Novak-Antolič Ž, Premru-Srsen T, Cizman M, Arnez M, Kraut A (2002): Prevention of congenital toxoplasmosis in Slovenia by serological screening of pregnant women. Scand J Infect Dis 34: 201-204.

[58] Logar J, Šoba B, Premru-Sršen T, Novak-Antolić Ž (2005): Seasonal variations in acute toxoplasmosis in pregnant women in Slovenia. Clin Microbiol Infect 11: 852–855.

[59] Logar J, Šoba B, Novak-Antolič Ž, Premru-Sršen T, Arneż M, Kraut A (2008): Serological screening for toxoplasmosis of pregnant women in Slovenia in the period 2000-2007. Toxoplasma Centennial Congress: From discovery to public health management, Búzios, Rio de Janeiro State, Brazil, September 20-24. Abstract book: p. 43.

[60] Maggi P, Volpe A, Carito V, Schinaia N, Bino S, Basho M, Dentico P (2009): Surveillance of toxoplasmosis in pregnant women in Albania. New Microbiol 32: 89-92.

[61] Marinculić A, Bosnić S, Rajković-Janje R (1997): [Seroepizootiological studies of toxoplasmosis among sheep from central Croatia]. Veterinarski dani '97, Cavtat, Croatia, October 15-18. Proceedings (Balenović T, ed.): pp. 311-314.

[62] Mišković M, Mijović G, Bujko M (2003): Anti-*Toxoplasma gondii* IgM and IgG antibody in a reproductive age female population in Montenegro during 2001-2002. In: Djurković-Djaković O, editor. Toxoplasmosis in human and veterinary medicine. Podgorica, Montenegro, October 14. Proceedings: pp. 54-58.

[63] Nowakowska D, Stray-Pedersen B, Śpiewak E, Sobala W, Małafiej E, Wilczyński J (2006): Prevalence and estimated incidence of *Toxoplasma* infection among pregnant women in Poland: a decreasing trend in the younger population. Clin Microbiol Infect 12: 913-917.

[64] Ntafis V, Xylouri E, Diakou A, Sotirakoglou K, Kritikos I, Georgakilas E, Menegatos I (2007): Serological survey of antibodies against *Toxoplasma gondii* in organic sheep and goat farms in Greece. J Hell Vet Med Soc 58: 22-33.

[65] Olariu TR, Darabus GH, Cretu O, Jurovits O, Giura E, Erdelan V Maricu I, Icobicu I, Petrescu C, Koreck A (2008): Prevalence of *Toxoplasma gondii* antibodies among women of childbearing age, in Timis County, Romania. Lucrâri Ştiinţifice MedicinâVeterinarâ 41: 367-371.

[66] Opsteegh M, Teunis P, Züchner L, Koets A, Langelaar M, van der Giessen J (2011a): Low predictive value of seroprevalence of *Toxoplasma gondii* in cattle for detection of parasite DNA. Intl J Parasitol 41: 343–354.

[67] Opsteegh M, Prickaerts S, Frankena K, Evers EG (2011b): A quantitative microbial risk assessment for meatborne *Toxoplasma gondii* infection in The Netherlands. Intl J Food Microbiol 150: 103–114.

[68] Prelezov P, Koinarski V, Georgieva D (2008): Seroprevalence of *Toxoplasma gondii* infection among sheep and goats in the Stara Zagora region. Bulg J Vet Med 11: 113–119.

[69] Rajković D, Vratnica Z (2008): Detection of immunoglobulin G (IgG) and IgM antibodies to *Toxoplasma gondii* with commercial immunoassay systems in Montenegro. In: Djurković-Djaković O, editor. Achievements and Perspectives (What we have done and where we are doing). Project Workshop (FP6-INCO-CT-043702-SERBPARZOON). Belgrade, Serbia, June 19-20. Proceedings: p. 51.

[70] Rajković-Janje R, Marinculić A, Jovanović-Bunta V, Živičnjak T (1993): Seroepidemiological survey for toxoplasmosis in goats in Republic of Croatia. Vet arhiv 63: 125-129.

[71] Rajković-Janje R, Marinculić A, Pauković Č, Kovač Z, Horvat J (1994): [Antibody findings for the *Toxoplasma gondii* protozoon in the sheep blood in the Republic of Croatia]. Vet Stanica 25: 145-150.

[72] RZS, Statistical office of the Republic of Serbia: Bulletins of the Household budget surveys 2006–2010, http://webrzs.stat.gov.rs/WebSite/Public/PageView.aspx?pKey=431&URL=http://pod2.stat.gov.rs/ElektronskaBiblioteka2/Pretraga.aspx?pubType=3%26areaId=01 (consulted 18 May 2012).

[73] Šibalić D (1977): [Incidence of *Toxoplasma gondii* infection in man and in various animals in some areas of Serbia]. Acta Parasitol Iugoslav 8: 13-18.

[74] Sibley LD, Khan A, Ajioka JW, Rosenthal BM (2009): Genetic diversity of *Toxoplasma gondii* in animals and humans. Philos Trans R Soc Lond B Biol Sci. 364: 2749-2761.

[75] Simitch T, Bordjoški A, Petrovitch Z, Tomanovitch B, Savin Ž (1961): [Toxoplasmose of birds. I. Natural infection of domestic poultry with *Toxoplasma gondii* in Yugoslavia]. Arch Inst Pasteur d'Algerie 39: 135-139.

[76] Simić T, Bordjoški A, Šibalić D (1967): [The role of domestic mammals meat and poultry in the infestation of men with toxoplasmosis]. Hrana i ishrana 8; 327-333.

[77] Smith JL (1993): Documented outbreaks of toxoplasmosis: Transmission of *Toxoplasma gondii* to humans. J Food Protect 56: 630-639.

[78] Szénási Z, Ozsvár Z, Nagy E, Jesenszky M, Szabo J, Gellen J, Vegh M, Verhofstede C (1997): Prevention of congenital toxoplasmosis in Szeged, Hungary. Int J Epidemiol 26: 428-435.

[79] Tenter AM, Heckeroth AR, Weiss LM (2000): *Toxoplasma gondii*: from animals to humans. Int J Parasitol 30: 1217-1258.

[80] Thulliez P (1992): Screening programme for congenital toxoplasmosis in France. Scand J Infect Dis 84 (Suppl.): 43-45.

[81] Tonkić M, Punda-Polić V, Sardelić S, Capkun V (2002): [Occurrence of *Toxoplasma gondii* antibodies in the population of Split-Dalmatia County]. Liječ Vjesn 124: 19-22.

[82] Vidić B, Savić-Jevđenić S, Grgić Ž, Bugarski D, Maljković M (2007): Infectious abortion in sheep. Biotechnol Anim Husband 23: 383-389.

[83] Vilibić-Čavlek T, Ljubin-Sternak S, Ban M, Kolarić B, Sviben M, Mlinarić-Galinović G (2011): Prevalence of TORCH infections in women of childbearing age in Croatia. J Matern Fetal Neonatal Med 24: 280-283.

[84] Vranić-Ladavac M, Markotić A, Pfeifer D, Ladavac R (2002): Clinical interpretation of serologic tests in diagnostic procedures in toxoplasmosis. 3rd Croatian Congress on Infectious Diseases with international participation, Dubrovnik, Croatia, October 12-15. Abstract book: p. 59-60.

[85] Vujanić M, Ivović V, Kataranovski M, Nikolić A, Bobić B, Klun I, Villena I, Kataranovski D, Djurković-Djaković O (2011): Toxoplasmosis in naturally infected rodents in Belgrade, Serbia. Vector Borne Zoonotic Dis 11: 1209-1211.

[86] Weigel RM, Dubey JP, Siegel AM, Hoefling D, Reynolds D, Herr L, Kitron UD, Shen SK, Thulliez P, Fayer R, Todd KS (1995): Prevalence of antibodies to *Toxoplasma gondii* in swine in Illinois in 1992. J Am Vet Med Assoc 206: 1747-1751.

[87] Wikerhauser T, Džakula N, Kovač Z (1983): [Isolation of the parasite *Toxoplasma gondii* from pork in Croatia]. Vet Arhiv 53: 11-16.

[88] Wikerhauser T, Kutičić V, Marinculić A, Majurdžić D (1988): [A survey of porcine and ovine diaphragms for viable toxoplasms]. Vet. Arhiv 58: 205-208.

[89] Živković J, Arežina Lj (1991): [Evidence and hygienic significance of *Toxoplasma gondii* sporozoa in the flesh of hens]. Vet Stanica 22: 323-330.

[90] Zufferey J, Di Mito C, Auckenthaler R (2007): Evaluation of the new Vidia toxoplasmosis IgG and IgM assays in women of childbearing age. Clin Microbiol Infect 13 (Suppl 1): p. 124.

Chapter 3

Toxoplasmosis in Animals in the Czech Republic – The Last 10 Years

Eva Bartova and Kamil Sedlak

Additional information is available at the end of the chapter

http://dx.doi.org/10.5772/50022

1. Introduction

Toxoplasmosis is a significant zoonosis that affects humans and warm blooded animals. The definitive hosts of parasite *Toxoplasma gondii* are cats and other felids. Many species of domestic, wild or zoo animals may serve as intermediate hosts.

In humans, clinical form of toxoplasmosis is rare in immunocompetent people, while it may leads to eye diseases, CNS or generalized infection in immunocompromissed individuals as well as interfere with the course or outcome of pregnancy. In Europe, *T. gondii* seroprevalence in humans ranges from 8% to 77% (Dubey 2010). In the Czech Republic, *T. gondii* antibodies were detected in 35% and 25% pregnant women by Sabin-Feldman Test (SFT) and Complement Fixation Test (CFT), respectively (Hejlicek et al. 1999). Repeated prevalence studies in humans in some European countries (France, Belgium, Sweden and Norway), revealed an evident trend of a decrease in *T. gondii* seroprevalence (Welton and Ades 2005). The same trend is observed in the Czech Republic. The prevalence of infection varies among ethnic groups due to sanitary and cooking habits. Consumption of raw or almost raw, dried, cured or smoked meat from domestic animals, unpasteurized goat milk or consumption of meat from wild animals may be associated with ingestion of the parasite (Kijlstra and Jongert 2008, Jones et al. 2009). Higher prevalence was found also in people who had frequent contact with animals and soil, such as abattoir workers, garbage handlers and waste pickers (Dubey and Beattie 1988). Children playing with dogs and cats can be infected by direct contact because animals can act as mechanical vectors (Etheredge et al. 2004).

In animals, *T. gondii* infection is a frequent cause of early embryonic death and resorption, fetal death and mummification, abortion, still birth and neonatal death. Thus, toxoplasmosis in domestic and farm animals is a disease of great importance for veterinary medicine and husbandry since it can cause productive and economic losses.

T. gondii antibodies have been found in animals worldwide. Seroprevalence to *T. gondii* varies among countries, within different areas of a country and within the same city. Dubey (2010) summarized the results of seroprevalence studies performed on different groups of animals from several countries.

In the Czech Republic, some important studies concerning *T. gondii* in animals were done in past years. The seroprevalence of *T. gondii* infection in domestic animals obtained by different serological methods is summarized in Table 1.

Animal	Prevalence	Assay	Reference
Cat	17 – 91%	SFT, CFT, MPA, IFAT	Havlik and Hubner 1958, Zastera et al. 1966, Zastera et al. 1969, Svoboda and Svobodova 1987, Svoboda 1988
Dog	15 – 58%	SFT, CFT, MPA	Havlik and Hubner 1958, Zastera et al. 1966, Zastera et al. 1969, Svoboda and Svobodova 1987, Hejlicek et al. 1995, Hejlicek et al. 1995
Sheep	4 – 77%	SFT, CFT, MPA, IHA, IFAT	Zastera et al. 1966, Zastera et al. 1969, Arnaudov et al. 1976, Kozojed et al. 1977, Hejlicek and Literak 1994c
Goat	20 – 86%	SFT, CFT, IFAT	Havlik and Hubner 1958, Zastera et al. 1966, Zastera et al. 1969, Hejlicek and Literak 1994b, Literak et al. 1995, Slosarkova et al. 1999
Cattle	2 – 42%	SFT	Havlík and Hubner 1958, Zastera et al. 1969, Kozojed et al. 1977
Pig	0.1 – 38%	SFT, CFT, MPA	Havlik and Hubner 1958, Zastera et al. 1969, Kozojed et al. 1977, Hejlicek and Literak 1993, Hejlicek and Literak 1994b, Vostalova et al. 2000
Horse	4 – 11%	SFT, CFT	Havlik and Hubner 1958, Zastera et al. 1969, Kozojed et al. 1977, Hejlicek and Literak 1994a, Zastera et al. 1966
Gallinaceous bird	0 – 20%	SFT	Zastera et al. 1965, Zastera et al. 1969, Kozojed et al. 1977, Literak and Hejlicek 1993
Water fowl	2 – 33%	SFT	Zastera et al. 1965, Zastera et al. 1969, Literak and Hejlicek 1993
Rabbit	6 – 95%	SFT, CFT	Havlik and Hubner 1958, Havlik and Hubner 1960, Zastera et al. 1969 , Kunstyr et al. 1970, Hejlicek and Literak 1994d

SFT – Sabin-Feldman Test, CFT – Complement Fixation Test, MPA – Microprecipitation in Agar, IHA –Indirect Hemaglutination Assay, IFAT – Indirect Fluorescent Antibody Test

Table 1. *Toxoplasma gondii* prevalence and assays used in different groups of domestic animals in the Czech Republic until year 2000

In a group of game animals, a prevalence of 15% was found in wild boars by SFT (Hejlicek et al. 1997), 4 – 31% in hares by SFT or Microprecipitation in Agar (MPA) (Havlik and Hubner 1958, Zastera et al. 1966, Vosta et al. 1981, Hejlicek et al. 1997), and 14 – 58% prevalence in wild ruminants by SFT (Havlik and Hubner 1958, Zastera et al. 1966, Hejlicek et al. 1997).

These studies were performed by one or by a combination of methods such as SFT, CFT, MPA and Indirect Hemaglutination Assay (IHA). Nowadays, these methods are less frequently used; it is preferred to use Modified Agglutination Test (MAT), and/or Indirect Fluorescent Antibody Test (IFAT), and/or an Enzyme-Linked Immunosorbent Assay (ELISA), and/or a Latex Agglutination Test (LAT). This trend is also evident from a recent review summarized worldwide prevalence of *T. gondii* infection in animals and humans (Dubey 2010).

Based on the results of examination of different groups of animals in the State Veterinary Institute Prague in years 2003 – 2006, it is evident that lethal toxoplasmosis in the Czech Republic is the most important in some species of zoo animals; while in domestic animals it was not proved (Sedlak and Bartova 2007). Contrary, the sera of cats and dogs were the most frequently examined. Insufficient attention is paid to small ruminants that can abort or have reproduction disorders due to toxoplasmosis with subsequent economic losses.

That is why during the last 10 years, our research team focused on *T. gondii* serosurveys in different groups of animals to obtain actual data and to evaluate which group of animals is the most affected by *T. gondii* infection. Following parts of chapter summarises the results of seroprevalence studies in domestic, game and zoo animals tested by using IFAT, ELISA and LAT with the possibility to compare the results with those obtained from other countries with the same methods used. The results of experimental studies and cases of clinical toxoplasmosis recorded in the Czech Republic are mentioned too.

2. Toxoplasmosis in domestic animals

2.1. Recent data from the Czech Republic

Serological studies

During years 1995-2012, the samples of blood were collected from different groups of animals and examined for specific *T. gondii* antibodies. The animals tested for *T. gondii* antibodies were clinically healthy, no case of abortion or other symptoms of toxoplasmosis were recorded. The blood samples were collected by veterinarians on farms, zoo or during hunting seasons and sent to State Veterinary Institute Prague for routine examination.

In a group of domestic animals, in total 4254 animals were tested with the following number of animals used: 286 cats, 413 dogs, 547 sheep, 251 goats, 546 cattle, 551 pigs, 552 horses and 1108 poultry (217 chickens and 293 broilers, 60 turkeys, 178 geese and 360 ducks). The animals came from 2 – 14 different districts of the Czech Republic (Figure 1).

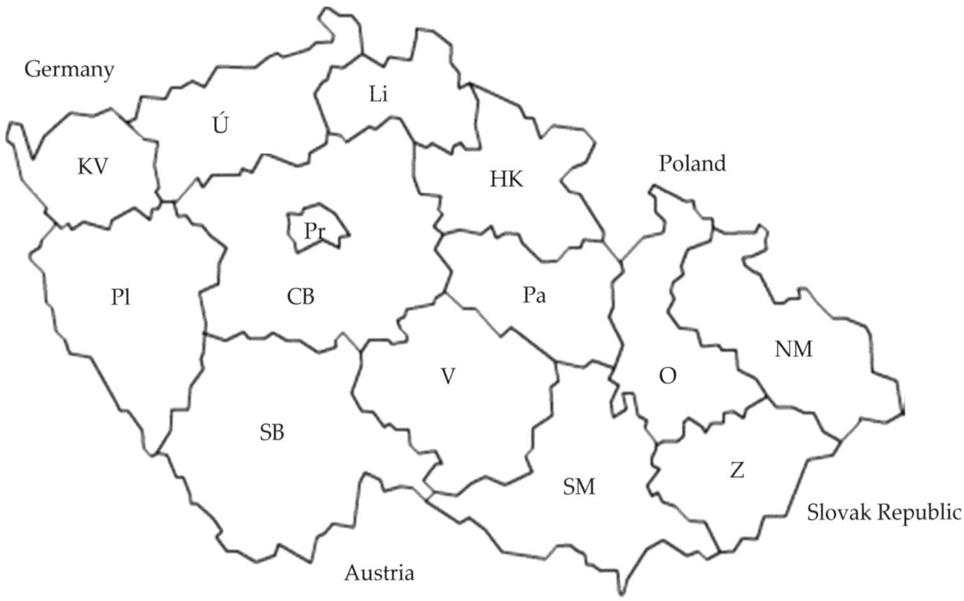

CB – Central Bohemia (cat, dog, sheep, goat, cattle, pig, horse, poultry, wild boar, hare, wild ruminant), HK – Hradec Králové (goat, cattle, pig, horse, poultry, wild boar), KV – Karlovy Vary (goat, cattle, pig, horse, poultry, wild boar, wild ruminant), Li – Liberec (goat, cattle, pig, horse, poultry, wild boar, wild ruminant), Pa – Pardubice (goat, horse, poultry), Pl – Plzeň (goat, cattle, pigs, horse, poultry, wild boar, wild ruminant), Pr – Prague (goat, cattle, horse, poultry, wild ruminant), O – Olomouc (poultry, hare, wild ruminant), NM – North Moravia (cat, dog, poultry, wild ruminant), SB – South Bohemia (horse, pig, poultry, wild boar, wild ruminant), SM – South Moravia (poultry, hare, wild ruminant), Ú – Ústí nad Labem (sheep, goat, cattle, pig, horse, poultry, wild boar, wild ruminant), V – Vysočina (pig, poultry, wild ruminant), Z – Zlín (poultry)

Figure 1. Map of the Czech Republic showing the sampled area with domestic and game animals tested for *T. gondii* antibodies.

Sera of domestic animals were tested for *T. gondii* antibodies by an indirect fluorescent antibody test (IFAT), using the Sevatest Toxoplasma Antigen IFR (Sevac, Prague, Czech Republic) and specific conjugates, by an ELISA (Institut Pourquier, Montpellier, France), or by a latex agglutination test (Pastorex TM Toxo, Biorad, France). The data on the method and cut-off used, specific conjugate for IFAT and producer are summarized in Table 2.

In a group of domestic animals, *T. gondii* antibodies were found in 66% goats, 59% sheep, 44% cats, 36% pigs, 26% dogs, 23% horses, 12% poultry (43% goose, 14% ducks, and 0.3% in broiler; turkeys and chickens were negative) and 9.7% cattle. The results of serological examination including the number of samples tested, the method and cut-off used, the number and percentage of positive samples, titres or %S/P obtained in positive samples and reference about published data are summarized in Table 3.

Animal	Assay (cut-off)	Conjugate for IFAT	Producer
Cat	IFAT (≥40)	anti-cat IgG	Sigma Aldrich, USA
Dog	IFAT (≥40)	anti-dog IgG	Sigma Aldrich, USA
Sheep	ELISA (≥50%S/P)	–	Sigma Aldrich, USA
Goat	ELISA (≥50% S/P)	–	Sigma Aldrich, USA
Cattle	ELISA (≥50% S/P)	–	Sigma Aldrich, USA
Pig	ELISA (≥50% S/P)	–	Sigma Aldrich, USA
Horse	LAT	anti-horse IgG	VMRD, Pulman, USA
Chicken Broiler	IFAT (≥40)	anti-chicken IgG	Sigma Aldrich, USA
Turkey	IFAT (≥40)	anti-chicken IgG	Sigma Aldrich, USA
Goose	IFAT (≥40)	anti-duck IgG	KPL, USA
Duck	IFAT (≥40)	anti-duck IgG	KPL, USA

IFAT – Indirect Fluorescent Antibody Test, ELISA – Enzyme-Linked Immunosorbent Assay, LAT – Latex Agglutination Test

Table 2. Serologic method, cut-off, specific conjugates for IFAT and producer used in domestic animals.

Animals	*T. gondii*			Assay (cut-off)	Titres or %S/P	Reference
	n	positive	%			
Cat	286	126	44	IFAT (40)	40 – 81920	Sedlak and Bartova 2006b
Dog	413	107	26	IFAT (40)	40 – 10240	Sedlak and Bartova 2006b
Sheep	547	325	59	ELISA (50%S/P)	50 – 200	Bartova et al. 2009a
Goat	251	166	66	ELISA (50%S/P)	56 – 191	Bartova et al. 2012
Cattle	546	53	9.7	ELISA (50%S/P)	50 – 200	Bartova et al. (unpublished)
Pig	551	198	36	ELISA (50%S/P)	50 – 337	Bartova and Sedlak 2011
Horse	552	125	23	LAT	–	Bartova et al. 2010a
Poultry						
Chicken	510	0	0	IFAT (40)	–	Bartova et al. 2009a
Broiler	293	1	0.3	IFAT (40)	40	Bartova et al. 2009a
Turkey	60	0	0	IFAT (40)	–	Bartova et al. 2009a
Goose	178	77	43	IFAT (40)	40 – 2560	Bartova et al. 2009a
Duck	360	52	14	IFAT (40)	40 – 320	Bartova et al. 2009a

IFAT – Indirect Fluorescent Antibody Test, ELISA – Enzyme-Linked Immunosorbent Assay, LAT – Latex Agglutination Test

Table 3. The result of serological examination of domestic animals with method used, cut-off, titres and %S/P in positive samples

Experimental studies

In the Czech Republic, two experimental studies were conducted on domestic poultry.

The first study was conducted on chickens (*Gallus domesticus*) that were inoculated *per os* with two different doses of *T. gondii* oocysts (Sedlak et al. 2000b). Antibodies to *T. gondii* were detected by IFAT first on day 14 p.i.; all chickens were serologically positive on days 21 and 28 p.i. No clinical symptoms were recorded. Parasite *T. gondii* was isolated from heart, muscle, spleen and brain. In one case, no *T. gondii* was isolated from any organ. Based on this experiment chickens seems highly resistant to *T. gondii* infection.

The second experimental study was conducted on domestic ducks (Bartova et al. 2004). Ducks were inoculated *per os* with different doses of *T. gondii* oocysts. Antibodies to *T. gondii* were detected in all ducks by IFAT on day 7 p.i. Antibody titres were found in the range of 20–640 depending on the infectious dose of the oocysts. From day 14 p.i., antibody titres increased to 80–20 480. Bioassay in mice revealed *T. gondii* in the breast and leg muscles, heart, brain, liver and stomach. The infected ducks showed no clinical symptoms, however, the results of bioassay indicate that, compared to gallinaceous birds, domestic ducks are relatively susceptible to *T. gondii* infection.

2.2. Comparison of data obtained

Cats

Clinical signs of toxoplasmosis in cats include fever, anorexia, dyspnea, uveitis, pneumonitis and others. Kittens can develop acute toxoplasmosis and die from it. The seropositivity increases with the age of cat, indicating postnatal transmission of infection. *T. gondii* antibodies have been found worldwide (Dubey 2010). Seroprevalence varies among countries, within different areas of a country and within the same city. In Europe, the highest prevalence 76% was found by SFT in Turkey (Karatepe et al. 2008), while the lowest 17% in Israel by ELISA (Salant and Spira 2004). In the Czech Republic, we found 44% prevalence by IFAT. In the previous studies from the Czech Republic, 17% – 91% prevalence was found by SFT, CFT and MPA. During the last 20 years, there is a trend of decreasing seroprevalence especially in cats staying at home and fed with commercial diet.

Dogs

T. gondii antibodies have been found in canine sera worldwide. Seroprevalence increases with age indicating postnatal infection, is higher in dogs from rural areas, in dogs housed exclusively outdoors, in dogs eating birds, small mammals, meat, viscera and home-cooked meals (Lopes et al. 2011b). In Europe, the highest prevalence 75% was found by SFT in Turkey (Aktas et al. 1998), while the lowest 5% in Sweden by ELISA (Lunden et al. 2002). In the Czech Republic, we found 26% prevalence by IFAT. In the previous studies from the Czech Republic, 4% – 58% prevalence was found by SFT or CFT. The lower prevalence is recorded in dogs staying at home and fed with commercial diet.

Sheep

T. gondii has been recognized as one of the main cause of infective ovine abortion in New Zealand, Australia, the United Kingdom, Norway and the United States. In the Czech

Republic, not yet a case of toxoplasmic abortion has been recorded in sheep herds. Seroprevalence was shown to increase with age, suggesting that animals acquire infection postnatally, however transplacental transmission of *T. gondii* may be more common than previously believed. Antibodies to *T. gondii* have been found in sheep worldwide (Dubey 2010). There is no validation of any serological test for the detection of *T. gondii* infection in sheep; different methods and cut-off are used.

In Europe, the highest prevalence 96% was found by ELISA in Turkey (Mor and Arslan 2007), while the lowest 10% was found in Slovak Republic by SFT (Kovacova 1993). We found 59% prevalence by ELISA. In the Czech Republic, 4% – 77% prevalence was found in past years.

Based on experimental studies, *T. gondii* was more frequently detected in brain and heart than in muscles; however *T. gondii* was detected also in milk (Camossi et al. 2011). Attention should be paid to meat or milk consumed without sufficient temperature treatment.

Goats

T. gondii antibodies have been found in goats worldwide (Dubey 2010). In Europe, the highest prevalence 91% was found by LAT in Netherland (McSporran et al. 1985), while no antibodies were found in Poland by IFAT (Gerecki et al. 2005). We found 66% prevalence by ELISA. In the Czech Republic, 20% – 86% prevalence was found in past years.

Goats appear to be more susceptible to clinical toxoplasmosis compared to other domestic animals, and even adult goats could die of acute toxoplasmosis. In the Czech Republic, toxoplasmosis was diagnosed in two Angora goat herds in South Moravia with an outbreak of abortions and births of weak kids; the goats showed also iodine deficiency (Slosarkova et al. 1999). Based on several experimental studies conducted on goats, *T. gondii* was detected in liver, muscles, heart, diaphragm, brain, kidneys and could be excreted in semen and milk. Attention should be paid to raw goat meat and milk if consumed without sufficient temperature treatment.

Cattle

Serum antibodies to *T. gondii* have been found in cattle in many surveys worldwide (Dubey 2010). In Europe, the highest seroprevalence 92% was found by MAT in Italy (Avezza et al. 1993), while no antibodies were found in Slovak Republic (Pleva et al. 1997) and Turkey (Oz et al. 1995). Actual prevalence rates are likely to be lower than indicated because of problem with the specifity of the tests used. The SFT test gives false or erratic results with cattle sera; on the other hand a titer of 1:100 or higher in the MAT appears to be indicative of *T. gondii* infection in cattle (Dubey 2010). We found 9.7% seroprevalence by ELISA. In the previous studies in the Czech Republic, 2% – 42% seroprevalence was found by SFT and DT.

There are no confirmed reports of clinical toxoplasmosis in adult cattle. In cattle, *T. gondii* can be transplacentally transmitted resulting in aborts; but it is probably a rare occurrence. There is more important parasite *Neospora caninum* leading to abortion in cattle. In the Czech Republic, there is very low prevalence of *N. caninum* in herds of cattle. The ingestion of beef or dairy products is not considered important in the epidemiology of *T. gondii* because cattle are not a good host for this parasite. Attempts to isolate *T. gondii* from cattle tissues have been unsuccessful, that is why it does not present risk of infection for humans.

Pigs

Clinical manifestation of toxoplasmosis in pigs could include diarhea, encephalitis, pneumonitis, necrotic hepatitis and abortion. Surveys based on the presence of *T. gondii* antibodies in blood sera of pigs have been reported worldwide (Dubey 2010). In Europe, *T. gondii* prevalence declined in the last decade especially because of good management system. There is a different sensitivity and specifity of the assays used for serosurveys in the following order MAT, IHA, LAT and ELISA starting with the most sensitive one. Good correlation was obtained between ELISA and MAT. In Europe, the highest prevalence 64% was found by IFAT in Italy (Genchi et al. 1991), while only 1% prevalence was found by the same method used in Austria (Edelhofer 1994). In the Czech Republic, we found 36% prevalence by ELISA. In the previous studies from the Czech Republic, 0 – 38% prevalence was found by SFT, CFT or MPA.

The higher prevalence is found among pigs from small backyard operations, while the prevalence among pigs from traditional large farms and modern large-scale farms is usually lower. Attention should be paid if pork meat is consumed nearly raw or without sufficient temperature treatment.

Horses

Horses have been shown to be susceptible to *Toxoplasma* infection (Tassi 2006) however there is no confirmed report of clinical toxoplasmosis. Serum antibodies to *T. gondii* have been found in horses in many surveys worldwide (Dubey 2010). In Europe, the highest prevalence 37% was found by SFT in Turkey (Gazayagci et al. 2011), while the lowest 1% in Sweden by DAT (Jakubek et al. 2006). In the Czech Republic, we found 23% by LAT. In the previous studies from the Czech Republic, 4 – 11% prevalence was found by SFT or CFT.

By reason that equine meat represents an important source of food in many human communities, infected equine meat could represent potential risk of *T. gondii* infection for humans.

Poultry

In general, there is a different sensitivity of birds to *T. gondii* infection. Owls and other predatory birds and domestic poultry seem to be resistant to *T. gondii* infection, while e.g. rock partridge (*Alectoris graeca*), pigeons and canaries are highly susceptible to toxoplasmosis. In Europe, there were some reports of birds (galliformes, columbiformes, psittaciformes and passeriformes) that died due to toxoplasmosis (Dubey 2010). Toxoplasmosis can also lead to drop in egg production and high mortality in embryonated eggs. In the Czech Republic, confirmed clinical toxoplasmosis has not been recorded in birds. Little is known concerning the validity of the serologic tests for the detection of *T. gondii* antibodies in avian sera. It is preferred to use MAT, nevertheless other methods such as SFT, CFT, ELISA and IFAT have been used worldwide.

We found higher prevalence in water fowls (43% and 14% in goose and ducks, respectively) compared to gallinaceous poultry (0.3% in broiler; turkeys and chickens were negative). In Europe, higher prevalence 36% was found in chicken from Austria by MAT (Dubey et al. 2005), or 20% in turkeys by ELISA in Germany (Koethe et al. 2011).

T. gondii have been isolated from brain, heart and leg muscles, but not from the pectoral muscle and liver (Dubey et al. 1993).

3. Toxoplasmosis in game animals

3.1. Recent data from the Czech Republic

Serological studies

In majority of game animals, the course of infection is subclinical. However, considering the high prevalence of *T. gondii* infection in game animals, they should be taken into account as the possible source of infection for human.

A total of 1618 game animals were tested, including 720 wild ruminants or ruminants living in reservations (377 red deer, 79 roe deer, 14 sika, 143 fallow deer, 105 mouflon and 2 reindeer), 565 wild boars and 333 hares. The animals came from 3 – 11 districts of the Czech Republic (Figure 1).

Sera of game animals were tested for *T. gondii* antibodies by an IFAT, using the Sevatest Toxoplasma Antigen IFR (Sevac) and specific conjugates (Table 4). Sera with titer ≥40 were marked as positive.

Animal	Conjugate for IFAT	Producer
Wild boar	anti-swine Ig G	Sigma, Praha
Hare	anti-rabbit Ig G	Sigma Aldrich, USA
Red deer	anti-deer Ig G	KPL Inc. Maryland
Sika	anti-deer Ig G	KPL Inc. Maryland
Fallow deer	anti-deer Ig G	KPL Inc. Maryland
Roe deer	anti-deer Ig G	KPL Inc. Maryland
Mouflon	anti-goat Ig G	VMRD, USA
Reindeer	anti-deer Ig G	KPL Inc. Maryland

IFAT – Indirect Fluorescent Antibody Test

Table 4. Specific conjugates for IFAT and producer used in game animals.

In a group of game animals, *T. gondii* antibodies were detected in 32% wild ruminants (50% in sika, 45% red deer, 24% roe deer, 17% fallow deer, 9% mouflon, and in one reindeer), 26% wild boars and 20% hares. The results of serological examination including the number of samples tested, the method and cut-off used, the number and percentage of positive samples, titres obtained in positive samples and reference about published data are summarized in Table 5.

Animals	*T. gondii*			Assay (cut-off)	Titres	Reference
	n	positive	%			
Wild boar	565	148	26	IFAT (40)	40 – 1280	Bartova et al. 2006
Hares	333	71	20	IFAT (40)	40 – 640	Bartova et al. 2010b
Wild ruminants						
Red deer	377	169	45	IFAT (40)	40 – 640	Bartova et al. 2007
Roe deer	79	19	24	IFAT (40)	40 – 160	Bartova et al. 2008
Sika	14	7	50	IFAT (40)	80 – 320	Bartova et al. 2009
Fallow deer	143	24	17	IFAT (40)	40 – 160	Bartova et al. 2010
Mouflon	105	9	9	IFAT (40)	40 – 320	Bartova et al. 2011
Reindeer	2	1		IFAT (40)	80	Bartova et al. 2012

IFAT – Indirect Fluorescent Antibody Test, ELISA – Enzyme-Linked Immunosorbent Assay, LAT – Latex Agglutination Test

Table 5. The result of serological examination of game animals with the sample number, the method and cut-off used, titres in positive samples and references.

Experimental studies

In the Czech Republic, two experimental studies were conducted on game animals.

The first study was conducted on hares (Sedlak et al. 2000a). Hares were experimentally infected with *T. gondii* oocysts. Most infected hares demonstrated behavioural changes, and all of them died between 8 and 19 days. In all hares, parasitemia was demonstrated on days 7 and 12 p.i. *T. gondii* was isolated from liver, brain, spleen, kidney, lung, heart and skeletal muscles. Based on this result, hares seem to be very sensitive species to *T. gondii* infection.

The second study was conducted on gallinaceous game birds (Sedlak et al. 2000b). Partridges (*Perdix perdix*), chukars (*Alectoris chukar*), wild guineafowl (*Numida meleagris*) and wild turkeys (*Meleagris gallopavo*) were inoculated *per os* with two doses of *T. gondii* oocysts. Antibodies to *T. gondii* were detected in the birds by IFAT first on day 7 p.i. Two of five partridges fed 10^3 oocysts and six of eight partridges fed 10^5 oocysts died between day 6 and 16 p.i. No clinical symptoms were observed in surviving birds, however enteritis was the most striking lesion in partridges that died. Bioassay in mice revealed *T. gondii* in the brain, liver, spleen, heart and leg muscles of all partridges and chukars. These results indicate that partridges are highly susceptible to toxoplasmosis, while chukars, wild guineafowls and turkeys seem to be less susceptible.

3.2. Comparison of data obtained

Wild boars

In Europe, the highest seroprevalence 100% was found in wild boars from Portugal (Lopes et al. 2011b) or 44% in wild boars from Spain (Closa-Sebastia et al. 2011); while the lowest prevalence 8% was found in wild boars from Slovak Republic (Antolova et al. 2007). In the Czech Republic we found 26% prevalence by IFAT. This prevalence was higher compared to 0% – 15% prevalence found by SFT in the previous studies from the Czech Republic.

The meat of wild boars may harbour tissue cysts of *T. gondii* and may represent a vehicle of human toxoplasmosis infection. Hejlicek et al. (1997) found tissue cysts in 2% examined wild boars from the Czech Republic, while in the neighbouring Slovakia, *T. gondii* was isolated from 31% of wild boars (Catar 1972). Hunters and their families consuming meat from wild boars should be aware of *T. gondii* infection and advised to take precautions. It is highly recommended to cook meat from wild boars thoroughly before human consumption.

Hares

There are several reports of *T. gondii* infection in hares from Europe (Dubey 2010). The highest seroprevalence 46% was found in hares from Germany (Frolich et al. 2003); in contrast no antibodies were detected in hares from Sweeden (Gustafsson and Uggla 1994). In the Czech Republic, we found 20% prevalence by IFAT. This result is comparable with 4% – 31% prevalence found in previous studies by SFT or MPA. Based on the results of experimental infection, hares seem to be sensitive to *T. gondii* infection; *T. gondii* was isolated from liver, brain, spleen, kidney, lung, heart and skeletal muscles (Sedlak et al. 2000).

Wild ruminants

T. gondii infection in game animals is of epidemiological significance. Deer are strictly herbivores and that is why the high prevalence of *T. gondii* in deer suggests widespread contamination of the environment with *T. gondii* oocysts. In red deer, the highest seroprevalence 32% was found by SFT in Scotland (Williamson and Williams 1980), while the lowest 8% by DAT in Norway (Vikoren et al. 2004). We found relatively high prevalence 45% by IFAT in red deer from the Czech Republic. In roe deer, the highest prevalence 63% was found in Norway and Sweden by SFT (Kapperud 1978), while the lowest 13% prevalence was found in Austria by IHA (Edelhofer et al. 1989). In the Czech Republic, we found 24% prevalence by IFAT that was also in range 14% – 58% prevalence found in our country in previous studies. In fallow deer, we found 17% prevalence that is comparable with 24% prevalence found in Spain by MAT (Gauss et al. 2006). In the Czech Republic, we found 9% prevalence in mouflon that is lower compared to 23% prevalence found in France (Aubert et al. 2010). In case of reindeer, only two animals were examined in the Czech Republic. This is very low number that is why it is not possible to compare it with 1% prevalence found in Norway by DAT (Vikoren et al. 20004).

Deer are popular game animals in several countries. The meat of deer may harbour tissue cysts of *T. gondii* and may represent a vehicle of human toxoplasmosis infection. Toxoplasmosis infection in men was documented after consummation of raw or nearly raw deer meat in USA (Sacks et al. 1983, Ross et al. 2001).

4. Toxoplasmosis in zoo animals

4.1. Recent data from the Czech Republic

Serological studies

In a group of zoo animals, 556 animals belonging to 114 species were tested (5 species of primates, 28 species of carnivores, 8 species of perissodactyla and 73 species of artiodactyla). The animals came from 12 zoo and 4 small private exotic centres in the Czech Republic.

Sera of zoo animals were tested for *T. gondii* antibodies by an IFAT, using the Sevatest Toxoplasma Antigen IFR (Sevac) and specific conjugates (Table 6). Sera with titer ≥40 were marked as positive.

Order and family	Indirect Fluorescent Antibody Test (IFAT)	
	Conjugate for IFAT	Producer of conjugate
Primates		
Cercopithecidae	anti-monkey IgG	Sigma-Aldrich s.r.o., Praha
Hominidae	anti-human IgG	Sevapharma, Praha
Carnivora		
Canidae	anti-dog IgG	Sigma-Aldrich s.r.o., Praha
Felidae	anti-cat IgG	Sigma-Aldrich s.r.o., Praha
Hyaenidae	anti-cat IgG	Sigma-Aldrich s.r.o., Praha
Mustelidae	anti-cat IgG	Sigma-Aldrich s.r.o., Praha
Otariidae	anti-cat IgG	Sigma-Aldrich s.r.o., Praha
Ursidae	anti-cat IgG	Sigma-Aldrich s.r.o., Praha
Viveridae	anti-cat IgG	Sigma-Aldrich s.r.o., Praha
Perissodactyla		
Equidae	anti-horse IgG	VMRD, Pullman, USA
Artiodactyla		
Bovidae	anti-bovine IgG, anti-goat IgG	VMRD, Pullman, USA
Cameliae	anti-llama IgG	VMRD, Pullman, USA
Cervidae	anti-deer IgG	KPL, Gaithersburg, Maryland
Suidae	anti-swine IgG	Sigma-Aldrich s.r.o., Praha

Table 6. Specific conjugates for Indirect Fluorescent Antibody Test and their producer used in zoo animals.

In a group of zoo animals, *T. gondii* antibodies were detected in 193 of 556 (35%) animals, representing 72 of 114 species tested (Sedlak and Bartova, 2006a). According to order, *T. gondii* antibodies were found in 90% carnivorous, 45% primates, 33% perissodactyles and 22% artiodactyles. According to families, *T. gondii* antibodies were found in ursidae (100%), felidae (93%), canidae (88%), hominidae (73%), equidae (33%), suidae (29%), cervidae (27%), camelidae (26%), bovidae (20%), cercopithecidae (18%) and in 3 animals of hyeenidae, 2 animals of mustelidae and 2 animals of viveridae. The highest prevalence 100% was found in Eurasian wolf (*Canis l. lupus*), Maned wolf (*Chrysocyon brachyurus*) and Sumatran tiger (*Panthera t. sumatrae*). The highest titre 40960 was found in Pallas's cat (*Otocolobus manul*). The results of serological examination of zoo animals are summarized in Table 7.

Order and Family	n	*T. gondii*	
		Positive	%
Primates	22	10	45
Cercopithecidae	11	2	18
Hominidae	11	8	73
Carnivora	87	78	90
Canidae	32	28	88
Felidae	41	38	93
Hyaenidae	3	3	
Mustelidae	2	2	
Otariidae	2	0	
Ursidae	5	5	100
Viveridae	2	2	
Perissodactyla			
Equidae	46	15	33
Artiodactyla	401	90	22
Bovidae	265	53	20
Cameliae	19	5	26
Cervidae	110	30	27
Suidae	7	2	29

Table 7. The result of serological examination of zoo animals

4.2. Experimental studies and cases of clinical toxoplasmosis

In the Czech Republic, experimental infection was conducted on budgerigars (*Melopsittacus undulatus*) that were orally inoculated with *T. gondii* oocysts with different doses (Kajerova et al. 2003). *T. gondii* antibodies were found by LAT in all birds. The birds showed no apparent signs of disease. *T. gondii* was isolated by bioassay in mice from all birds fed 10^3 or more oocysts. The results show that budgerigars are resistant to *T. gondii* infection.

Cases of clinical toxoplasmosis in the Czech Republic were recorded in nilgais (*Boselaphus tragocamelus*) and saiga antelope (*Saiga tatarica*) (Sedlak et al. 2004). Three captive female nilgais aborted two fetuses and two of their newborn calves died within two days of birth. Parasite *T. gondii* was demonstrated in the brains and livers of both fetuses and in one of the two neonates by single-stage polymerase chain reaction (PCR) with TGR1E and by semi-nested PCR with B1 gene. Retrospectively, antibodies titers ≥640 were found by IFAT in the sera of all three female nilgais and in one male nilgai used to breed them. Fatal toxoplasmosis was diagnosed in one captive adult female saiga antelope. Tissues cysts of *T. gondii* were found in the liver, lung, spleen, kidney, and intestine of saiga antelope. Toxoplasmosis was confirmed also by PCR with TGR1E and immunohistochemically. Toxoplasmic hepatitis and pneumonia were considered to be a primary cause of death.

The other cases of fatal toxoplasmosis were recorded in year 2004 in seven Pallas cats in several zoos in the Czech Republic (Sedlak and Vodicka 2005).

4.3. Comparison of data obtained

There are many reports on toxoplasmosis in zoo animals. Marsupials, New World monkeys, hares and some small ruminants belong to the most sensitive to clinic toxoplasmosis. Fatal toxoplasmosis was also recorded e.g. in captive dik-dik and Pallas cats from zoo in USA (Riemann et al. 1974; Dubey et al. 2002), in lions from a zoo in Africa (Ocholi et al. 1989) and in a Siberian tiger from a zoo in Belgium (Dorny et al. 1989). In the Czech Republic, fatal toxoplasmosis was recorded in saiga and nilgais antelopes from Prague and Chomutov zoos (Sedlak et al. 2004) and in Pallas cats (Sedlak and Vodicka 2005).

In our study, antibodies to *T. gondii* were found in 90% carnivora, 45% of primates, 33% perissodactyla and 22% artiodactyla. When compared to other similar study concerning zoo animals, *T. gondii* antibodies were found in 47% carnivora, 25% artiodactyla and 23% primates (Gorman et al. 1986). We found 93% prevalence in felids; that is higher when compared with 32%, 64.9% or 75.8% prevalence found in felids from zoo in California (Riemann et al. 1974), Brazil (Silva et al. 2001) and Florida (Lappin et al. 1991), respectively.

The potential source of *T. gondii* infection for carnivores is meat contaminated with *T. gondii* tissue cysts; herbivores can be infected by food contaminated with *T. gondii* oocysts and omnivorous animals by both ways. To prevent spreading of *T. gondii* infection among zoo animals, cats, including all wild felids should be housed in buildings separated from other animals, particularly the most sensitive marsupials and New World monkeys. There must be protection against free access of domestic cats to sources of food and water or into the buildings with animals, especially those that are the most sensitive to toxoplasmosis. Feline faeces should be removed daily to prevent sporulation of oocysts.

5. Further research

Further work should focus on serological studies in other animal groups that are neglected but may represent a risk of infection for humans in case of consumption of their meat or other products. Such animals include, for example, rabbits, ostriches, pigeons, pheasants and mallard ducks. In addition, rodents, wild birds and wild carnivores (foxes, marten and others) may play an important part in the circulation of *T. gondii* infection in nature and thus represent a risk of infection for wildlife, domestic animals and human people alike. Serological studies should be supplemented with an evaluation of the infection risk factors and with the use of molecular methods to detect *T. gondii* in animal products, as well as to characterize *T. gondii* genotypes circulating in animal populations in the Czech Republic.

Author details

Eva Bartova

Department of Biology and Wildlife Diseases, Faculty of Veterinary Hygiene and Ecology, University of Veterinary and Pharmaceutical Sciences, Brno, Czech Republic

Kamil Sedlak

Department of Virology and Serology, State Veterinary Institute Prague, Prague, Czech Republic

Acknowledgement

The results obtained in last 10 years were supported by the Ministry of Education, Youth and Sports of the Czech Republic (Grant No. MSM6215712402). We would like thank to R. Vodička, J. Váhala and F. Treml for their assistance in the collection of the serum samples and thank to students (V. Říhová, Z. Satková, H. Michnová, M. Syrová, M. Šíblová, H. Říhová, A. Šedivá, J. Drastíková) for their assistance with serological examinations.

6. References

[1] Aktas M, Babur C, Karaer Z, Dumanli N, Koroglu E (1998) Seroprevalence of Toxoplasmosis on Stray Dogs in Elazig. Vet. bil. dergisi. 14: 47-50.

[2] Antolova D, Reiterova K, Dubinsky P (2007) Seroprevalence of *Toxoplasma gondii* in Wild Boars (*Sus scrofa*) in the Slovak Republic. Ann. agric. environ. med. 14: 71-73.

[3] Arnaudov D, Kozojed V, Jira J, Stourac L (1976) Imunoepizootic Study of Ovine Toxoplasmosis (in Czech). Vet. med. 21: 375-384.

[4] Aubert D, Ajzenberg D, Richomme C, Gilot-Fromont E, Terrier ME, Gevigney C, Game Y, Maillard D, Gibert P, Darde ML, Villena I (2010) Molecular and Biological Characteristics of *Toxoplasma gondii* Isolates from Wildlife in France. Vet. par. 171: 346-349.

[5] Avezza F, Greppi G, Agosti M, Belloli A, Faverzani S (1993) Bovine Toxoplasmosis: the Results of Sero-Epidemiologic Study (in French). Att. soc. ital. buiatria. 25: 621-624.

[6] Bartova E, Dvorakova H, Barta J, Sedlak K, Literak I (2004) Susceptibility of the Domestic Duck (*Anas platyrhynchos*) to Experimental Infection with *Toxoplasma gondii* Oocysts. Avian pathol. 33: 153-157.

[7] Bartova E, Sedlak K (2011) Seroprevalence of *Toxoplasma gondii* and *Neospora caninum* in Slaughtered Pigs in the Czech Republic. Parasitology 138: 1369-1371.

[8] Bartova E, Sedlak K, Literak I (2006) Prevalence of *Toxoplasma gondii* and *Neospora caninum* Antibodies in Wild Boars in the Czech Republic. Vet. par. 142: 150-153.

[9] Bartova E, Sedlak K, Literak I (2009a) Serologic Survey for Toxoplasmosis in Domestic Birds from the Czech Republic. Avian pathol. 38: 317-320.

[10] Bartova E, Sedlak K, Literak I (2009b) Presence of *Toxoplasma gondii* and *Neospora caninum* Antibodies in Sheep in the Czech Republic. Vet. par. 161: 131-132.

[11] Bartova E, Sedlak K, Literak I (2012) *Neospora caninum* and *Toxoplasma gondii* Antibodies in Goats in the Czech Republic. Acta vet. med (Czech) 57 (3): 111-114.

[12] Bartova E, Sedlak K, Pavlik I., Literak I (2007) Prevalence of *Neospora caninum* and *Toxoplasma gondii* Antibodies in Wild Ruminants from the Countryside or Captivity in the Czech Republic. J. parasitol. 93: 1216-1218.

[13] Bartova E, Sedlak K, Syrova M, Literak I (2010a) *Neospora* spp. and *Toxoplasma gondii* Antibodies in Horses in the Czech Republic. Par. res. 107: 783-785.

[14] Bartova E, Sedlak K, Treml F, Literak I (2010b) *Neospora caninum* and *Toxoplasma gondii* Antibodies in Hares in the Czech Republic, Slovakia and Austria. Vet. par. 171: 155-158.

[15] Camossi LG, Greca-Junior H, Correa APFL, Richini-Pereira VB, Silva RC, Da Silva AV, Langoni H (2011) Detection of *Toxoplasma gondii* DNA in the Milk of Naturally Infected Ewes. Vet. par. 177: 256-261.

[16] Catar G (1972) Studies on Toxoplasmosis as Regards its Natural Focality in Slovakia. Folia parasitol. prague 19: 253-256.

[17] Closa-Sebastia F, Casas-Diaz E, Cuenca R, Lavin S, Mentaberre G, Marco I (2011) Antibodies to Selected Pathogens in Wild Boars (*Sus scrofa*) from Catalonia (NE Spain). Eur. j. wildl. res. 57: 977-981.

[18] Dorny P, Fransen J (1989) Toxoplasmosis in a Siberian Tiger (*Panthera tigris altaica*). Vet. rec. 23: 647 pp.

[19] Dubey JP (2010) Toxoplasmosis of Animals and Humans. 2nd ed. Boca Raton: CRC Press, 313 pp.

[20] Dubey JP, Beattie CP (1988) Toxoplasmosis of Animals and Man. Boca Raton, Fl: CRC Press.

[21] Dubey JP, Edelhofer R, Marcet P, Vianna MCB, Kwok OCH, Lehmann T (2005) Genetic and Biologic Characteristics of *Toxoplasma gondii* infections in free-range chickens from Austria. Vet. par. 133: 299-306.

[22] Dubey JP, Ruff MD, Camargo ME, Shen SK, Wilkins GL, Kwok OCH, Thulliez P (1993) Serologic and Parasitologic Responses of Domestic Chickens after Oral Inoculation with *Toxoplasma gondii* Oocysts. Am. j. vet. res. 54: 1668-1672.

[23] Dubey JP, Tocidlowski ME, Abbitt B, Llizo SY (2002) Acute Visceral Toxoplasmosis in Captive Dik-Dik (*Madoqua guentheri smithi*). J. par. 88: 638-641.

[24] Edelhofer R (1994) Prevalence of Antibodies Against *Toxoplasma gondii* in Pigs in Austria – an Evaluation of Data from 1982 and 1992. Par. res. 80: 642-644.

[25] Edelhofer R, Heppe-Winger EM, Haßi A, Aspock (1989) *Toxoplasma*-Infections in Game in Eastern Austria. Mitt. oster. gest. trop. parasit. 11: 119-123.

[26] Etheredge GD, Michael G, Muehlenbein MP, Frenkel JK (2004) The Roles of Cats and Dogs in the Transmission of *Toxoplasma* Infection in Kuna and Embera Children in Eastern Panama. Rev. panam. salud. publica 16: 176-186.

[27] Frolich K, Wisser J, Schmuser H, Fehlberg U, Neubauer H, Grunow R, Nikolaou K, Primer J, Thiede S, Streich WJ, Speck S (2003) Epizootiologic and Ecologic Investigations of European Brown Hares (*Lepus europaeus*) in Selected Populations from Schleswig-Holstein, Germany. J. wildlife. dis. 39, 751-761.

[28] Gauss CBL, Dubey JP, Vidal D, Cabezon O, Ruiz-Fons F, Vicente J, Marco I, Lavin S, Gortazar C, Almeria S (2006) Prevalence of *Toxoplasma gondii* in Red Deer (*Cervus elaphus*) and Other Wild Ruminants from Spain. Vet. par. 136: 193-200.

[29] Gazaygci S, Macun HC, Babur C (2011) Investigation of Seroprevalance of Toxoplasmosis in Mares and Stallions in Ankara Province, Turkey. Iran j. vet. res. 12: 354-356.

[30] Genchi G, Polidori GA, Zaghini L, Lanfranchi P (1991) A Survey of *Toxoplasma* Infection in Pig Intensive Breeding. Arch. vet. ital. 42: 105-111.

[31] Gerecki MT, Andrzejewska I, Steppa R (2005) Prevalence of *Toxoplasma gondii* in Sheep and Goats. Med. wet. 61: 98-99.

[32] Gorman TR, Rivoros V, Alcaino HA, Salas DR, Thiermann ER (1986) Helminthiasis and Toxoplasmosis Among Exotic Mammals at the Santiago National Zoo. J. am. vet. med. assoc. 189: 1068-1070.

[33] Gustafsson K, Uggla A (1994) Serologic Survey for *Toxoplasma gondii* Infection in the Brown Hare (*Lepus europaeus* P.) in Sweden. J. wildlife dis. 30: 201-204.

[34] Havlik O, Hubner J (1958) Serological Detection of Toxoplasma in Some Domestic and Wildlife Animals (in Czech). Českoslov. epidem. mikrob. imunol. 6: 396-402.

[35] Hejlicek K, Literak I (1993) Prevalence of Toxoplasmosis in Pigs in the Region of South Bohemia. Acta vet. Brno 62: 159-166.

[36] Hejlicek K, Literak I (1994a) Prevalence of Antibodies to *Toxoplasma gondii* in Horses in the Czech Republic. Acta par. 39: 217-219.

[37] Hejlicek K, Literak I (1994b) A Contribution to the Epizootiology and Ecology of Toxoplasmosis in Pigs. Wien. tier. monat. 81: 170-174.

[38] Hejlicek K, Literak I (1994c) Incidence and Prevalence of Toxoplasmosis Among Sheep and Goats in Southern and Western Bohemia. Acta vet. Brno 63: 151-159.

[39] Hejlicek K, Literak I (1994d) Prevalence of Toxoplasmosis in Rabbits in South Bohemia. Acta vet. Brno 63: 145-150.

[40] Hejlicek K, Literak I, Lhotak M (1995) Prevalence of Antibodies to *Toxoplasma gondii* in Army Dogs in the Czech Republic and Slovak Republic. Vet. med. (Czech) 40: 137-140.

[41] Hejlicek K, Literak I, Nezval J (1997) Toxoplasmosis in Wild Mammals from the Czech Republic. J. wild. dis. 33: 480-485.

[42] Hejlicek K, Literak I, Vostalova E, Kresnicka J (1999) *Toxoplasma gondii* Antibodies in Pregnant Women in the Ceske Budejovice District (in Czech). Epidemiol. mikrobiol. imunol. 48: 102-105.

[43] Jakubek EB, Lunden A, Uggla A (2006) Seroprevalence of *Toxoplasma gondii* and *Neospora* sp. Infections in Swedish Horses. Vet. par. 138: 194-199.

[44] Jones JL, Dargelas V, Roberts J, Press C, Remington JS, Montoya JG (2009) Risk Factors for *Toxoplasma gondii* Infection in the United States. Clin. infect. dis. 49: 878-884.

[45] Kajerova V, Literak I, Bartova E, Sedlak K (2003) Experimental Infection of Budgerigars (*Melopsittacus undulates*) with a Low Virulent K21 Strain of *Toxoplasma gondii*. Vet. par. 116: 297-304.

[46] Kapperud G (1978) Survey for Toxoplasmosis in Wild and Domestic Animals from Norway and Sweeden. J. wild. dis. 14: 157-162.

[47] Karatepe B, Babur C, Karatepe M, Kilic S, Dundar B (2008) Prevalence of *Toxoplasma gondii* Antibodies and Intestinal Parasites in Stray Cats from Nigde, Turkey. It. j. anim. sci. 7: 113-118.

[48] Kijlstra A, Jongert E (2008) Toxoplasma-Safe Meat: Close to Reality? Trends parasitol. 25: 18-22.

[49] Koethe M, Pott S, Ludewig M, Bangoura B, Zoller B, Daugschies A, Tenter AM, Spekker K, Bittame A, Mercier C, Fehlhaber K, Staubinger RK (2011) Prevalence of Specific IgG-Antibodies Agains *Toxoplasma gondii* in Domestic Turkeys Determined by Kinetic ELISA Based on Recombinant GRA7 and GRA8. Vet. par. 180: 179-190.

[50] Kovacova D (1993) Serologic Prevalence of *Toxoplasma gondii* in sheep (in Slovak). Veterinarstvi 43: 51-54.

[51] Kozojed V, Roudna V, Jira J, Hodkova Z (1977) Surveillance of Toxoplasmosis in Animal Host Spheres (in Czech). Zprávy československ. zool. spol. 52: 10-12.

[52] Lappin MR, Jacobson ER, Kollias GV, Powell CC, Stover J (1991) Comparison of Serologic Assays for the Diagnosis of Toxoplasmosis in Nondomestic Felids. J. zoo wildl. med. 22: 169-174.

[53] Literak I, Hejlicek K (1993) Incidence of *Toxoplasma gondii* in Populations of Domestic Birds in the Czech Republic. Avian pathol. 22: 275-281.

[54] Literak I, Skrivanek M, Skalka B, Celer V (1995) Antibodies to Some Infections on Large Goat Farms in the Czech Republic. Vet. med. Czech 40: 133-136.

[55] Lopes AP, Sargo R, Rodigues M, Cardoso L (2011a) High Seroprevalence of Antibodies to *Toxoplasma gondii* in Wild Animals from Portugal. Parasitol. res. 108: 1163-1169.

[56] Lopes AP, Santos H, Neto F, Rodrigues M, Kwok OCH, Dubey JP, Cardoso L (2011b) Prevalence of Antibodies to *Toxoplasma gondii* in Dogs from Northeastern Portugal. J. parasitol. 97: 418-420.

[57] Lunden A, Lind P, Engvall EO, Gustavsson K, Uggla A, Vagsholm I. (2002) Serological Survey of *Toxoplasma gondii* Infection in Pigs Slaughtered in Sweden. Scan. j. inf. dis. 34: 362-365.

[58] McSporran KD, McCaughan C, Currall JHS, Demsteegt A (1985) Toxoplasmosis in Goats. New zel. vet. j. 33: 39-40.

[59] Mor N, Arslan MO (2007) Kar Yoresindeki Koyunlarda *Toxoplasma gondii* nin Seroprevalansi. Kafkas univ. vet. fak. derg. 13: 165-170.

[60] Ocholi RA, Kalejaiye JO, Okewole PA (1989) Acute Disseminated Toxoplasmosis in Two Captive Lions (*Panthera leo*) in Nigeria. Vet. rec. 124: 515-516.

[61] Oz I, Ozyer M, Corak R (1995) A Study on the Prevalence of Toxoplasmosis in Cattle, Sheep and Goats in Adana Region by Using ELISA and IHA Tests J. etlik vet. microb. 8: 87-89.

[62] Pleva J, Sokol J, Cabadaj R, Saladiova D (1997) Epizootologic and Epidemiologic Importance of Toxoplasmosis (in Czech). Slov. vet. čas. 22: 127-129.

[63] Riemann HP, Behymer DE, Fowler ME, Schulz T, Lock A, Orthoeferr JG, Silverman S, Franti CE (1974) Prevalence of Antibodies to *Toxoplasma gondii* in Captive Exotic Mammals. J. am. vet. med. assoc. 165: 798-800.

[64] Ross RD, Stec LA, Werner JC, Blumenkranz MS, Glazer L, Williams GA (2001) Presumed Acquired Ocular Toxoplasmosis in Deer Hunters. Retina 21: 226-229.

[65] Sacks JJ, Delgado DG, Lobel HO, Parker RL (1983) Toxoplasmosis Infection Associated with Eating Undercooked Venison. Am. j. epidemiol. 118: 832-838.

[66] Salant H, Spira DT (2004) A Ccross-Sectional Survey of anti-*Toxoplasma gondii* Antibodies in Jerusalem Cats. Vet. par. 124: 167-177.
[67] Sedlak K, Bartova E (2006a) Seroprevalences of Antibodies to *Neospora caninum* and *Toxoplasma gondii* in Zoo Animals. Vet. par. 136: 223-231.
[68] Sedlak K, Bartova E (2006b) The Prevalence of *Toxoplasma gondii* IgM and IgG Antibodies in Dogs and Cats from the Czech Republic. Vet. med. (Czech) 51: 555-558.
[69] Sedlak K, Bartova E (2007) Toxoplasmosis of Animals and its Laboratory Diagnosis in the Czech Republic (in Czech). Veterinářství 9: 562-566.
[70] Sedlak K, Bartova E, Literak I, Vodicka R, Dubey JP (2004) Toxoplasmosis in Nilgais (*Boselaphus tragocamelus*) and a Saiga Antelope (*Saiga Tatarica*). J. zoo wild. med. 35: 530-533.
[71] Sedlak K, Literak I, Faldyna M, Toman M, Benak J (2000a) Fatal Toxoplasmosis in Brown Hares (*Lepus europaeus*): Possible Reasons of Their High Susceptibility to the Infection. Vet. par. 93: 13-28.
[72] Sedlak K, Literak I, Vitula F, Benak J (2000b) High Susceptibility of Partridges (*Perdix perdix*) to Toxoplasmosis Compared with Other Gallinaceous Birds. Avian pathol. 29: 563-569.
[73] Sedlak K, Vodicka P (2005) Feeding Rations and its effect on the Health Status of Pallas Cats (*Otocolobus manul*) in Captivity. Proceedings from VI. Seminar of Exots, wild animals and zoo animals – Nutrition and metabolic disorders, 1.-2. 10. 2005, Lešná, Czech Republic.
[74] Silva JCR, Ogassawara S, Marvulo MFV, Ferreira-Neto JS, Dubey JP (2001) *Toxoplasma gondii* Antibodies in Exotic Wild Felids from Brazilian Zoos. J. zoo wildl. med. 32: 349-351.
[75] Slosarkova S, Literak I, Skrivanek M, Svobodova V, Suchy P, Herzig I. (1999) Toxoplasmosis and Iodine Deficiency in Angora Goats. Vet. par. 81: 98-97.
[76] Svoboda M (1988) The Occurence of Antibodies to *Toxoplasma gondii* in Cats Living in the City of Brno and Its Vicinity. Vet. med. Czech 33: 45-54.
[77] Svoboda M, Svobodova V (1987) Effects of Breed, Sex, Age, Management and Nutrition on the Incidence of *Toxoplasma gondii* Antibodies in Dogs and Cats. Acta vet. Brno 56: 315-330.
[78] Tassi P (2006) *Toxoplasma gondii* Infection in Horses – a Serological Survey in Horse Slaughtered for Human Consumption in Italy. In: Proceedings of the Conference Toxo and Food, pp. 96-97.
[79] Vikoren T, Tharaldsen J, Fredriksen B, Handeland K (2004) Prevalence of *Toxoplasma gondii* Antibodies in Wild Red Deer, Roe Deer, Moose, and Rindeer from Norway. Vet. par. 120: 159-169.
[80] Vosta J, Hanak P, Rehacek J, Brezina R, Gresikova M (1981) The Field Hare (*Lepus europaeus* Pallas, 1778) as a Reservoir of Zoonoses. Folia venat. 10-11: 163-177.
[81] Vostalova E, Literak I, Pavlasek I, Sedlak K (2000) Prevalence of *Toxoplasma gondii* in Finishing Pigs in a Large-scale Farm in the Czech Republic. Acta vet. Brno 69: 209-212.
[82] Welton NJ, Ades AE (2005) A Model of Toxoplasmosis Incidence in the UK: Evidence Synthesis and Consistency of Evidence. Appl. statist. 54: 385-404.

[83] Williamson JMW, Williams H (1980) Toxoplasmosis in Farmed Red Deer (*Cervus elaphus*) in Scotland. Res. vet. sci. 29: 36-40.
[84] Zastera M, Hubner J, Pokorny J, Seeman J (1966) Rabbits as a Possible Source of Toxoplasmic Infection of Man (in Czech). Českoslov. epidem. 15: 172-177.
[85] Zastera M, Hubner J, Pokorny J. Valenta Z (1965) Isolation of *Toxoplasma gondii* from chicken (*Gallus gallus* dom.) (in Czech). Českoslov. epidem. mikrob. imunol. 14: 168-169.
[86] Zastera M, Pokorny J, Hubner J (1969) Toxoplasmosis in Human and Animals in ČSR (in Czech). Zprávy epidem. mikrob. 11: 1-30.

Chapter 4

Toxoplasmosis in Livestock and Pet Animals in Slovakia

Lenka Luptakova, Eva Petrovova, David Mazensky,
Alexandra Valencakova and Pavol Balent

Additional information is available at the end of the chapter

http://dx.doi.org/10.5772/47810

1. Introduction

The health status of livestock largely reflects on the human population. Livestock is important in terms of production of safe foodstuffs or breeding purposes.

Infections caused by pathogenic protozoa give rise to frequent problems mainly in tropical and subtropical regions, where they are widespread. It is reported that up to 4000 protozoa live as parasites. Worldwide, the most prevalent protozoan infection is malaria, while the most prevalent infection in the Slovak Republic is toxoplasmosis, by which the 30% of population are infected on average.

Parasitic pathogenic protozoa largely parasitize intracellularly, the course of these infections is acute, often cause the death. On the other hand, they can progress subclinically. The latent respectively chronic stage can follow the acute form and infections can persist throughout the whole life of the host. The course of the disease mostly depends also on the pathological agents. They stimulate the innate and adaptive immune response of the host. In mostly protozoan infections the immune response is not so sufficiently effective for a complete destruction of the parasite. This situation ensures the survival of the parasite and it is the characteristic feature for mostly protozoan infections.

Since a total elimination of the influence of negative factors (including pathogens) in each animal species is impossible, in the case of an unexpected outbreak of disease the solution is in its rapid and reliable diagnostics. The detection of pathogens as infection agents is carried out in laboratories using multiple techniques. The direct proof of parasite is usually microscopically and it is clear confirmation of infection. In systematic infections where the direct proof of parasite is unlikely serological methods are carried out in diagnostics for detection of antigen or antibody present in the biological samples. Serological methods often don´ t solve the problems of diagnosis in the early stage of infection or in the case of latent infection. For diagnostics of these stages are required more sensitive laboratory methods. In At present molecular methods based on the detection of the nucleic acid are used in the laboratories. A polymerase chain reaction (PCR - standard or quantitative) has wide range of using in the detection of parasites.

Toxoplasmosis is an acute parasitic infection monitored based on the epidemiological situation in the country. Therefore it is necessary to interconnect an epidemiological monitoring of infection in humans and animals because of a zoonotic character of this infection.

We here review the information available on the seroprevalence of *T. gondii* infection in livestock and pet animals in Slovakia. In addition we discuss the various serological and molecular methods available for the diagnosis of toxoplasmosis (in animals) and suggest a diagnostic approach based our data.

2. Basic characteristics about *T. gondii*

Toxoplasma gondii is a protozoan parasite of great medical and veterinary importance. Toxoplasmosis is one of the most common parasitic zoonoses in the world afflicting a broad range of both mammals and birds. The aetiological agent is *T. gondii* whose definite hosts are representatives of the family of *Felidae* infected by oocysts from the environment, or by tachyzoites and bradyzoites from intermediary hosts, such as all kinds of vertebrates, including humans. It is a pantropical cosmopolite and facultative heterogenic coccidia. *T. gondii* causes a mild infection in immuno-competent hosts, but in the immuno-compromised hosts, foetus and neonates, toxoplasmosis is severe even leading to death [1].

Toxoplasmosis may affect a number of organs, but it primarily affects lungs, the CNS (central nervous system) and eyes. Canine and feline toxoplasmosis is a multi-systemic disease; however a latent form of the disease usually develops. Dogs may act as a mechanical factor in transmitting toxoplasmosis to humans by rolling in foul-smelling substances and by ingesting fecal material. Just remember that 50% of stray dogs and dogs carry *T. gondii* antibodies, which means that they have been infected and may transmit the parasite. Cats are very important hosts in the epidemiological cycle of *T. gondii*, a zoonotic protozoan parasite that can infect humans and many other animal species worldwide. People and especially immuno-compromised individuals and pregnant women should observe the hygienic principles not only after contact with soil, cats, before eating, but also after contact with dogs. In gravid animals, particularly in sheep and goats, the *T. gondii* infection causes embryonic mortality, foetus death or abortion depending on the stage of gravidity in which the infection occurred. Variation in the clinical presentation and severity of disease has been attributed to several factors, including the heterogeneity of the host and the genotype of the infective parasite. The sources of the contamination by oocysts are mainly moist and shady places with the occurrence of cats where are suitable conditions for surviving of oocysts for a long period in the external environment [2]. Sheep were in fact the first mammals in which congenital toxoplasmosis were proven with abortions, dead-born fetuses and frequent manifestations of infection including infertility. The first case of manifest toxoplasmosis in sheep with symptoms of encephalomyelitis and tachycardia was described by Olafson and Monlux [3]. Sheep are most frequently infected with *T. gondii* from environment, i.e. from feed and pasture.

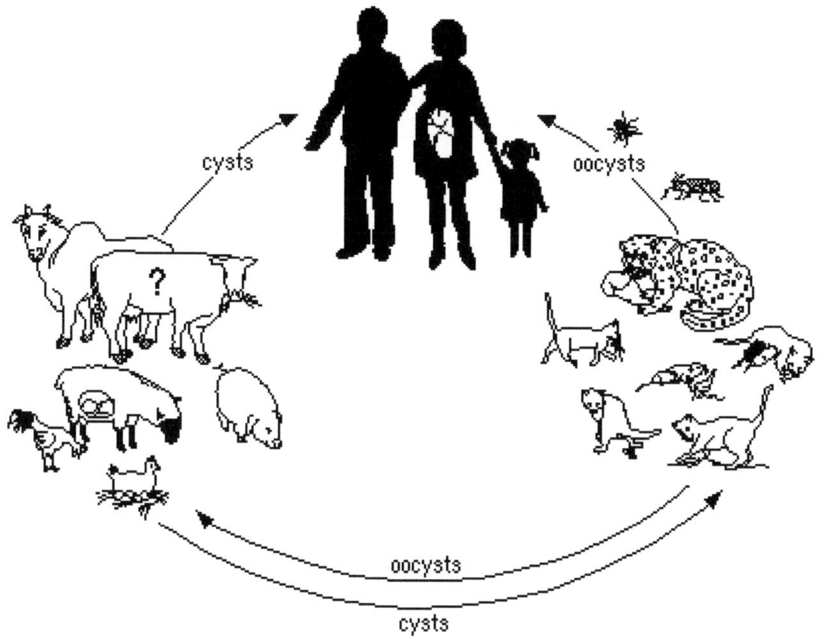

Figure 1. *T.* gondii - life cycle

3. *T.* and the immune system

T. gondii is able to survive and persist in immuno-competent intermediate hosts for the host's life. This is despite the induction of a vigorous humoral and more importantly cell-mediated immune response during infection. *T. gondii* has evolved multiple strategies to avoid or to interfere with potentially efficient anti-parasitic immune responses of the host immune evasion includes indirect mechanisms by altering the expression and secretion of immunomodulatory cytokines or by altering the viability of immune cells and direct mechanisms by establishing a lifestyle within a suitable intracellular niche and by interference with intracellular signaling cascades, thereby abolishing a number of antimicrobial effector mechanisms of the host [4].

4. Non-specific immune response

In immuno-competent hosts this parasite activates asymptomatic chronic infection, what make possible its transmission and survival. The infection of *T. gondii* may be lethal for immuno-compromised patients. At the beginning of immune response parasite changes to bradyzoites, which persist in tissue cyst for life. *T. gondii* is capable of triggering the non-specific activation of macrophages and natural killer cells (NK-cells) along with other haematopoietic and non-haematopoietic cells. This activation is intended to limit parasite proliferation due to its direct or indirect cytotoxic action and to trigger a specific immune response due to the presentation of *T.* antigens. Non-specific response begins immediately following the first contact between the parasite and the host [5]. NK-cells take part in early phase of immune response. During the early phase of the infection, it is through the combined and synergetic action of the NK-cells and the macrophages, activated by IFN-γ. In activated macrophages vacuoles of lived tachyzoites merge with lysosomes and then follow out the destruction of parasites. Neutrophils and, very probably, eosinophils, and mast cells rapidly interfere to the infection and are involved in setting up a non-specific early immune response *via* the production of IL-12 and various proinflammatory factors [6].

5. Specific immune response

The non-specific immune response has led to differentiation of macrophages and B-lymphocytes into antigen presenting cells. The effector cells are stimulated by dendritic cells presenting the antigen to T-lymphocytes. This mechanism requires a close interaction between the antigen presenting cell and the T-lymphocytes [7]. The interaction of parasite with mechanisms of non-specific immune response is important to orientation of progress of specific immunity. The induction of IL-12 and then IFN-γ stimulate the progression of Th1 subpopulations so that polarize the immune response for behoof cellular immunity. After acute infection, the cells presenting antigens (macrophages) are exciting to produce IL-12 and initiate differentiation of immature CD4 T-lymphocytes to Th1. The cellular immunity initiates the production of IFN-γ. This cytokine effects as a major mediator of cellular immunity during toxoplasmosis. The key function in specific immune response plays T-lymphocytes. These effector cells, which are involved in resistance to *T.* infection, then exert their function via a cytotoxic activity and/or the secretion of cytokines involved in the regulation of immune response [8].

$CD4^+$ and $CD8^+$ T-lymphocytes are the main players involved in resistance of the host to *T.* infection $CD4^+$ T-lymphocytes are required for the development of resistance during the early phase of the infection, and for immunity during vaccination. The $CD8^+$ T-lymphocytes exert a cytotoxic activity against tachyzoites or cells infected with *T. gondii* [9].

6. Humoral immune response

Antibodies play a minor role but remain the essential means for diagnosing toxoplasmosis. The production of specific IgG antibodies usually begins 4 weeks after the infection and can continue for several months while the dynamics of antibody production does not yield substantial change during the course of disease. IgG are the second immunoglobulins to appear in toxoplasmosis. They play a role in protection of the foetus because they are capable of crossing the placenta. The main target antigens of IgG are the surface antigens of the parasite [6].

IgM antibodies may appear earlier and decline more rapidly than IgG antibodies. The serum IgM only appears at the end of the first week following infection. These immunoglobulins are the best activators of the complement system. Due to their structure, they enable excellent agglutination and have a high level of cytotoxicity. This phenomenon is used especially in serological diagnosis techniques. Their persistence is subject to a high level of individual variation and can be as much as a year in most cases, thanks to the use of increasingly sensitive detection techniques [6].

IgA may be detected in sera of actuely infected adults and congenitally infected infants. In acquired toxoplasmosis, the appearance of IgA is not systematic. In immunodepressed subjects, IgA is thought to be an early marker in 50 % of cases. In congenital toxoplasmosis, the detection of IgA is valuable, since these can be detected in the absence of IgM. IgA (like IgM) do not cross the placenta and are actively involved in the diagnosis of congenital toxoplasmosis [2,13].

IgE antibodies are detectable in sera of actually infected adults, congenitally infected infants and children with congenital toxoplasmic chorioretinitis. The appearance on IgE in acute or congenital toxoplasmosis is random. The presence of this isotype is correlated with the beginning of complications, such as adenopathies, chorioretinitis, and *T.* reactivations in immunodepressed subjects [1].

7. Acute and chronic infection

Cell-mediated immune responses are essential for host control of intracellular infections. *T. gondii* is a protozoan parasite that infects multiple vertebrate species and invades multiple cell types. Upon initial encounter with the immune system, the parasite rapidly induces production of the protective cytokine IL-12 most likely from a subpopulation of dendritic cells. NK and T-lymphocytes are then activated and triggered to synthesize IFN-γ, the major mediator of host resistance during the acute and chronic phases of infection. Cytokine (IFN-γ and TNF-alpha) rather than cytotoxicity-based effector functions are more critical for protective immunity both during the acute and chronic phases of *T. gondii* infection. [10].

The T-lymphocytes, macrophages, and activity of interleukin IL-12 and IFN-γ is necessary for maintaining quiescence of chronic *T gondii* infection. IFN-γ stimulates anti-*T. gondii* activity, not only of macrophages, but also of nonphagocytic cells. TNF-alpha is another cytokine essential for control of chronic infection with *T. gondii* [11].

8. Congenital infection

Congenital toxoplasmosis poses a public health problem, being capable of causing foetal death and ocular and neurological sequelae in congenitally infected children. Congenital infection occurs only when mothers first encounter *T. gondii* during pregnancy. Resistance to *T. gondii* is mainly mediated by protective cytokines, such as IFN-γ and interleukin 2 (IL-2), whereas regulatory cytokines, such as IL-4 and IL-10, are associated with increased susceptibility to infection. Susceptibility of the pregnant host to toxoplasmosis may be due to a regulatory cytokine bias that is maintained during gestation. This cytokine pattern of pregnancy enhances susceptibility to toxoplasmosis, together with the risk of placental infection and congenital transmission. Cell-mediated immune responses involving CD4 and CD8 T cells and NK-cells play a protective role in *T. gondii* primary infection [12].

9. Diagnosis of toxoplasmosis

The diagnosis of *T. gondii* infection may be establishes by serologic test, amplification of specific nucleic acid sequences (i. e. polymerase chain reaction), histological demonstration of the parasite antigens (i. e. imunoperoxidase stain) or isolation of the organism. Biological diagnostics of infections caused by *T. gondii* can be provided by: direct methods (microscopic analysis, in vitro isolation on cell cultures, histological methods, detection of DNA of *T. gondii*) and by indirect serological methods to indicate the presence of specific antibodies in serum. Suitable combination of complementary techniques (detection of antibodies in serum and manifestation of parasite), must lead in majority of cases to precise diagnostics of congenital toxoplasmosis. The use of serologic tests for demonstration of specific antibody to *T. gondii* is the initial and primary method of diagnosis. Serological diagnostics of active infection is not reliable, because reactivation is not always accompanied by changes in the level of antibodies and presence of IgM does not indicate present infection. There are several serological tests available for the detection of *T. gondii* antibodies. In one type of test the observer judges the given colour of tachyzoites under a microscope, such as with the dye test (DT) and IFA test. Another depends on the principle of agglutination of *T.* tachyzoites, red blood cells or latex particles, such as with the direct agglutination test (DAT) and indirect haemagglutination test (IHA) and latex agglutination (LA) test, respectively. With the enzyme-linked immunosorbent assay (ELISA), the degree of colour change defines the quantity of specific antibody in a given solution. The most frequently used method for detection of *T. gondii* infection is complement fixation test for antibody detection of IgG class and ELISA tests for detection of the markers of acute infection in IgM, IgA and IgE classes. IFAT method demands intact tachyzoites and it is more sensitive and more specific compared with IHA, LA, ELISA tests, because during infection the first significant rise of IgM and IgG antibodies was observed against cuticular antigens. Diagnostics of acute infection during gravidity in women is difficult. IgM antibodies can be detected a long time after acute phase, IgA rise has higher diagnostic value because it can be detected in 6-7 months in the time when short kinetics of IgE can be useful only for dating of the onset of infection. IgG seroconversion is necessary for diagnostics. Serological diagnostics of prenatal infection is difficult from the time when maternal IgG passively transmit into fetus and interpretations of IgM and IgA results must be cautious [1,2,14]

Histological examination of biological samples shows insufficient reliability if animals are infected by a few parasites. Mouse inoculation is the most reliable method even in the case if detection of cysts in mouse brain demands 40 days. Tachyzoites of virulant strains can be isolated from peritoneal exudate 3-4 days after inoculation. Inoculation of samples in cell cultures (VERO, human fibroblasts) demands specialised laboratories [2].

The most reliable method for prenatal diagnostics are PCR, mouse inoculation, cell techniques with usage of amniotic fluid, blood of fetus and peripheral maternal blood in pregnant serologically positive individuals. Utilization of quantitative PCR has developed sensitive, specific and rapid method for detection of *T. gondii* DNA in amniotic fluid, blood, samples of tissues and cerebrospinal fluid. Molecular methods do not rely on immune response and enable direct detection of parasites in biological samples. They can be used for diagnostics of the disease also in the case if serological tests are not sufficient. In molecular tests are especially useful sequences specific for *T. gondii* e.g. B1 gene or 529 bp sequence. PCR is very sensitive and is promising technique for obtaining of quantitative results. Molecular methods are used also for genotypization. Molecular methods do not rely on immune response and enable direct detection of a parasite in biological samples. They can be used for diagnostics of a disease even in the case ig serological tests are not sufficient. Sequences specific for *T. gondii* e. g. B1 gene that repeats in genome 35 times, TGR1 gene, 529 bp sequence are useful in molecular tests. Immediate PCR is very sensitive and it is very promising technique for obtaining of quantitave results [15].

Diagnostics of acute, postnatally achieved primary toxoplasmosis will be based on serological methods. Acute infection caused by *T. gondii* will be diagnosed by detection of parasite directly using histological and immunological methods, isolation of *T. gondii* from blood, body fluids or tissues on cell cultures. Combination of methods is needed for diagnostics of congenital infection and its late secondary consequences or reactivation of latent infection in immunodeficient patients. In these cases rapid and exact diagnostics is needed to start therapy. PCR method will be used for diagnostics of primary toxoplasmosis in pregnant women to prevent transmission of parasites into fetus but also for diagnostics of toxoplasmosis encephalitis in immunodeficient patients, in which cerebral biopsy is up to now the only diagnostic method and also in the eye form of toxoplamosis. Utilization of quantitative PCR will bring sensitive, specific and rapid method for detection of *T. gondii* DNA in amniotic fluid, in blood, in tissue samples and in cerebrospinal fluid. Specific sequence for *T. gondii* e.g. B1 gene or 529-bp sequence will be used in molecular tests. They can be used for diagnostics of the disease also in the case, when serological test are not sufficient. Prompt PCR is very sensitive and is promising technique for obtaining of quantitative results [16].

We obtained data about seroprevalence of anti-*T. antibodies* and occurrence of *T.* DNA from 698 animal serum samples and 256 animla uncoagulated blood samples. For this Examined blood samples were taken from asymptomatic animals, out of which 233 were sheep, 41 goats, 76 cattle, 63 pigs, 91 wild boars, 32 hens, 102 dogs, 39 cats and 21 rabbits. Blood samples were taken from *vena jugularis* of the beef cattle, sheep and goats, from *vena cava cranialis* of pigs, form *vena cephalica* in dogs and cats, *vena auricularis* in rabbits, and in wild boars and hens the blood was taken immediately after death when animals were bled.

For obtaining serological data about seroprevalence we used two serological tests: complement fixation test (CFT) and ELISA. CFT was performed by the micromodified method after Zástěra *et al.* [17] published as a supplement to the standard method in Acta

Hygienica, Epidemiologica et Microbiologica. The test is performed in two steps. The first step resides in the incubation of the mixture of antigen and antibody together with complement (its optimum concentration is tested advance). The second step consists of the detection of free or not fixed complement after its reaction with the immunity complex, while the suspension ready-to-use haemolytic system is used as an indicator. The activity of the complement is determined quantitatively as 50 % hemolysis of haemolytic system. The basic dilution was 1:32 and this titer was considered positive. For diagnosis *T.* antigen (Virion, Switzerland), complement (made from guinea pig serum, Virion, Swizerland; work dilution 1:47.5), *T.* positive and negative serum (Imuna a. s., the Slovak Republic), and Hemolytic system (ready to use; Virion, Switzerland) were used.

An enzyme-linked immunosorbent assay (ELISA) was carried out for the detection of IgG and IgM antibodies to *T. gondii* according to the manufacturer´s instructions (Test-Line, Czech Republic). In the first step, specific IgG or IgM antibodies in serum were bound to the *T. gondii* antigen coated on the surface of reagent wells and then, the rabbit anti-species IgG or IgM antibodies (sheep, dog, rabbit, cattle, and wild boar) labelled with peroxidase (Sigma- Aldrich, USA) were applied to the complex formed between the *T. gondii* antigen and circulating antibodies. After addition of the enzyme substrate, TMB (3,3´,5,5´-tetramethylbenzidine), the absorbance was read at 450 nm using a Dynex spectrophotometer (Dynex Technologies, USA). Positive and negative serum controls previously tested by conventional serological test were included on each plate. For each sample, the index of positivity (IP) was calculated according to the schema provided by the manufacturer: IP= sample absorbance/average absorbance of cut-off serum (cut-off serum is a serum sample which contains antibodies to *T. gondii* in limiting concentration). Samples with IP < 0.8 were considered to be negative, samples with IP between 0.8-1.0 were considered to be dubious and samples with IP>1.0 were considered to be positive [18].

For molecular analysis total DNA was then purified from white blood cells by using the commercial kit QIAamp DNA Mini Kit (QIAGEN, Germany) according to the manufacturer´s instructions. Amplification of the isolated DNA was carried out by the standard PCR and real time PCR method from the *T. gondii* gene region TGR1E, repeated in the genome 30-35 times, using the specific primers TGR1E-1 and TGR1E-2 [19].

Standard PCR was executed in 25 μL reaction volume containing 0.2 μM of each primer (TGR1E-1, TGR1E-2), 0.2 mM of each dNTP, 1.5 mM $MgCl_2$ and 2.5 U of *Taq* DNA polymerase and the reaction was conducted in a thermocycler (Genius, UK) with the following temperature profile: initial denaturation at 94°C for 3 min., 40 cycles of amplification (94°C 1 min., 60°C 1 min., 72°C 1 min.) and final extension at 72°C for 7 min. The PCR products were visualized in 3% agarose gel and stained with ethidium bromide [20]. The final positive PCR product has 191 bp in size.

For quantitative real time cloned *T. gondii* TGR gene (GenExpress, Germany) diluted to 10^4-10^9 was used for the calibration curve. In each reaction, a melting analysis (comparison of the melting temperature (Tm) of PCR products) was determined to differentiate specific and non-specific PCR products. The reaction volume was 25 ul, which contained commercial

FastStart Universal SYBR Green Master (Roche, Germany) and 0.2 uM primers (TGR1-1 and TGR1E-2). Real-time PCR was completed using a thermocycler Line GeneK with the software Line GeneK Fluorescent Quantitative Detection system (BIOER Technology, China). After incubation at 50°C for 2 minutes and initial denaturation at 95°C for 10 minutes, 40 amplification cycles were performed (95°C for 15 s, 60°C for 1 minute). Melting analysis was carried out at temperatures ranging from 60°C to 95°C, in which the temperature was gradually increased by 0.5°C and the period of measurement at individual steps was 15 s. Every PCR run included a control without DNA (containing the reaction mix alone and nuclease-free water).

The examined animals were divided into groups for better understanding of the relationship between the seroprevalence of toxoplasmosis and the age of animals. Each group of examined animals was divided into subgroups according to the age (sheep: female and male lambs up to 4 months of age, rams and ewes; goats: kids - young goats up to 4 months of age, adults - from 7 months of age; pigs: suckling piglets, sows; cattle: calves - up to 6 months of age, heifers, dairy cows; wild boars under 1 year old and adult; Table 1).

Animals	N	Groups	n
sheep	233	lambs	40
		rams	64
		ewes	129
goats	41	kids	15
		goats	26
pigs	63	sucking piglets	20
		sows	43
cattle	76	calves	25
		heifers	10
		dairy cows	41
wild boars	91	young (<1year)	29
		adults	62
dogs	102	dog shelter	38
		professional breeders	32
		households	32
cats	39	mixed	39
rabbits	21	mixed	21
hens	32	mixed	32
Total	698		698

Table 1. Groups of animals including in serological testing

For PCR analysis (standard PCR and quantitative real time PCR) each sample was examined by ELISA for detection of IgM and IgG specific antibodies to *T. gondii*. After serological examination samples were divided into three froups: Group I contained samples only positive to IgM antibodies (acute infection), group II contained samples positive only to IgG antibodies (chronic infection) and group III contained samples without IgM or IgG antibodies (no infection).

Fisher´s exact test was used to compare the success of real-time PCR depending on the presence of IgM or IgG antibodies.

During our study we obtained following data in serological analysis. By CFT 698 animals were examined for the presence of overall anti-*T.* antibodies. A sample with a titre 1:32 and higher was considered to be positive. Out of all specimens, the presence of antibodies to *T. gondii* was detected in 206 cases (29.5%). out of 233 examined sheep sera 26 (11.1%) of lambs, 37 (15.9%) of rams and 51 (21.9%) of ewes were positive. The frequency of *T. gondii* contamination was significantly higher in group of ewes than in other two groups of animals ($\chi 2$ test: $p < 0.01$). In group of goats, out of 41 serum samples, 5 (12.2%) were positive in subgroup of kids and 7 (14.1%) in subgroups of adult goats. From 63 examined pigs, only 2 (3.2%) sucking piglets were positive. From 76 examined cattle only 2 (2.6%) of calves were positive for presence of antibodies to *T. gondii*. From 91 examined wild boars, 18 (19.8%) exhibited a positive serological reaction to *T. gondii*. The occurrence of anti-*T.* antibodies was higher in young animals (less than 1 year; 10 positive animals - 10.9%) than in adults (2 positive animals - 2.2%). Out of 102 examined dog sera, 17 (16.7%) were positive in group of dogs from dog shelters, 15 (14.7%) dogs from professional breeders and 10 (9.8%) dogs keeping in households. In group of cats, out of 39 examined sera, 13 (33.3%) were considered as positive, out of 21 rabbits, 3 (14.3%) were positive. In group of 32 hens, no positive animal was found (Table 2).

For comparison of CFT and ELISA 102 dog serum specimens were examined for the presence of antibodies to *T. gondii* by two serological tests (CFT and ELISA). The presence of antibodies to *T. gondii* was detected in 75 cases (73.5%). Anti-*T.* IgG antibodies were found in 51 (50%) by ELISA. Samples positive only with CFT was 39 (38.2%), only in ELISA 14 (13.7%), positive in both tests 37 (36.3%) and negative in both tests 12 (11.8%). The titres of latent infection (1:8 – 1:128) in CFT were recorded in 75 dogs: 13 dogs (12.7%; 1:8), 20 dogs (19.6%; 1:16), 20 dogs (19.6%; 1:32), 20 dogs (19.6%; 1:64) and 1 dog (1%; 1:128). The prevalence of acute infection (1:256 and higher) was recorded in 1 dog (1%; 1:256). The coincidence of CFT and IgG antibodies was recorded in 37 samples (36.3 %). Comparison of detection of antibodies by these two tests was statistically significant ($p<0.001$, Figure 2).

In molecular analysis by standard PCR and quantitative PCR at first IgM antibodies which appear at the beginning of infection and which are characteristic for acute infection were detected in 45 of 256 (17.6%) by ELISA. IgG antibodies which corresponded with chronic infection were detected in 120 of 256 (46.8%). In 91of 256 (35.5%) animals neither IgM nor IgG were detected by ELISA. The occurrence of IgM or IgG antibodies in each species is summarized in Table 3.

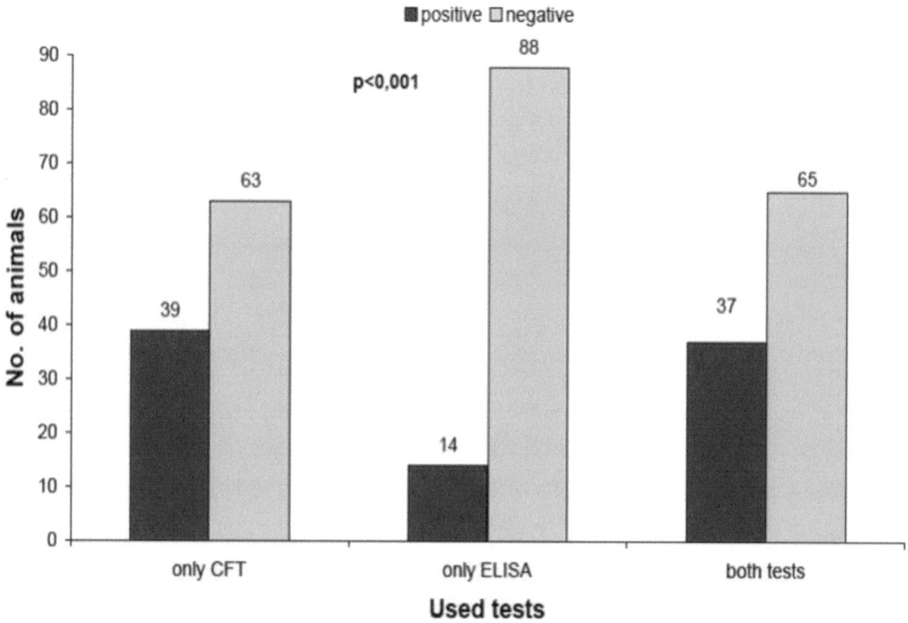

P*value were obtained by comparing results obtained by CFT to results obtained only by ELISA

Figure 2. Number of animals positive only in CFT, only in ELISA and in both tests ($p<0.001$)

Animals	n	Groups	N/SP %
sheep	233	lambs	26/11.1
		rams	37/15.9
		ewes	51/21.9*
goats	41	kids	5/12.2
		goats	7/14.1
pigs	63	sucking piglets	2/3.2
		sows	0/0
cattle	76	calves	2/2.6
		heifers	0/0
		dairy cows	0/0
wild boars	91	young (<1year)	10/10.9
		adults	2/2.2
dogs	102	dog shelter	17/16.7
		professional breeders	15/14.7
		households	10/9.8
cats	39	mixed	13/33.3
rabbits	21	mixed	3/14.3
hens	32	mixed	0/0
Total	**698**		**206/29.5**

n - number of examined samples; N - number od positive samples; SP - seroprevalence (%)

Table 2. Occurrence of overall antibodies to *T. gondii* by CFT in different animal species

Animals	IgM		IgG		Negative
	N/n	%	N/n	%	
sheep	27/50	54%	23/50	46%	0
cattle	4/32	12.5%	20/32	62.5%	8
rabbits	7/36	19.4%	24/36	66.6%	5
wild boars	5/9	15.5%	18/91	19.8%	68
dogs	2/47	4.3%	35/47	74.5%	10
Total	**25/256**	**17.6%**	**120/256**	**46.9%**	**91**

N – number of positive samples; n – number of examined samples; % seroprevalence

Table 3. Occurence of IgG and IgM antibodies *to T. gondii* by ELISA in different animal species

According to the serological results animals were divided into three groups: animals with suspicion of acute (group I, n=45) or chronic toxoplasmosis (group II, n=120) and without infection (group III, n=91). For statistical analysis, we considered group I (acute infection, IgM positive) and group II (chronic infection, IgG positive).

By standard PCR the presence of DNA *T. gondii* was detected in ten samples of non-coagulated blood (6 sheep, 1 wild boar and 3 rabbits) with the DNA product length 191 bp (Figure 3).

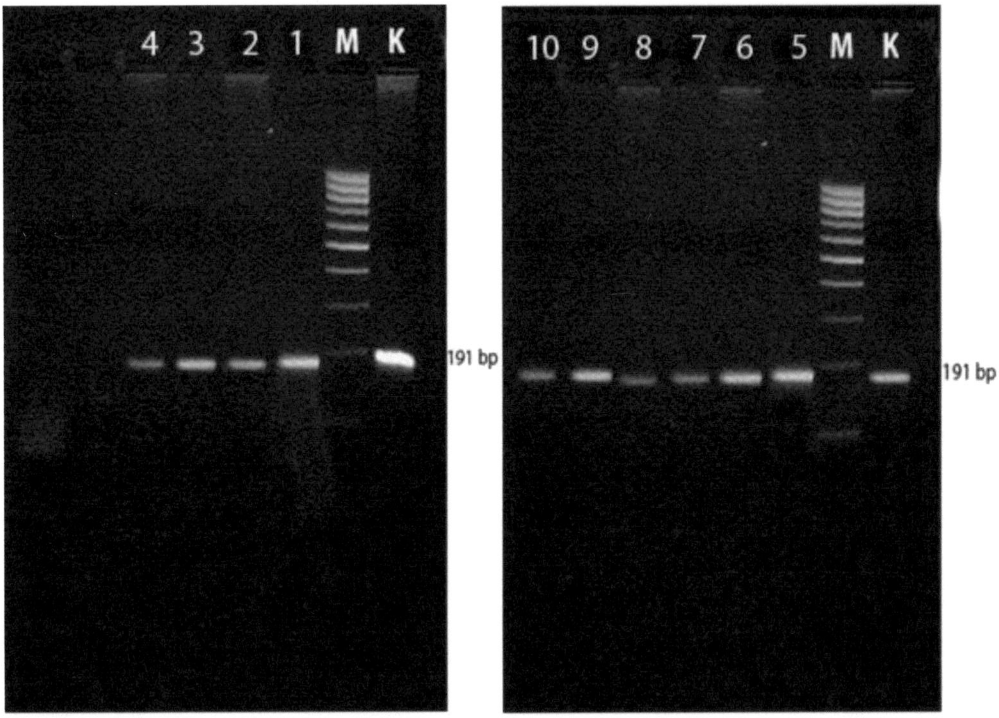

Figure 3. PCR fragment of *T. gondii* DNA (191 bp) in a 3% agarose gel. K: positive control, M: marker of size (100bp plus DNA ladder, Fermentas, Germany); lane 1: positive wild boar sample, lanes 2-4: positive rabbit samples; lanes 5-10: positive sheep samples

Using quantitative real time PCR the presence of DNA *T. gondii* was detected and the number of their copies quantified in the 256 non-coagulated animal blood samples. Using real time PCR *T. gondii* DNA was detected and quantified in ten samples of non-coagulated blood (6 sheep, 1 wild boar and 3 rabbits; Table 4). For animals presenting acute toxoplasmosis (group I), the presence of *T. gondii* DNA was detected in 9 of 45 (20%), whereas in chronic group (group II) only one sample was positive (1/120; 0.8%). In group III which contained animals without IgM or IgG antibodies no DNA of *T. gondii* (0/91) was detected by real time PCR. The proof of DNA by real time PCR in IgM positive samples was statistically significant in comparison to IgG positive samples ($P<0.0001$).

Standards with the known dilution of *T.* DNA were used to determine the detection limit of a modified real time PCR and to create a calibration curve that ranged from 10^9 to 10^4 copies of *T.* DNA. The correlation coefficient of the calibration curve was 0.998. As SYBR Green a fluorescent dye, was used as a detection system, a melting analysis was a part of the real-time PCR to distinguish between specific and non-specific products. During the melting analysis the melting temperature (Tm) of a positive control and positive samples was 84 °C (Figure 4). In quantifying the examined samples within a 40-cycle protocol for the real time PCR, the number of copies detected in the positive samples ranged from 1.07×10^2 to 1.49×10^5 (Table 5).

	N	Real time PCR		P value
		positive	negative	
Group I (IgM+)	45	9	36	<0.0001*
Group II (IgG+)	120	1	119	-

Group I-acute toxoplasmosis; Group II-chronic toxoplasmosis; P*value were obtained by comparison of the proof of *T.* DNA by qPCR in group I (acute infection, IgM positive) and group II (chronic infection, IgG positive)

Table 4. Relation between the presence of *T. gondii* DNA and serological results

Sample	Number of copies	Group
Sheep 1	5.92×10^4	IgM+
Lamb 1	1.49×10^5	IgM+
Sheep 3	3.67×10^4	IgM+
Sheep 4	5.75×10^2	IgM+
Sheep 5	3.89×10^4	IgM+
Sheep 6	2.56×10^3	IgM+
Wild boar	1.05×10^5	IgM-
Rabbit 1	1.07×10^2	IgM+
Rabbit 2	2.09×10^2	IgM+
Rabbit 3	3.17×10^2	IgM+

Table 5. The number of *T. gondii* DNA copies in the examined samples in a 25 µl-volume

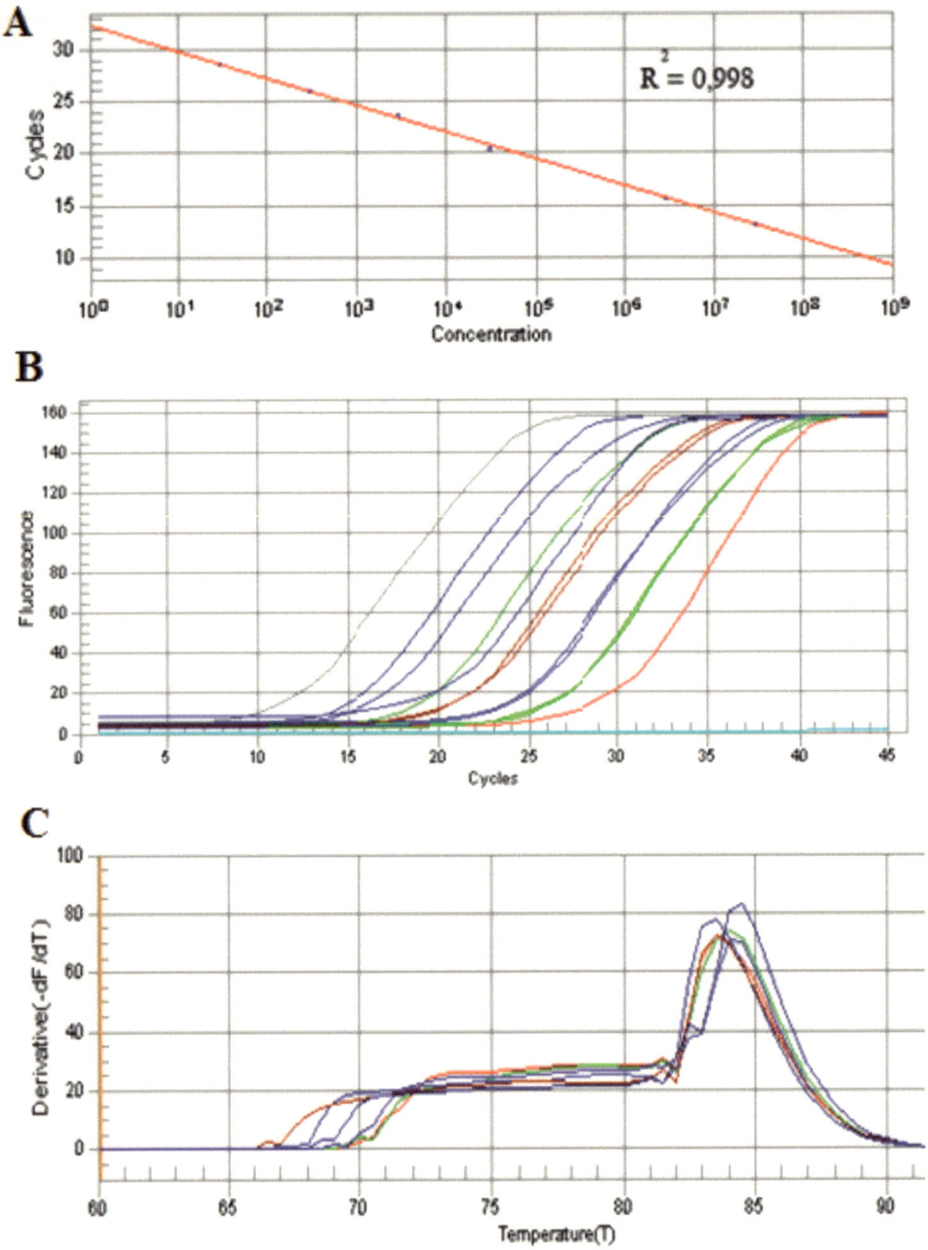

Figure 4. Quantitative real time PCR - A-Calibration curve; B - Samples; C - Melting analysis

The diagnosis of toxoplasmosis may be established by serological tests, polymerase chain reaction (PCR), histological demonstration of the parasite and/or its antigens (i.e. immunoperoxidase stain), or isolation of the organism. The serological tests are able to show the presence of IgM antibodies which can represent the acute infection as well as these IgM antibodies can be residual. Avidity tests may help in this setting by distinguishing between

IgG of high and low affinity, corresponding to either chronic or acute toxoplasmosis. Results of serological tests don't reflect the course of infection. The presence of specific serum antibodies is possible to detect in organism of each potential host who come in the contact with the pathogen. Based on the serological prevalence in the population is possible to suppose only the certain relationship between population and morbidity. The advantage of serological tests is that specific antibodies can be detected two week before histological proof of parasite in pathological lesions and 4 weeks before the molecular proof of parasites in infected tissues. The positive serological result is only indicative of infection, whereas direct detection of *T. gondii* in blood or other clinical samples categorically confirms the parasite presence in the organism [15,21]. Several indirect methods have been proposed for the detection of antibodies to *T.* in animals, generally in samples of serum and plasma. In addition, thoracic fluid of aborted fetuses, milk and samples of fluid obtained by freezing and thawing portions of muscular tissue (meat juice) can be tested as well for antibodies. However, data from different studies may not always be directly comparable due to discrepancies in the procedures used for the detection of antibodies. For example, the modification of protocols, the different strains of *T.*, and the different cut-off points of tests. Not all assays are suitable for every animal species and cross reactions with antibodies to related parasites may result in false positives. Serological methods of *T.* diagnostics are still very important. They are required for quick and reliable results about epizootological situations in countries because of the zoonotic character of *T.* infection. Toxoplasmosis belongs to the majority of prevalent infections in livestock. The prevalence of this protozoan disease has been demonstrated by studies carried out to detect antibodies to *T. gondii* in farms of domestic animals in other European countries. It can be demonstrated by Fusco et al. [22] and Masala et al. [23] who have detected the presence of antibodies to *T. gondii* in their work using serological methods in sheep and goats. Fusco et al. [22] examined 117 flocks of sheep bred in pastures in the region of Campania, southern Italy. Blood and milk specimens were collected from 10 adult sheep from each of the flocks (sheep aged more than 18 months). A total of as many as 1,170 sheep were examined. The serum specimens were examined for the presence of IgG antibodies by means of an IFAT method (an indirect immunofluorescence antibody test). Out of the 1,170 examined sheep, 333 specimens were positive to *T.* infection (28.5%). Between 1999 and 2002 Masala et al. [23] analyzed 9,639 serum specimens and 815 abortion specimens (670 aborted fetuses and 145 placentas) from 964 sheep and goat farms in Sardinia. The collected sera were examined for the detection of IgG and IgM specific antibodies to *T. gondii* using the indirect immunofluorescence method. Specific IgG antibodies were diagnosed in 652 sheep (9%). In France, the presence of specific IgG antibodies to *T. gondii* was detected in 22 % of lambs and 65.6% of gravid sheep; in Sicily, the seroprevalence ranges between 70 and 90%; in Switzerland, it is in approximately 58.6% of sheep; while in Germany, it is only 19.1% [24]. Seroprevalence of toxoplasmosis were determined in 87 goats of the eastern Slovakia. From these animals antibodies were found out in 43 goat sera (49.43%). Statistically significant correlation ($P < 0.0001$) was found between the prevalence of antibodies against *T. gondii* and animal age in comparing age groups – goats up to 36 months of age and above 37 months of age [25]. In view of the prevalence of toxoplasmosis in pigs in the Czech Republic, an interesting result occurred from the examination of 787 pigs in 1999. They came from a modern large-capacity breeding farm in southern Bohemia. They were all examined using a complement fixation test and out of a total of 787 animals, the antibodies were detected only in 4 cases [26]. In the Slovak republic were detected antibodies to *T. gondii* by ELISA in 840 serum samples of pigs and 21 samples (2.5%) were considered as positive [27]. Pleva et al. [28] published the results of examination of 582 serum samples of cattle in 1996 and in no sample antibodies against *T. gondii* was found. In 2008 were examined 85 samples of cattle from Slovakia by ELISA. Anti-*T.* antibodies were detected only in 2 (2.35%) samples [29]. In 2009 they examined 312 serum samples of cattle from Slovakia. From all examined samples they found out the presence of antibodies to *T. gondii* in 31 (9.94%) samples. The risk of infection of domestic animals with *T. gondii* is very high. Among the measures that can be taken are keeping meat-producing animals in captivity on farms during the whole feeding period, maintaining the stables without rodents, birds or insects, paying closer attention to feeding the animals with non-contaminated fodder. By taking these measures it is possible to run farms with low prevalence of toxoplasmosis [30]. Wild boar is an autochthonous species of leafy exploitation of the Slovak republic. Due to the agricultural exploitation of landscape, disseminating of maize production, intensive forest management and low mortality of piglet during snow and absence of big carnivores, the wild boar population started to increase from the second half of the 20th century. The rising number of wild boars causes economic losses and may represent a source of dissemination of different diseases. Tissue cysts of *T. gondii* in meat of different game species are potential sources of human infection [31]. The overall *T. gondii* seroprevalence in wild boars was 19.8% in the present study and was significantly higher in young animals (37.9%). This corresponds to the fact that toxoplasmosis is most commonly seen in young animals, especially in neonates and in immuno-compromised animals. Toxoplasmosis in young animals causes severe damage such as intra-uterine growth restriction, icterus, hepato-splenomegaly, myocarditis, pneumonitis, and various rashes. Neurologic involvement, often prominent, includes chorio-retinitis, hydrocephalus, intracranial calcifications, microcephaly, and seizures [31]. In Europe, anti-*T. gondii* antibodies were found in 8.1% (26/320) or 38.5% (5/13) of wild boars from Slovakia [32], 26.2% (148/565) from the Czech Republic [33], 16.6% (2/12) from Bulgaria [34] and 21.1% (11/52) from Eastern Poland [35]. In France Richomme et al. [36] tested 148 sera and tissues of wild boars for *T.* infection from two French regions, one continental and one insular. Antibodies to *T. gondii* were found in 26 (17.6%) of 148 wild boars using the modified agglutination test (MAT, positivity threshold: 1:24). Seroprevalence was 45.9% when considering a threshold of 1:6. Hearts of individuals with a positive agglutination (starting dilution 1:6) (n = 60) were bioassayed in mice for isolation of viable *T. gondii*. In total, 21 isolates of *T. gondii* were obtained. In other wildlife from France Aubert et al. [37] *T. gondii* antibodies were found in 14 of 19 (73.7%) red foxes, with titers between 1:25 and 1:6400 and parasite isolation was successful in 9/13 seropositive animals (69.2%). Thirty-six of the 60 roe deer (60%) showed antibodies with titers between 1:6 and 1:6400. Thirty-three bioassays were performed, 12 isolates were obtained from animals with antibodies titers between 1:25 and 1:6400. *T. gondii* antibodies were found in 4 of 24 red deer (17%) with titers of 1:6 (2), 1:10 (1) and 1:25 (1) and a viable parasite was isolated from the heart of one red deer with a titer of 1:6. No parasite was isolated from fallow deer with only one positive with a titer of 1:25. *T. gondii* antibodies were found in 7 of 31 mouflons (23%) with titers between 1:6 and 1:6400 and the isolate was detected only in one samples. The brown hare (*L. europaeus*) is a common species of wild mammals in Europe where they are extensively hunted. They detected *T. gondii* antibodies in only 9% of sera from brown hares but failed to isolate viable parasites. In households animals (such as cats, dogs and rabbits) *T. gondii* represent a health hazard and can have the impact for the owners. Toxoplasmosis of pet animals as dogs, cats and rabbits is also important source of infection. In dogs, toxoplasmosis is a rare primary disease of dogs. Martins and Viana [38] highlight the importance of dogs in the epidemiological chain of the disease, through the habit of ingesting, and rolling in cat feces, thus permitting transmission of oocysts by contact of the contaminated hide. Lindsay et al. [39] demonstrated that after ingestion of *T. gondii* non-sporulate oocysts, these could pass through the intestinal tract of dogs, and be excreted in their infectious stage, re-enforcing the theory that dogs act as mechanical vectors of oocysts. The sources of the contamination by oocysts are mainly moist and shady places with the occurrence of cats where are suitable conditions for surviving of oocysts for a long period in the external environment [40]. Serological diagnosis of *T. gondii* infections in dogs and cats has been evaluated by many investigators. The tests used include the Sabin-Feldman, the complement fixation, the indirect haemagglutination, the direct agglutination, the indirect fluorescent antibody and the enzyme immunoassay. The demonstration of antibodies by these serological tests just indicates previous infection by *T. gondii.* A laboratory diagnosis defined to toxoplasmosis-disease requires the demonstration of high titers of specific antibodies and increasing levels in two serum samples taken 2 to 4 weeks apart. The prevalence of antibodies to *T. gondii* was determined in sera from dogs in Grenada, West Indies. Using a modified agglutination test, antibodies to *T. gondii* were found in 52 (48.5 %) of the 107 dogs, with titers of 1:25 in 17, 1:50 in 19, 1:100 in 7, 1:1,600 in 5, and 1:3,200 or higher in 4 [41]. Lopes et al. [42] reported a serological survey of antibodies to *T. gondii* in domestic cats from northeastern Portugal, by means of the modified agglutination test. Three cats had titres of 20 (3.9%), 18 had titres of 40 (23.7%) and 55 animals had titres of ≥800 (72.4%). Infection levels were also significantly different between cats that lived totally indoors (7.7%) and those that had access to outdoors (45.4%), as well as between cats living alone (13.8%) and those that had contact with other cats (39.4%). Seroprevalence values in cats fed only commercial canned or dried food (22.9%) and animals whose diet included raw or undercooked viscera and/or meat (53.5%) were also significantly different. Age, habitat and diet were identified as risk factors for the feline *T. gondii* infection by logistic regression analysis. Some control measures are suggested based on these findings [42]. Samples of serum taken during 1986 and 1987 from 244 pet cats, 303 dogs, were screened by enzyme-linked immunosorbent assay (ELISA) for antibodies to *T. gondii* 42% of cats, 23% of dogs examined were found seropositive [43]. Five hundred and sixty seven sera of healthy house cats were examined for the presence of anti-*T.* antibodies by indirect immunofluorescence assay. Twenty-five percent of cats tested positive for IgG and/or IgM. Seroprevalence increased with age from 2% below 12 months of age up to 44% at age 7.

These results suggest that *T. gondii* infections are common in house cats and that there is a high chance for a negative cat to seroconvert in its second life-year [44]. Sera of 413 dogs and 286 cats from the Czech Republic were tested for antibodies to *T. gondii* by the indirect fluorescent antibody test. The IgM antibodies to *T. gondii* were found in 10 dogs (2.4%) and 8 cats (2.8%); IgG antibodies were found in 107 dogs (25.9%) and 126 cats (44.1%). Of the dogs, the most exposed group were pet dogs, followed by police dogs; no antibodies were found in laboratory dogs. No statistically significant differences in prevalence were observed between clinically healthy (n = 115) and diseased pet dogs (n = 80); compare 0.87% and 1.25% for IgM, and 33.9% and 33.75% for IgG, respectively. Although *T. gondii* is a common parasite in domestic cats and dogs, the clinical importance is low [45]. Figueroa-Castillo et al. [46] determined antibodies to *T. gondii* by indirect ELISA in serum samples from domestic rabbits from 3 rabbit farms in Mexico. Antibodies to *T. gondii* were found in 77 (26.9%) of 286 animals. On the farm with the higher rearing standards, the seroprevalence was 18.7%, whereas on the farm with medium standards and another managed by a family, seroprevalence was 39.7 and 33.3%, respectively. This report is the first report concerning the prevalence of antibodies to *T. gondii* in rabbits from Mexico. Although the prevalence found in the present study is within the range reported for other countries, 2 of the farms revealed a relatively high prevalence, which was probably associated with the presence of cats inside rabbit houses [46]. In term of infection spread is important animal breeding, contact with another animal and composition and processing of feed. In animals keeping in households the most important role is composition and processing of food. The feeding of raw or undercooked meat or offal plays the main role in spreading of infection in household animals. The important part of rabbit feeding is fruits and vegetables. The fruits and vegetables contaminated with infected soil and inadequately washed presents the important source of *T.* infection with infected oocysts. The role of domestic rabbit in epidemiology of toxoplasmosis in humans has not been established in detail, but is probably important. Although some authors treat this role marginally, others place the rabbit among the animal species posing a major source of infection for man [47]. Ishikawa et al. [48] described the case of cervical toxoplasmosis transmitted from rabbit to man. Nevertheless, there is a lack of controlled epidemiological studies on the degrees of a correlation between the prevalence of toxoplasmosis in rabbits and in humans having contacts with these animals [48].

Among laboratory diagnostic techniques, a complement fixation test is one of the most frequently employed techniques for detecting antibodies to *T. gondii.* Results acquired in complement fixation tests in examinations for the presence of antibodies against *T. gondii* antigens in the serum specimens of infected animals facilitate the interpretation of such results. The level of overall antibodies in a CFT significantly correlates with the dynamics of IgM and IgA antibodies. A titre of 1:256 - 512 is significant for the acute phase of infection, whereas titres below 1:128 point to the chronic or latent course of the disease. With respect to the determination of *T.* infection in a serological examination, a CFT is of greater informative value in comparison to the same requirement related to IgG antibodies. Specific IgG antibodies detected by ELISA are a reliable substitution of quantitative results that can be assessed by CFT but due to the fact that the dynamics of CFT antibodies is more significantly associated with course of the disease, the assessment of the phase of infection must be supported also by parallel examination of IgM or IgA antibodies [49]. So CFT should be the first part of basic examination procedures in the laboratory diagnosis of toxoplasmosis. The complement fixation test is the basic method in the diagnosis of toxoplasmosis. Despite its standard and reproducible results, it is rarely used in routine diagnosis of toxoplasmosis where the detection of IgG by means of ELISA is widely used. Our results suggested that CFT is reliable indicator of *T.* infection because was found a correlation between CFT and IgG ELISA. In our study were positive 36.3% of samples in both tests and 38.2 % of examined samples were positive only in CFT. A significant differences in results obtained by CFT and ELISA could be influenced also by the higher positive titer established in ELISA (1:100). Also it is possible that this difference is due to the fact that by CFT we detected overall antibodies (characteristic for acute and chronic reaction) but by ELISA we detected only IgG antibodies (characteristic mainly for chronic infection) not overall antibodies. Ondriska et al. [49] analyzed 1705 samples of serum from human patients by CFT and IgA, IgM and IgG ELISA. They found a dependence when comparing the CFT titres and concentrations of IgG antibodies ($r=0.549$, $p<0.05$). A higher correlation was found when compared the CFT titres and concentrations of IgA antibodies ($r=0.956$) [49]. The limiting criterion for the evaluation of laboratory results is the assessment of the limiting cut-off value for the substance being assessed in reaction. In view of individual immunoreactivity and reactivity implying from organ localization of infection, the determination of CFT value is problematic and therefore it is more suitable to use the term of "diagnostically significant value". For example, while Feldner [50] considers CFT titer equal to or over 1:10 in the correlation with positive IgM antibodies to be characteristic for acute infection, according to Catár et al. [51] this titre is more frequent in latent infections. Flegr and Havlíček [52] consider the titres as high as 1:128 to be significant. The titres equal to or below 1:64 according to these authors are detected mostly in patients with chronic or latent infection. In our study were found mostly titres characterized for latent infection and only one sample was in titer 1:256 responsible for acute infection.

Gene amplification methods (PCR, LCR, NASBA, etc.) are now used widely in the diagnosis of infectious diseases. Key advantages are their relative speed, the potential to detect very low numbers of pathogens (or, more precisely, specific nucleic acid sequences from pathogens) and the ability to discriminate accurately at the species or sub-species level. In the case of non-persistent pathogens that are cleared from the body, a positive PCR finding is usually significant. The diagnosis of toxoplasmosis by PCR, however, is complicated by the fact that the parasite persists (principally in heart, brain and skeletal muscle in the form of quiescent tissue cysts) for many years after active infection has ceased. Thus, the presence of *T. gondii* in such tissues does not necessarily equate to active toxoplasmosis. Therefore is possible to find discrepancy between the serological results and results of molecular methods [2]. Molecular tests detecting circulating parasites would be helpful in the final diagnosis. Direct methods, such as PCR need biopsy samples [2,53]. Methods of sampling of the brain and other internal organ tissues in animals are not as sophisticated as in humans. This is particularly true of large animals meat-producing animals (e.g. cattle, sheep, goats and pigs), which pose the greatest risk of toxoplasmosis transmission to humans. In our study we decided to use blood as the main sample for isolation and detection of *T. gondii*

DNA. The purpose of this study was to find out the relationship between the phase of infection acute or persist and the ability of quantitative PCR to detect DNA *T. gondii* in circulating leukocytes in the blood stream. Our study has shown that PCR analysis of animal blood can only detect DNA of *T. gondii* in acute phase of infection. At this time in infection parasites are hidden within leukocytes and that are circulating in the blood stream. At this stage, we are able to capture parasites and isolate DNA of *T. gondii*. After initiation of the chronic phase, parasites are hidden within cysts in the tissues and organs of the animals and it is not possible to detect their presence in the blood. DNA of *T. gondii* was confirmed in 10 animals from the total of 256 animals sampled. Of the ten PCR-positive animals DNA was detected in nine individuals with ongoing acute phase of infection (confirmed by ELISA). Hitt and Filice [54] detected *T. gondii* DNA in 12 of 32 (37%) rabbit blood samples by PCR. The decreased PCR sensitivity in blood samples was believed to be influenced by localization of leukocytes. In their study leukocytes in heparinised blood were not localized in leukocyte layer but they were distributed widely, mostly in erythrocyte layer. Therefore, the choice of the genome area which is amplified is important for efficiency of PCR analysis. Hitt and Filice believed that the B1 gene of genome enhanced the sensitivity of PCR techniques from blood samples [54]. Other investigators have been unable to detect *T. gondii* DNA in bone marrow from humans or whole blood from mice with toxoplasmosis. Heme, heparin, and other poorly characterized substances have been reported to decrease sensitivity [55]. Kompalic-Cristo et al. [56] examined 183 buffy coat samples from serologically examined patients, of the IgM seropositive patients 48.6% presented parasiteamia proven by PCR, whereas 3.6% positivity was achieved in individuals with chronic infection [56]. Lamoril et al. [57] examined 19 patients with confirmed cerebral toxoplasmosis and in only three cases samples were PCR positive. In the case of generalized toxoplasmosis, the lymph nodes, liver, spleen could be affected by infection and in this situation there is higher possibility to detect *T.* DNA by PCR [57]. Truppel et al. [58] examined Capybaras, *Hydrochaeris hydrochaeris*, by serological test and also examined lymph node, liver, spleen, heart and blood samples for the detection of *T.* DNA. *T.* DNA has been detected in the same samples of liver and blood [58]. In general PCR techniques are less sensitive in diagnosis of toxoplasmosis. One of the main problems is missing standardization of PCR performance according to laboratory conditions. The other problem is the kind of tested tissue (e.g. blood, liver, spleen, cerebrospinal fluid etc.). Each study has different sensitivity in the PCR with different tissues. Comparison studies, that compare PCR using different tissue samples give us the better view on sensitivity of PCR and help us to choose the best tissue samples with regard to easy and the least invasive for the animals.

10. Conclusion

All mammals and birds that are consumed by humans may serve as intermediate hosts for *T. gondii* and thus may be a potential source of infection for humans. In the life cycle of *T. gondii* are three infectious stages i.e. tachyzoites, bradyzoites contained in tissue cysts and sporozoites contained in sporulated oocysts. All three stages are infectious for both intermediate and definitive hosts which may acquire a *T. gondii* infection horizontally by oral ingestion of infectious oocysts from the environment, horizontally by oral ingestion of tissues cysts contained in raw and undercooked meat or primary offal of intermediate hosts and vertically by transplacental transmission of tachyzoites [1]. From the animal point of view, meat-producing animal represent the source of tissue cysts for humans. Tissue cysts of *T. gondii* have a high affinity for neural and muscular tissues. They are located predominantly in the central nervous system, the eye, as well as skeletal and cardiac muscles. Therefore, tissue cysts of *T. gondii* contained in meat, meat derived products or offal may be importance sources of infections for humans. Although the potential for transmission of the parasite to humans via food has been known for several decades, it is not known which routes are most important from a public health point of view. It is likely that transmission of the parasite to humans is influenced not only by the potential contamination of various food sources, but also by the individual behavior of consumers in different ethnic groups and geographical regions. Most current methods for detection of *T. gondii* in meat-producing animals, in products of animal origin, or in the environment are insufficient because they do not allow quantification of infectious stages. Hence, most studies report only qualitative data from which it is difficult to assess the true risk of infection in individual cases. There is a need for quantitative data so that efficient strategies to reduce food-borne transmission of *T. gondii* to humans can be developed [59]. For public health purposes it is important to note that the organotropism of *T. gondii* and the number of tissue cysts produced in a certain organ vary with the intermediate and host species. Therefore, not all animals used for human consumption are of the same public health significance. In livestock, *T. gondii* tissue cysts are most frequently observed in various tissues of infected pigs, sheep and goats, and less frequently in infected poultry, rabbits, dogs and horses. By contrast, tissue cysts are found only rarely in skeletal muscles of cattle or buffaloes. Usually, the consumption of raw or undercooked pork or mutton is regarded as a major factor in food-borne transmission to humans. However, it is possible to significantly reduce the risk of *T. gondii* infection in livestock using intensive farm management with adequate measures of hygiene, confinement and prevention. These measures include: keeping meat-producing animals indoors throughout their life-time; keeping the sheds free of rodents, birds and insects; feeding meat-producing animals on sterilised food and controlling access to sheds and feed stores, i.e., no pet animals should be allowed inside them. Using such preventive measures, it is economically possible to produce pigs and poultry free of *T. gondii* infection. By contrast, production of free-ranging livestock will inevitably be associated with *T. gondii* infection. Animals such as sheep and goats kept on pastures have an increased risk of infection due to contamination of the environment with sporulated oocysts. Such animals show high levels of seropositivity in many areas of the world, i.e. up to 92% and 75%, respectively [1]. This is of particular importance because tissue cysts have been found in many edible parts of sheep [60,61] and small ruminants are important in both milk and meat production throughout the world. Seropositivity is distinctly lower and more varying in horses, rabbits and poultry. This may reflect epidemiological factors such as different types of confinement, hygiene of stables and different types of feed. By contrast, seropositivity is usually high in dogs, indicating their continuous exposure to a natural environment and the cumulative effect of age. All of these animals may harbour a considerable number of tissue cysts in their organs, including skeletal muscles, and thus have importance in food-borne transmission to humans who consume their meat [1,62].

Tissue cysts of *T. gondii* in venison and other meat of wild animals, including hares, wild boars, deer and other cervids, kangaroos and bears are other potential sources of infection for humans [1,63]. In addition to higher environmental pressure of infection, there is a cumulative effect of age in many wild animals that results in a very high prevalence of infection. Some wild animals, such as Australian native marsupials, have evolved in the absence of *T. gondii* until cats were introduced to their environment only a few hundred years ago. As a consequence, these animals are highly susceptible to the parasite. Although seropositivity of *T. gondii* infection in marsupials is usually lower than in placental mammals, kangaroo meat in particular has been recognised as a potential source of infection for humans, because it is very lean with little fat and, thus, is usually consumed rare or undercooked [64]. It is important to know that seropositivity of meat-producing animals does not necessarily reflect the risk that those animals pose for their consumers. For example, the meat of cattle and buffaloes rarely contains tissue cysts, although in some area more than 90% of these animals are seropositive for *T. gondii*. By contrast, seropositive pigs, sheep and goats can be assumed to harbor large number of tissue cysts in their meat [63,65]. On the basis of the abovementioned facts, it is assumable that the prevalence of the infection with *T. gondii* mainly in livestock is closely related to the method of breeding these animals. In animals which are bred extensively and are grazed in pastures, the risk of infection is higher than in animals bred on farms with no contact with the outside environment. While grazing, the animals are exposed for long periods to the possibility of infection from the environment. Infected green fodder, soil and water are the most frequent sources of infection in these animals. In farm breeding, where zoohygienic conditions are maintained, animal contact with the environment is prevented and the fodder is well-stored, possibilities of infection are lowered to the minimum and thus the seroprevalence is considerably lower. So it is possible to reduce the risk of *T. gondii* infection in meat-producing animals using intensive farm management with adequate measures of hygiene, confinement and preventions, such as keeping the sheds free of rodents, birds, and insects, keeping meat-producing animals indoors throughout their life-time, feeding meat-producing animals on sterilized food, controlling of access to sheds and feed stores (no pet animals).

Author details

Lenka Luptakova, Alexandra Valencakova and Pavol Balent
Department of Biology and Genetics,
University of Veterinary Medicine and Pharmacy, Kosice, The Slovak Republic

Eva Petrovova and David Mazensky
Department of Anatomy, Histology and Physiology,
University of Veterinary Medicine and Pharmacy, Kosice, The Slovak Republic

Acknowledgement

The paper is a result of research work done within the frames of grant projects VEGA of the Ministry of Education of the Slovak Republic No. 1/0271/11

11. References

[1] Tenter AM, Heckeroth AR, Weiss LM (2000) *T. gondii*: from animals to humans. Internat. j. parasitol. 30: 1217-1258.

[2] Montoya JG (2002) Laboratory diagnosis of *T. gondii* infection and toxoplasmosis. J. infect. dis. 185 Suppl 1: 73-82.

[3] Olafson P, Monlux WS (1942) *T.* infections in animals. Cornell vet. 32: 16-190.

[4] Lang C, Gross U, Luder CG (2007) Subversion of innate and adaptive immune responses by *T. gondii*. Parasitol. res. 100: 191-203.

[5] Gross U, Ros T, Appoldt D, Heeseman J (1992) Improved serological diagnosis *of T. gondii* infection by detection of immunoglobulin A (IgA) and IgM antibodies against P30 by using the immunoblot technique. J. clin. microbiol. 30: 1436-1441.

[6] Filisetti D, Candolfi E (2004) Immune response to *T. gondii*. Ann. ist. super sanità 40: 71-80.

[7] Reichmann G, Walker W, Villegas EN, Craig L, Cai G, Alexander J, Hunter, CA (2000) The CD40/CD40 ligand interaction is required for resistance to toxoplasmic encephalitis. Infect. immun. 68: 1312-1318.

[8] Hunter CA, Candolfi E, Subauste C, Van Cleave V, Remington J (1995) Studies on the role of interleukin-12 in acute murine toxoplasmosis. Immunol. 84: 16-20.

[9] Gazzinelli RT, Hakim FT., Hieny S, Shearer GM, Sher A (1991) Synergistic role of CD4+ and CD8+ T-lymphocytes in IFN-gamma production and protective immunity induced by attenuated *T. gondii* vaccine. J. immunol. 146: 286-292.

[10] Yap GS, Sher A (1999) Cell-mediated immunity to *T. gondii*: initiation, regulation and effector function. Immunobiology. 201: 240-247.

[11] Subauste CS (2002) CD154 and type-1 cytokine response: from hyper IgM syndrome to human immunodeficiency virus infection. J. infect. dis. 15 Suppl 1: 83-89.

[12] Abou-Bacar A, Pfaff AW, Georges S, Letscher-Bru V, Filisetti D, Villard O, Antoni E, Klein JP, Candolfi E (2004) Role of NK cells and gamma interferon in transplacental passage of *T. gondii* in a mouse model of primary infection. Infect. immun. 72: 1397-1401.

[13] Pinon JM, Dumon H, Chemla C, Franck J, Petersen E, Lebech M, Zufferey J, Bessieres MH, Marty P, Holliman R, Johnson J, Luyasu V, Lecolier B, Guy E, Joynson DH, Decoster A, Enders G, Pelloux H, Candolfi E (2001) Strategy of diagnosis of congenital toxoplasmosis: evaluation of methods comparing mothers and newborns and standard methods for postnatal detection of immunoglobulin G, M and A antibodies. J. clin. microbiol. 39: 2267-2271.

[14] Davidson MG (2000) Toxoplasmosis. Vet. clin. north. am. small. anim. pract. 30: 1051-1062.

[15] Bastien P (2002) Molecular diagnosis of toxoplasmosis. Trans. r. soc. trop. med. hyg. 96: 205-215.

[16] Cassaing S, Bessières MH, Berry A, Berrebi A, Fabre R, Magnaval JF (2006) Comparison between two amplification sets for molecular diagnosis of toxoplasmosis by real-time PCR. J. clin. microbiol. 44: 720-724.

[17] Zástera M, Pokorný J, Jíra J, Valkoun A (1986) Addition of standard methods of laboratory diagnostics of toxoplasmosis. [in Czech]. Acta hyg. epidem. microbiol. Annex 3/87: 3-14.

[18] Horváth KN, Szénási Z, Danka J, Kucsera I (2005) Value of the IgG avidity in the diagnosis of recent toxoplasmosis: A comparative study of four commercially available anti-*T. gondii* IgG avidity assays. Acta parasitol. 50: 255-260.

[19] Cristina N, Liaud MF, Santoro F, Oury B, Ambroise-Thomas P (1991) A family of repeated DNA sequences in *T. gondii*: cloning, sequence analysis, and use in strain characterization, Exp. Parasitol. 73: 73-81.

[20] Cermáková Z, Rysková O, Plísková L (2005) Polymerase chain reaction for detection of *T. gondii* in human biological samples. Folia microbiol. 50: 341-344.

[21] Prelezov, P., Koinarski, V., Georgieva, D., Seroprevalence of *T. gondii* infection among sheep and goats in the Stara Zagora Region. Bulgarian Journal of Veterinary Medicine, 2008, 11, 113-119.

[22] Fusco G, Rinaldi L, Guarino A, Proroga YTR, Pesce A, Giuseppina DM, Cringoli G (2007) *T. gondii* in sheep from the Campania region (Italy). Vet. parasitol. 149; 1-4.

[23] Masala G, Porcu R, Madau L, Tanda A, Ibba B, Satta G, Tola S (2003) Survey of ovine and caprine toxoplasmosis by IFAT and PCR assays in Sardinia, Italy. Vet. parasitol. 117: 15-21.

[24] Vesco G, Buffolano W, La Chiusa S, Mancuso G, Caracappa S, Chianca A, Villari S, Currò V, Liga F, Petersen E (2007) *T. gondii* infections in sheep in Sicily, southern Italy. Vet. parasitol. 146: 3-8.

[25] Spisak F, Turceková L, Reiterová K, Spilovská S, Dubinsky P (2010) Prevalence estimation and genotypization of *T. gondii* in goats. Biologia 65: 670-674.

[26] Vostalová E, Literák I, Pavlásek I, Sedlák K (2000) Prevalence of *T. gondii* in finishing pigs in large-scale farm in the Czech Republic. Acta vet. Brno 69: 209-212.

[27] Spisak F, Turceková L, Reiterová K, Spilovská S, Kelemenová B, Dubinský P (2009) Epizoolotogical monitoring of toxoplasmosis in livestock in Slovakia [in Slovak]. Slovak veterinary journal 6: 384-386.

[28] Pleva J, Sokol J, Cabadaj R, Saladiová D (1997) Epizootological and epidemiological importance of toxoplasmosis [in Slovak] Slovak veterinary journal 3: 127-129.

[29] Spisak F, Turceková L, Reiterová K, Spilovská S, Dubinsky P (2010) The occurrence of *T. gondii* in cattle. In Proceedings of the International Conference "IX. Slovenské a české parazitologické dni [in Slovak]", May 24.-28, Liptovský Ján, 72-73.

[30] Spilovská S, Reiterová K (2008) Seroprevalence of *Neospora caninum* in aborting sheep and goats in the Eastern Slovakia. Folia Veterinaria 52: 33-35.

[31] Frank RK (2001) An outbreak of toxoplasmosis in farmed mink (*Mustela vison S*). J. vet. invest. 13: 245-249.

[32] Antolová D, Reiterová K, Dubinský P (2007) Seroprevalence of *T. gondii* in wild boars (*Sus Scrofa*) in the Slovak Republic. Ann. agric. environ. med. 14: 71-73.
[33] Bártová E, Sedlák K, Literák I (2006) Prevalence of *T. gondii* and *Neospora caninum* antibodies in wild boars in the Czech Republic. Vet. parasitol. 142: 150-153.
[34] Arnaudov D, Arnaudov A, Kirin D (2003) Study on the toxoplasmosis among wild animals. Exp. pathol. parasitol. 6: 51-54.
[35] Sroka J, Zwoliński J, Dutkiewicz J (2007) Seroprevalence of *T. gondii* in farm and wild animals from the area of Lublin province. Bull. vet. inst. Pulawy 51: 535-540.
[36] Richomme C, Aubert D, Gilot-Fromont E, Ajzenberg D, Mercier A, Ducrot C, Ferté H, Delorme D, Villena I (2009) Genetic characterization of *T. gondii* from wild boar (*Sus scrofa*) in France. Vet. parasitol. 14: 296-300.
[37] Aubert D, Ajzenberg D, Richomme C, Gilot-Fromont E, Terrier ME, De Gevigney C, Game Y, Maillard D, Gibert P, Dardé L, Villena I (2010) Molecular and biological characteristics of *T. gondii* isolates from wildlife in France. Vet. parasitol.171: 346-349.
[38] Martins CS, Viana JA (1988) Toxoplasmose – O que todo professional de saúde deve saber. Revista clín. vet. 15: 33-37.
[39] Lindsay DS, Dubey JP, Butler JM, Blagburn BL (1997) Mechanical transmission of *T. gondii* oocysty by dogs. Vet. parasitol. 73: 27-33.
[40] Valencáková A, Malceková B (2008) Detection of oocysts *T. gondii* in environmental samples. Proceedings of international conference „Actual questions oj animal bioclimatology [in Slovak]", 9th-10th december, Brno, 100-102.
[41] Dubey JP, Stone D, Kwok OC, Sharma RN (2008) *T. gondii* and *Neospora caninum* antibodies in dogs from Grenada, West Indies. J. parasitol. 94: 750-751.
[42] Lopes AP, Cardoso L, Rodrigues M (2008) Serological survey of *T. gondii* infection in domestic cats from northeastern Portugal. Vet. parasitol. 155: 184-189.
[43] Uggla A, Mattson S, Juntti N (1990) Prevalence of antibodies to *T. gondii* in cats, dogs and horses in Sweden. Acta veter. scand. 31: 219-222.
[44] De Craeye S, Francart A, Chabauty J, De Vriendt V, Van Gucht S, Leroux I, Jongert E (2008) Prevalence of *T. gondii* infection in Belgian house cats. Vet. parasitol. 157: 128-132.
[45] Sedlák K, Bártová E (2006) The prevalence of *T. gondii* IgM and IgG antibodies in dogs and cats from the Czech Republic. Vet. Med-Czech 51: 555-558.
[46] Figueroa-Castillo JA, Duarte-Rosas V, Juarez-Acevedo M, Luna-Pasten H, Correa D (2006) Prevalence of *T. gondii* antibodies in rabbits (*Oryctolagus cuniculus*) from Mexico. J. parasitol. 92: 394-395.
[47] Sroka J, Dutkiewicz J, Toś-Luty S, Latuszyńska, J (2003) Toxoplasmosis in rabbits confirmed by strain isolation: a potential risk of infection among agricultural workers. Ann. Agric. Environ. Med. 10: 125-128.
[48] Ishikawa T, Nishino H, Ohara M, Shimosato T, Nanba K, (1990) The identification of a rabbit-transmitted cervical toxoplasmosis mimicking malignant lymphoma. Am. j. clin. pathol. 94: 107-110.
[49] Ondriska F, Catár G, Vozárov G (2003) The significance of complement fixation test in clinical diagnosis of toxoplasmosis. Bratisl. lek. listy 104: 189-96.
[50] Feldner J (1991) Toxoplasmose. Behringwerke AG. 3: 1-39 .

[51] Catár G, Hynie-Holková, R, Zachar M (1967) The comparison of an indirect immunofluorescence and complement fixation test [in Slovak]. Bratisl. lek. listy 47: 219-225.

[52] Flegr J, Havlícek J (1999) Change in the personality profile of young women with latent toxoplasmosis. Fol. parasitol. 46: 22-28.

[53] Shaapan RM, El-Nawawi FA, Tawfik MAA (2008) Sensitivity and specificity of various serological tests for the detection of *T. gondii* infection in naturally infected sheep. Vet. parasitol. 153: 359-362.

[54] Hitt JA, Filice GA (1992) Detection of *T. gondii* parasitemia by gene amplification, cell culture, and mouse inoculation. J. clin. microbiol. 30: 3181-3184.

[55] Van de Ven E, Melchers W, Galama J, Camps W, Meuwissen J (1991) Identification of *T. gondii* infections by B1 gene amplification. J. clin. microbiol. 29: 2120-2124.

[56] Kompalic-Cristo A, Frotta C, Suaárez-Mutis M, Fernandes O, Britto C (2007) Evaluation of real time PCR assay based on the repetitive B1 gene for detection of *T. gondii* in human peripheral blood. Parasitol. res.101: 619-625.

[57] Lamoril J, Molina JM, de Gouvello A, Garin YJ, Deybach JC, Modai J, Derouin F (1996) Detection by PCR of *T. gondii* in blood in the diagnosis of cerebral toxoplasmosis in patients with AIDS. J. clin. pathol. 49: 89-92.

[58] Truppel JH, Reifur L, Montiani-Ferreira F, Lange RR, de Castro Vilani RG, Gennari SM, Thomaz-Soccol V (2010) *T. gondii* in Capybara (Hydrochaeris hydrochaeris) antibodies and DNA detected by IFAT and PCR. Parasitol. res. 107: 141-146.

[59] Tenter AM (2009) *T. gondii* in animals used for human consumption. Mem Inst Oswaldo Cruz. 104: 364-369.

[60] Dubey JP, Kirkbride CA (1989) Economic and public health considerations of congenital toxoplasmosis in lambs. J. Am. vet. med. assoc. 195: 1715-1716.

[61] Lundén A, Uggla A (1992) Infectivity of *T. gondii* in mutton following curing, smoking, freezing or microwave cooking. Int. j. food microbial. 15: 357-363.

[62] Tassi P (2007) *T. gondii* infection in horses. A review. Parassitologia 49: 7-15.

[63] Dubey JP, Jones JL (2008) *T. gondii* infection in humans and animals in the United States. Int. j. parasitol. 38: 1257-1278.

[64] Robson JMB, Wood RN, Sullivan JJ, Nicolaides NJ, Lewis BR (1995) A probable foodborne outbreak of toxoplasmosis. Commun. dis. intell. 19: 517-522.

[65] Dubey JP (2000) The scientific basis for prevention of *T. gondii* infection: studies on tissue cyst survival, risk factors and hygiene measures. In: Ambroise-Thomas P, Petersen E, editors. Congenital toxoplasmosis: scientific background, clinical management and control. Paris: Springer-Verlag. pp. 271–5.

Section 2

Molecular Diagnosis and Epidemiology

Chapter 5

Molecular Detection and Genotyping of *Toxoplasma gondii* from Clinical Samples

Vladimir Ivović, Marija Vujanić, Tijana Živković, Ivana Klun and Olgica Djurković-Djaković

Additional information is available at the end of the chapter

http://dx.doi.org/10.5772/50830

1. Introduction

Over the past two decades, molecular diagnosis of toxoplasmosis, which is based on the detection of *T. gondii* DNA in clinical samples, became an indispensable laboratory test. This method is independent of the immune response, and depending on methodological approach, may facilitate more accurate diagnosis, especially in cases in which inadequacy of conventional methods is faced with deteriorating and potentially severe clinical outcome (congenital, ocular toxoplasmosis and cases of immunosuppression).

Molecular methods based on polymerase chain reaction (PCR) are simple, sensitive, reproducible and can be applied to all clinical samples (Bell and Ranford-Cartwright, 2002; Contini et al., 2005; Calderaro et al., 2006; Bastien et al., 2007). These methods are divided into two groups. The first group consists of techniques focused on detection of *T. gondii* DNA in biological and clinical samples, including conventional PCR, nested PCR and real-time PCR. The second group consists of molecular methods including PCR-RFLP, microsatellite analysis and multilocus sequence typing of a single copy *T. gondii* DNA and those are predominantly used for strain typing (Su et al., 2010).

However, it is important to emphasize that molecular diagnostics, being a constantly improving modern methodology, is not standardized even among the world's leading laboratories. The differences are substantial and numerous, and they extend to all segments of the methodology such as target genes for parasite detection and markers for genotyping, equipment manufacturers and different protocols (various sets of primers and probes and their concentration, different internal controls, etc...).

2. Molecular diagnostics

2.1. Methodology

Conventional PCR was, in the beginning, the molecular detection method of choice for the majority of laboratories dealing with the diagnosis of toxoplasmosis and it was based on both in-house protocols and commercial kits (Lavrard et al., 1995). To increase the sensitivity of molecular diagnostics of toxoplasmosis nested PCR was introduced, although in recent years real-time PCR has shown a significantly higher sensitivity as well as specificity (Jauregui et al., 2001; Reischl et al., 2003; Contini et al., 2005; Calderaro et al., 2006; Edvinsson et al., 2006). Real-time PCR detection also has the capability of quantification of *T. gondii* in biological samples, which has found wide application in monitoring the kinetics and outcome of infection in patients undergoing therapy, as well as in experimental models (Lin et al., 2000; Jauregui et al., 2001; Contini et al., 2005; Djurković-Djaković et al., 2012).

Molecular diagnostics of toxoplasmosis is generally based on the detection of a specific DNA sequence, using different assays and protocols, mostly from highly conserved regions such as the B1 gene repeated 35 times in the genome, 529 bp repetitive element with about 200-300 copies in the genome, ITS-1 (internal transcribed spacer) that exists in 110 copies and 18S rDNA gene sequences (Table 1). Qualitative PCR protocols for the detection of single copy genes such as the P30 gene appeared less sensitive and they are rarely used for diagnostic purposes (Jones et al., 2000).

Markers	No. of copies	References
B1	≈ 35	Wahab et al., 2010 Correia et al., 2010 Okay et al., 2009
529 bp (AF146527)	200-300	da Silva RC et al., 2011 Yera et al., 2009 Vujanić et al., 2011
ITS-1 or 18S rDNA	≈110	Truppel et al., 2010 Miller et al., 2004
P30	Single copy gene	Buchbinder et al., 2003 Eida et al., 2009 Cardona et al., 2009

Table 1. *T. gondii* DNA detection markers (latest and most significant data)

The first protocol for molecular detection of *T. gondii,* for conventional PCR targeting B1 gene, was developed in 1989 and has since been modified and optimized in many laboratories (Burg et al., 1989; Lopez et al., 1994; Liesenfeld et al., 1994; Reischl et al., 2003; Switaj et al., 2005). The B1 gene, although of unknown function, is widely exploited in a number of diagnostic and epidemiological studies because of its specificity and sensitivity. There are also some studies in which the detection of *T. gondii* parasites was based on amplification of ITS-1 and 18S rDNA fragments, whose sensitivity was similar to the B1 gene (Hurtado et al., 2001; Calderaro et al., 2006). However, the repetitive element of 529 bp in length, which was firstly identified by Homan, has showed a 10 to 100 times higher sensitivity compared to the B1 gene (Homan et al., 2000; Reischl et al., 2003). Nevertheless, there are several studies indicating that there are *T. gondii* strains in which either the whole or parts of the 529bp fragment have been deleted or mutated or in which the number of repeats vary. One report suggests that the 529bp repeat element, of unknown function as well, was not present in all isolates analyzed; 4.8% of the samples gave false-negative results compared to results from amplification of the B1 gene (Wahab et al. 2010.). Furthermore, some of the latest studies question its validity for quantification in clinical diagnostics since the number of copies of the 529 bp repetitive sequence in *Toxoplasma* genome appears to be 5 to 12 times lower than the previous estimations (Costa & Bretagne, 2012). Nevertheless, the detection of *T. gondii* DNA using the 529 bp repetitive element, and real-time PCR protocols that detect the presence of this element, is currently the most widely used molecular approach for the detection of *T. gondii* (Reischl et al., 2003; Kasper et al., 2009).

However, it can be of great methodological significance to further clarify the specificity of using a multicopy target of unknown function before the introduction of such protocol into the laboratory diagnostics (Edvinsson at al., 2006)

2.2. Clinical significance in various biological samples

Molecular detection of *T. gondii* in cases of suspected congenital toxoplasmosis may be performed in the amniotic fluid, and fetal and neonatal blood samples. Also, it is performed in the peripheral blood of immunosuppressed patients, and in samples of humor aqueous and cerebrospinal fluid of patients suspected of ocular and cerebral toxoplasmosis, as well as in bronchoalveolar lavage fluid (BAL). Furthermore, in our laboratory, peripheral blood of patients suspected of acute toxoplasmosis was also analyzed (Table 2).

Clinical sample	Real-time PCR	
	No. tested	No. positive (%)
Blood	91	28 (30.8)
Amniotic fluid	28	10 (35.7)
Fetal blood	9	3 (33.3)
BAL	1	1 (100)
Aqueous humor	10	6 (60)
Cerebrospinal fluid	7	4 (57.1)
Total	146	52 (35.6)

Table 2. Real-time PCR results on various clinical samples of patients suspected of active toxoplasmosis examined in the National Reference Laboratory for Toxoplasmosis, Belgrade, Serbia

2.2.1. Peripheral blood

In our laboratory, the presence of *T. gondii* DNA was shown in about one-third (31%) of all analysed cases. Similar research carried out on peripheral blood samples derived from patients with an acute *T. gondii*-related lymphadenopathy, resulted in the detection of parasite DNA in 35% of all samples (Guy & Joynson, 1995). In a study involving patients with acute toxoplasmosis in southeastern Brazil, the rate of parasite DNA-positive peripheral blood samples was 48.6% (17/35) (Kompalic-Cristo et al., 2007). Interestingly, both of these studies used B1 as the target gene, which is considered to be of lower sensitivity than the AF146527 marker that we used; however, the total number of analyzed samples was smaller and the patient selection criteria may have differed. In addition, in the Brazilian study DNA extraction was performed from the buffy coat instead of the whole blood, which may have contributed to the extraction of larger amounts of parasite DNA and higher success in its detection (Menotti et al., 2003; Jalal et al., 2004). Timely (early) sampling is also of particular importance, as detection of *T. gondii* DNA from the peripheral blood of patients with acute toxoplasmic lymphadenopathy has been shown to be very difficult 5.5 to 13 weeks after the onset of infection (Guy & Joynson, 1995). Successful PCR detection of *T. gondii* DNA should indicate recent infection. However, one must take into consideration that PCR detection of parasitic DNA alone does not necessarily mean that parasites are viable. The immune system rapidly kills circulating parasites but the *T. gondii* DNA could be retained for some period of time in the circulation. Also, it has been suggested that even in the chronic phase of infection it is possible, though very rarely, to detect in blood the DNA originating from cysts present in the muscles and nervous system (Guy & Joynson, 1995). On the other hand, negative PCR cannot exclude recent infection because of several reasons such as the small number of parasites circulating in the blood or short period of duration of parasitemia. Here it must be stressed that the exact kinetics of parasites in humans still remains unclear. Other reasons for negative PCR results include the small sample size from which DNA is extracted compared to the total volume of blood in the human body, as well as the fact that the blood contains components that may inhibit the PCR reaction, primarily heme, hemoglobin, lactoferrin and immunoglobulin G.

We have analyzed real-time PCR results from peripheral blood samples originating from patients suspected of acute toxoplasmosis according to the serological criteria for acute infection, i.e. avidity of specific IgG antibodies and the finding of specific IgM antibodies. The results showed that positive real-time PCR correlates better with the finding of specific IgM antibodies, than with low avidity of specific IgG antibodies (Vujanić, 2012).

Comparison of molecular detection and bioassay findings on peripheral blood samples of the patients with specific IgM antibodies and specific IgG antibodies of low avidity, suggesting acute toxoplasmosis, has been done as well. It was shown that in nearly one-third (29%) of the analyzed cases *T. gondii* DNA was detected in comparison to approximately 20% positive bioassays. This result undoubtedly indicates a higher sensitivity of the real-time PCR method in relation to the bioassay. However, molecular detection of parasite DNA in peripheral blood is of the greatest significance in immunosuppressed patients, where it may be the only method for both the diagnosis and monitoring of the therapeutic effect of the administered antiparasitic drugs. The significance of real-time PCR for monitoring the kinetics of the infection has been shown in immunosuppressed patients after bone marrow and liver transplantation (Costa et al., 2000; Botterel et al., 2002 ; Edvinsson et al., 2008; Daval et al., 2010). Using real-time PCR, we too have observed a decline in parasitemia in a patient with reactivated toxoplasmosis during specific treatment (Vujanić 2012).

Although the detection of parasite DNA in peripheral blood of adults may not always be direct evidence of active parasitemia, *T. gondii* DNA detected in fetal and neonatal blood samples is of the utmost clinical importance because there is no possibility of detection of DNA from earlier infections. Therefore, the most important application of molecular methods is in the diagnosis of congenital toxoplasmosis, as the isolation of the parasite in cell culture is insufficiently sensitive (Thulliez et al., 1992; Foulon et al., 1999) and the isolation by bioassay takes approximately 6 weeks.

2.2.2. *Amniotic fluid*

In the last two decades, the detection of *T. gondii* DNA in the amniotic fluid has become particularly important, as it allows for timely diagnosis of fetal infection, and subsequent implementation of appropriate therapy and infection control (Menotti et al., 2010; Wallon et al., 2010). We have so far studied a total of 28 amniotic fluid samples obtained from women suspected of infection in pregnancy. Real-time PCR revealed parasite DNA in 36% of the amniotic fluid samples whereas mouse bioassay was positive in 25%. A similar difference in the positivity rate between PCR (17/85, 20%) and bioassay (14/85, 16.5%) results was obtained in a study in Egypt (Eida et al., 2009).

Given that in many published studies real-time PCR and bioassay results from the amniotic fluid did not match, which is the case in our research as well, and as congenital infection cannot be excluded by negative PCR (Romand et al., 2001; Golab et al., 2002), for prediction of congenital toxoplasmosis it is optimal to combine both molecular detection and bioassay. In one study of prenatal diagnosis of congenital toxoplasmosis in patients from 6 European centers of reference it was shown that PCR from amniotic fluid has a higher sensitivity (81%) in regard to both bioassay (58%) and cell culture (15%) (Foulon et al., 1999). The combination of PCR and bioassay increases the sensitivity to 91%, and represents the best diagnostic approach (Foulon et al., 1999).

In European countries such as France and Austria regular serological monitoring of pregnant women for *T. gondii* is regulated by law, which allows for precise timing of seroconversion and timely prenatal diagnosis of fetal infection. This has also allowed for a vast experience with the diagnosis of congenital toxoplasmosis, and provided data on the superior sensitivity of molecular methods compared to conventional parasitological tests. Thus, one long-term study conducted in France showed that out of 2632 women in whom the infection occurred during pregnancy, congenital toxoplasmosis was confirmed by positive PCR in the amniotic fluid and/or fetal blood in 34 cases in which congenital infection was diagnosed by conventional methods, as well as in three fetuses in whom the infection was not diagnosed by other methods (Hohlfeld et al., 1994). Also, in a similar study in Austria, outcome of prenatally diagnosed children was followed-up during the first year of life to assess the validity of PCR results from the amniotic fluid. Of the 49 amniotic fluid samples analyzed, congenital infection was confirmed postnatally by serological monitoring in all 11 (22.4%) PCR-positive ones, whereas none of the 38 children in whom PCR of the amniotic fluid was negative was shown to be infected (Gratzl et al., 1998).

2.2.3. *Cord blood*

Cord blood is not considered the ideal sample for prenatal diagnosis of congenital toxoplasmosis. For example, the results of a survey carried out in France did not show any positive PCR result among 19 tested cord blood samples from children with proven congenital toxoplasmosis (Filisetti et al., 2003). Nevertheless, cord blood samples that are occasionally provided to our laboratory, have shown a rate of positivity in real-time PCR of 33%. All cord blood samples in our study were inoculated into mice and the rate of positivity of bioassay was 55.5%. A higher rate of isolation of viable parasites by bioassay compared to the detection of parasitic DNA by real-time PCR may be explained by a larger sample volume used for mouse inoculation in comparison to the amount used for DNA extraction, as well as by probable presence of PCR inhibitors. In one study performed on a representative sample of pregnant women in China a similar rate of real-time PCR positive results was obtained from the amniotic fluid and fetal blood samples (Ma et al., 2003).

It can be concluded that the diagnosis of congenital toxoplasmosis from fetal blood samples should be based on the results of both bioassay and molecular detection.

2.2.4. *Aqueous humor*

Prior to the introduction of molecular methods, the laboratory diagnosis of ocular toxoplasmosis has been based primarily on a comparison of the level of antibodies detected in the humor aqueous and serum in order to detect intraocular synthesis of specific antibodies (Witmer-Goldman's coefficient). Lately, molecular methods are becoming a standard diagnostic approach in the diagnosis of ocular toxoplasmosis as well. A number of studies has already shown that a positive PCR result is not always accompanied by positive serology indicating local synthesis of IgG antibodies (Villard et al., 2003; Talabani et al., 2009) and thus can be the only confirmation of the diagnosis (Okhravi et al., 2005).

We have so far studied 10 humor aqueous samples from patients clinically suspected of ocular toxoplasmosis of which 60% (6/10) were real-Time PCR positive. A similar result was obtained in a French study when 55% (22/40) of humor aqueous samples were positive by real-Time PCR using AF146527 as a marker (Talabani et al., 2009). Also, the detection of the same AF146527 marker by real-Time PCR in another French study, revealed somewhat lower rate of positive samples, 38.2% (13/34) (Fekkar et al., 2008). It is interesting that in the latter study the sample volume of 10 μL used for DNA extraction was unusually small, which certainly could affect the success of PCR reactions. However, in another study performed in Strasbourg, the amplification of 18S rRNA and B1 gene by conventional PCR resulted in the 28% (5/18) of the humor aqueous samples positive for the presence of *T. gondii* DNA (Villard et al., 2003).

2.2.5. Cerebrospinal fluid

Cerebral toxoplasmosis usually affects immunosuppressed patients and is mostly the result of reactivation of chronic infection which may be fatal if left untreated. Definitive diagnosis of toxoplasmosis can be made by the detection of tachyzoites in brain tissue samples obtained by biopsy, but this method, because of its invasiveness, is seldom applied, and certainly not since the PCR, giving consistent and quick result, has been introduced in the diagnostics (Vidal et al., 2004). A study of cerebral toxoplasmosis in HIV-infected patients infected in Brazil, showed that 27.4% (14/51) of cerebrospinal fluid samples were positive for *T. gondii* DNA (Mesquita et al., 2010). Noteworthy, DNA extraction was performed using phenol-chloroform method, in which the phenolic residues can often inhibit the PCR reaction. In our limited experience, of the 7 cerebrospinal fluid samples obtained from patients with different neurological conditions (including one case of congenital hydrocephalus) examined by real-time PCR, 4 (57%) were positive.

2.3. Comment

In summary, all above-mentioned results confirm the value of the use of molecular methods, due to their high sensitivity and specificity, in the diagnosis of toxoplasmosis. Coupled with conventional parasitological diagnostic methods, PCR-based methods allow for the timely diagnosis especially of congenital toxoplasmosis and of reactivated toxoplasmosis in immunosuppressed patients. Further advances of the technology itself along with its wide, (universal) use may be expected to markedly improve diagnostics and monitoring of the course of infection as well as of the therapeutic effect.

3. Genotyping

In the early days of strain designation, isolates of *T. gondii* have been grouped according to virulence in outbred mice. First phylogenetic studies of *T. gondii* strains indicated that their genetic complexity was much smaller than expected (Darde et al., 1992; Sibley & Boothroyd, 1992). Howe and Sibley's *T. gondii* population structure study (1995) performed on 106 isolates collected from both humans and animals from North America and Europe, showed the presence of three clonal types (type I, II and III) and very small differences between clonal lineages which is why it was concluded that *T. gondii* has a clonal population structure. Comparative sequence analysis of individual genes indicated extremely low allelic diversity within the clonal lines, and only 1% divergence at the DNA level. In addition, limited genetic diversity between and within clonal lines indicated that they have quite recently evolved from a common ancestor, 10,000 years ago at the most (Su et al., 2003).

Nevertheless, most recent phylogenetic studies indicate that the population structure of *T. gondii* is much more complex than initially considered. While it has been undeniably established that type II is predominant in Europe and North America (Darde et al., 1992; Howe & Sibley, 1995; Howe et al., 1997), there are significant regional differences. Thus, research in Portugal and Spain showed the presence of types I and III in this area (Fuentes et al., 2001; de Sousa et al., 2006), while genotyping of isolates from Crete and Cyprus showed the predominance of type III (Messaritakis et al., 2008); however it must be noted that these studies have been conducted using only one marker (SAG2 or GRA6). Also, phylogenetic analyses of *T. gondii* isolates, which have only recently begun in South America, Asia and Africa, have shown considerable genetic diversity of this parasite strains.

A realistic picture of the distribution of genotypes in Europe is also difficult to obtain because research on *T. gondii* is not performed to the same extent and using the same methods in all geographical areas. So far, the largest number of isolates has been genotyped in France, mainly thanks to the mandatory program of testing of pregnant women for toxoplasmosis in this country, which allows for the availability of research material. One French study has shown that of the 86 isolates from cases of suspected and confirmed congenital toxoplasmosis 85% were of type II (Ajzenberg et al., 2002). A predominance of the same type was indicated in Poland, where genotyping was also performed in samples originating from clinical cases of congenital toxoplasmosis (Nowakowska et al., 2006). In South-East Europe the first strain genotyped was isolated from a case of congenital toxoplasmosis in Serbia, and was also designated as type II (Djurković-Djaković et al., 2006).

Further work on the genotyping of *T. gondii* strains in Serbia showed another two type II isolates, originating from a case of congenital toxoplasmosis and a case of toxoplasmosis in pregnancy, respectively. However, another isolate from a peripheral blood sample of a neonate with suspected congenital toxoplasmosis had been typed to the clonal type I. Isolation of this genotype from cases of congenital toxoplasmosis has been described, but at a significantly lower rate than type II (Howe & Sibley, 1995), as results of research conducted in France have shown, where out of 86 genotyped isolates only 4 belonged to type I (Ajzenberg et al., 2002).

Sample number	Sample type	Clinical entity	Genotype
1	blood	toxoplasmosis in pregnancy	II
2	amniotic fluid	congenital toxoplasmosis	II
3	blood	congenital toxoplasmosis	I
4*	blood	bone marrow transplantation	II
5*	bronchoalveolar lavage fluid	bone marrow transplantation	II

*samples 4 and 5 are from the same patient

Table 3. Genotypes of human *T. gondii* isolates from clinical samples in Serbia

We have also genotyped isolates from both a blood and BAL sample from an immunosuppressed patient after bone marrow transplantation, which were found to belong to type II. In another study, genotyping of strains isolated from immunosuppressed patients, HIV infected or patients who had undergone organ transplantation, has shown predominance of type II in patients who were infected in Europe (Ajzenberg et al., 2009). On the other hand, isolates that do not belong to this type usually come from people who are infected with *T. gondii* out of Europe. In this group of patients type III was the second in abundance whereas type I was rare (Ajzenberg et al., 2009). In other studies carried out in immunosuppressed patients (patients with AIDS, lymphoma or patients with transplants), which mainly came from France, it was shown that type II isolates were also predominant, while types I and III were isolated rarely (Howe et al., 1997; Honore et al., 2000).

Furthermore, results of a study performed in the USA, based on genotyping of strains isolated from cerebrospinal fluid originating from eight HIV-positive patients showed that most of them were infected with type I strain or strains that have type I alleles (Khan et al., 2005). Although the possible association between clinical entities induced by *T. gondii* with specific *T. gondii* genotypes is yet unclear, it is likely that the resistance or susceptibility to a particular type, especially in immunosuppressed patients, is primarily dependent on individual factors (Ajzenberg et al., 2009). The greatest limitation in genotyping of isolates from clinical samples is the small number of parasites in original material; hence the amount of extracted *T. gondii* DNA is often also small. This problem can be partially eliminated by enriching the sample by bioassay or cell culture, but even the most sensitive molecular methods, such as a multiplex nested PCR, have a threshold of 50 and 25 parasites/mL, respectively (Khan et al., 2005; Nowakowska et al., 2006). The PCR-RFLP protocol by which genotyping was performed in our study has a sensitivity of approximately 170 parasites/mL, which is probably the major reason for the small number of successful genotypizations.

Numerous studies of the *T. gondii* population structure were based on genotyping using a single marker, mostly SAG2 (Howe et al., 1997; Fuentes et al., 2001; Sabaj et al., 2010) and particularly, due to its polymorphisms and sensitivity, GRA6 (Fazaeli et al., 2000; Messaritakis et al., 2008). However, genotyping with a single marker does not allow identification of nonclonal strains, and to determine more precisely the presence of polymorphisms in the population, application of multilocus PCR-RFLP and microsatellite analysis of multiple markers is necessary (Ajzenberg et al., 2005; Su et al., 2006). Although in our experience the GRA6 gene was, due to a small amount of *T. gondii* DNA, the only amplified marker in a blood sample of a neonate suspected of congenital toxoplasmosis (Table 3), that clearly indicated the presence of type I, in our laboratory genotyping is regularly performed using SAG1, SAG2, GRA6 and GRA7 as markers (Miller et al., 2004; Dubey et al., 2007; Prestrud et al., 2008; Richomme et al., 2009; Aubert et al., 2010).

But even the use of multiple markers does not always provide satisfactory results, mainly due to insufficient amounts of extracted parasite DNA. Therefore, there are cases when amplification of all markers in each sample is not successful, as it can be observed in studies performed in the United States and Poland, where PCR-RFLP analysis was carried out also using four genetic markers SAG2, SAG3, BTUB and GRA6 (Khan et al., 2005; Nowakowska et al., 2006). Using these genetic markers, it was possible to discriminate types I, II and III, but also strains that have a genotype with two allele types at the same locus. Such was the case with one sample in our study which, after the digestion of the product of the amplified GRA7 gene, turned out to possess alleles of both types I and II (Fig. 1, *Mbo* II and *Eco* RI).

Although PCR-RFLP has a limited ability to distinguish between closely related isolates within a clonal line as compared to microsatellite analysis, analysis of up to 9 or 10 genetic markers by this method has been successfully performed in world-class laboratories (Su et al., 2006; Dubey & Su, 2009). On the other hand, the microsatellite analysis is presumed to be more informative to distinguish recent mutations in closely related isolates of the same line, while the RFLP markers are better for detection of time period when the separation of distinct strains in different clonal group has occurred (Su et al., 2006). Multilocus PCR-RFLP genotyping is still the first method of choice in clinical research, mainly for its simplicity and favorable reagent prices, but the best approach for successful genotyping is the use of both methods.

Marker	SAG 1	SAG 2		GRA 6	GRA 7		
Restriction enzyme	*Dde I*	*Mbo I*	*Hha I*	*Tru I*	*Mbo II*	*Eco RI*	*Bse GI*

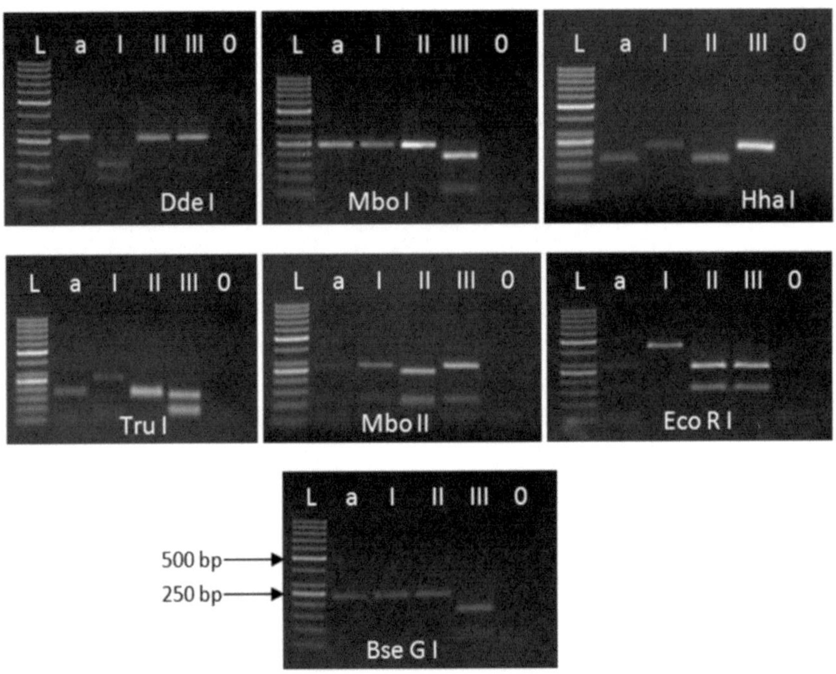

Figure 1. Genotyping pattern summary (markers and restriction enzymes used in genotyping protocol) – illustrative example

Along with the phylogenetic study of *T. gondii*, there is ongoing research aimed at explaining the possible link between the different genotypes and clinical forms of the disease. In spite of the results indicating lack of connection, or a much more complex one than some studies show, there are reported findings on population structure of *T. gondii* that are likely to have important clinical implications. Although it is generally accepted that type II is predominant in cases of congenital toxoplasmosis, at least in Europe and North America (Howe & Sibley, 1995; Howe et al., 1997; Ajzenberg et al., 2002; Darde et al., 2007), type I strains may also be associated with some severe forms of the disease (Howe et al., 1997; Fuentes et al., 2001). Furthermore, strains of atypical genotypes were isolated from immunocompetent patients with severe acquired toxoplasmosis in French Guiana (Carme et al., 2002; Demar et al., 2011), whereas type I and some recombinant strains were isolated from immunocompetent individuals suffering from severe or atypical ocular toxoplasmosis in United States (Grigg et al., 2001).

Even the generally accepted concept of major clinical importance that immunized mothers are resistant to reinfection thereby preventing infection of the offspring, have been recently challenged by insight into the strain variation at the genotype level. Six cases of reinfection among chronically infected pregnant women resulting in a vertical transmission and congenital infection either with a distinct typical or atypical strain have already been reported (Lindsay & Dubey, 2011).

Despite this significant new knowledge, the clinical relevance of the infecting genotypes is an issue that will continue to intrigue researchers in the coming years. Insight into the global population structure of *T. gondii* and its clinical implications, complicated by the growing rate of human migrations among continents, will require wide research efforts based on more standardized protocols, and should include not only clinically manifest cases, but also individuals with asymptomatic infection.

4. Conclusion

The introduction of highly sensitive molecular methods into the diagnosis of toxoplasmosis is of great importance and this paper emphasizes its practical importance and potential as a part of the standard laboratory protocols. Nevertheless, it can be concluded that, at the moment, the best diagnostic approach is a combination of both conventional and molecular methods.

We also present the very first and original phylogenetic data on the *T. gondii* population structure in Serbia. It is shown that in this area, as much as in the rest of the Europe, a clonal population structure is characterized by the predominance of genotype II and much less of genotype I. However, given the fact that the whole region of the Balkan Peninsula is an area of contact with Asia and Africa, where the *T. gondii* population structure is rather different, one may expect a larger diversity, including the presence of clonal type III or even atypical strains, particularly in wild animals.

Author details

Vladimir Ivović*, Marija Vujanić, Tijana Živković,
Ivana Klun and Olgica Djurković-Djaković
Serbian Centre for Parasitic Zoonoses , Centre of Excellence in Biomedicine, Institute for Medical Research, University of Belgrade, Serbia

Acknowledgement

The work was supported by a grant (project No. III41019) from the Ministry of Education and Science of Serbia.

5. References

Ajzenberg D, Cogne N, Paris L, Bessieres MH, Thulliez P, Filisetti D, Pelloux H, Marty P, Darde ML (2002): Genotype of 86 *Toxoplasma gondii* isolates associated with human congenital toxoplasmosis, and correlation with clinical findings. J Infect Dis 186, 5: 684-689.

Ajzenberg D, Dumetre A, Darde ML (2005): Multiplex PCR for typing strains of Toxoplasma gondii. J Clin Microbiol 43, 4: 1940-1943.

Ajzenberg D, Yera H, Marty P, Paris L, Dalle F, Menotti J, Aubert D, Franck J, Bessieres MH, Quinio D, Pelloux H, Delhaes L, Desbois N, Thulliez P, Robert-Gangneux F, Kauffmann-Lacroix C, Pujol S, Rabodonirina M, Bougnoux ME, Cuisenier B, Duhamel C, Duong TH, Filisetti D, Flori P, Gay-Andrieu F, Pratlong F, Nevez G, Totet A, Carme B, Bonnabau H, Darde ML, Villena I (2009): Genotype of 88 *Toxoplasma gondii* isolates associated with toxoplasmosis in immunocompromised patients and correlation with clinical findings. J Infect Dis 199, 8: 1155-1167.

Aubert D, Ajzenberg D, Richomme C, Gilot-Fromont E, Terrier ME, de Gevigney C, Game Y, Maillard D, Gibert P, Darde ML, Villena I (2010): Molecular and biological characteristics of *Toxoplasma gondii* isolates from wildlife in France. Vet Parasitol 171, 3-4: 346-349.

Bastien P, Jumas-Bilak E, Varlet-Marie E, Marty P (2007): Three years of multi-laboratory external quality control for the molecular detection of *Toxoplasma gondii* in amniotic fluid in France. Clin Microbiol Infect 13, 4: 430-433.

Bell A, Ranford-Cartwright L (2002): Real-time quantitative PCR in parasitology. Trends Parasitol 18, 8: 338.

Botterel F, Ichai P, Feray C, Bouree P, Saliba F, Tur Raspa R, Samuel D, Romand S (2002): Disseminated toxoplasmosis, resulting from infection of allograft, after orthotopic liver transplantation: usefulness of quantitative PCR. J Clin Microbiol 40, 5:1648-1650.

Buchbinder S, Blatz R, Rodloff AC (2003): Comparison of real-time PCR detection methods for B1 and P30 genes of *Toxoplasma gondii*. Diagn Microbiol Infect Dis 45, 4: 269-271.

* Corresponding Author

Burg JL, Grover CM, Pouletty P, Boothroyd JC (1989): Direct and sensitive detection of a pathogenic protozoan, *Toxoplasma gondii*, by polymerase chain reaction. J Clin Microbiol 27, 8: 1787-1792.

Caldearo A, Piccolo G, Gorrini C, Peruzzi S, Zerbini L, Bommezzadri S, Dettori G, Chezzi C (2006): Comparison between two real-time PCR assays and a nested-PCR for the detection of *Toxoplasma* gondii. Acta Biomed 77, 2: 75-80.

Cardona N, de-la-Torre A, Siachoque H, Patarroyo MA, Gomez-Marin JE (2009): *Toxoplasma gondii*: P30 peptides recognition pattern in human toxoplasmosis. Exp Parasitol 123, 2: 199-202.

Carme B, Bissuel F, Ajzenberg D, Bouyne R, Aznar C, Demar M, Bichat S, Louvel D, Bourbigot AM, Peneau C, Neron P, Darde ML (2002): Severe acquired toxoplasmosis in immunocompetent adult patients in French Guiana. J Clin Microbiol 40, 11: 4037-4044.

Contini C, Seraceni S, Cultrera R, Incorvaia C, Sebastiani A, Picot S (2005): Evaluation of a Real-time PCR-based assay using the lightcycler system for detection of *Toxoplasma gondii* bradyzoite genes in blood specimens from patients with toxoplasmic retinochoroiditis. Int J Parasitol 35, 3: 275-283.

Correia CC, Melo HR, Costa VM (2010): Influence of neurotoxoplasmosis characteristics on real-time PCR sensitivity among AIDS patients in Brazil. Trans R Soc Trop Med Hyg 104, 1: 24-28.

Costa JM, Bretagne S (2012): Variation of B1 gene and AF146527 repeat element copy numbers according to *Toxoplasma gondii* strains assessed using real-time quantitative PCR. J Clin Microbiol 50, 4: 1452-1454.

Costa JM, Pautas C, Ernault P, Foulet F, Cordonnier C, Bretagne S (2000): Real-time PCR for diagnosis and follow-up of Toxoplasma reactivation after allogeneic stem cell transplantation using fluorescence resonance energy transfer hybridization probes. J Clin Microbiol 38, 8: 2929-2932.

Darde ML, Bouteille B, Pestre-Alexandre M (1992): Isoenzyme analysis of 35 *Toxoplasma gondii* isolates and the biological and epidemiological implications. J Parasitol 78, 5: 786-794.

Darde M, Ajzenberg D, Smith J (2007): Population Structure and Epidemiology of *Toxoplasma gondii*. In: Weiss, L.M., Kim, K. (Eds.) *Toxoplasma gondii* The Model Apicomplexan: Perspectives and Methods. Elsevier, pp. 49-76.

Daval S, Poirier P, Armenaud J, Cambon M, Livrelli V (2010): [Development of a real-time PCR assay for quantitative diagnosis of Toxoplasma gondii after allogeneic bone marrow transplantation]. Pathol Biol (Paris) 58, 1: 104-109.

Demar M, Hommel D, Djossou F, Peneau C, Boukhari R, Louvel D, Bourbigot AM, Nasser V, Ajzenberg D, Darde ML, Carme B (2011): Acute toxoplasmoses in immunocompetent patients hospitalized in an intensive care unit in French Guiana. Clin Microbiol Infect doi: 10.1111/j.1469-0691.2011.03648.x.

Djurković-Djaković O, Djokić V, Vujanić M, Zivković T, Bobić B, Nikolić A, Slavić K, Klun I, Ivović V (2012): Kinetics of parasite burdens in blood and tissues during murine toxoplasmosis. Exp Parasitol 131, 3: 372-6.

Djurkovic-Djakovic O, Klun I, Khan A, Nikolic A, Knezevic-Usaj S, Bobic B, Sibley LD (2006): A human origin type II strain of *Toxoplasma gondii* causing severe encephalitis in mice. Microbes Infect 8, 8: 2206-2212.

Dubey JP, Su C (2009): Population biology of *Toxoplasma gondii*: what's out and where did they come from. Mem Inst Oswaldo Cruz 104, 2: 190-195.

Dubey JP, Sundar N, Gennari SM, Minervino AH, Farias NA, Ruas JL, dos Santos TR, Cavalcante GT, Kwok OC, Su C (2007): Biologic and genetic comparison of *Toxoplasma gondii* isolates in free-range chickens from the northern Para state and the southern state Rio Grande do Sul, Brazil revealed highly diverse and distinct parasite populations. Vet Parasitol 143, 2: 182-188.

Edvinsson B, Lappalainen M, Evengard B (2006): Real-time PCR targeting a 529-bp repeat element for diagnosis of toxoplasmosis. Clin Microbiol Infect 12, 2: 131-136.

Edvinsson B, Lundquist J, Ljungman P, Ringden O, Evengard B (2008): A prospective study of diagnosis of *Toxoplasma gondii* infection after bone marrow transplantation. APMIS 116, 5: 345-351

Eida OM, Eida MM, Ahmed AB (2009): Evaluation of polymerase chain reaction on amniotic fluid for diagnosis of congenital toxoplasmosis. J Egypt Soc Parasitol 39, 2: 541-550.

Fazaeli A, Carter PE, Darde ML, Pennington TH (2000): Molecular typing of *Toxoplasma gondii* strains by GRA6 gene sequence analysis. Int J Parasitol 30, 5: 637-642.

Fekkar A, Bodaghi B, Touafek F, Le Hoang P, Mazier D, Paris L (2008): Comparison of immunoblotting, calculation of the Goldmann-Witmer coefficient, and real-time PCR using aqueous humor samples for diagnosis of ocular toxoplasmosis. J Clin Microbiol 46, 6: 1965-1967.

Filisetti D, Gorcii M, Pernot-Marino E, Villard O, Candolfi E (2003): Diagnosis of congenital toxoplasmosis: comparison of targets for detection of *Toxoplasma gondii* by PCR. J Clin Microbiol 41, 10: 4826-4828.

Foulon W, Pinon JM, Stray-Pedersen B, Pollak A, Lappalainen M, Decoster A, Villena I, Jenum PA, Hayde M, Naessens A (1999) Prenatal diagnosis of congenital toxoplasmosis: a multicenter evaluation of different diagnostic parameters. Am J Obstet Gynecol 181, 4: 843-847.

Fuentes I, Rubio JM, Ramirez C, Alvar J (2001) Genotypic characterization of *Toxoplasma gondii* strains associated with human toxoplasmosis in Spain: direct analysis from clinical samples. J Clin Microbiol 39, 4: 1566-1570.

Guy E, Joyson D (1995): Potential of the Polymerase Chain Reaction in the Diagnosis of Active *Toxoplasma* Infection by Detection of Parasite in Blood. J Infect Dis 172, 1: 319-322.

Golab E, Nowakowska D, Waloch M, Dzbenski TH, Szaflik K, Wilczynski J (2002): [Detection of congenital toxoplasmosis in utero with a polymerase chain reaction on amniotic fluid]. Wiad Parazytol 48, 3: 311-315.

Gratzl R, Hayde M, Kohlhauser C, Hermon M, Burda G, Strobl W, Pollak A (1998): Follow-up of infants with congenital toxoplasmosis detected by polymerase chain reaction analysis of amniotic fluid. Eur J Clin Microbiol Infect Dis 17, 12: 853-858.

Grigg ME, Ganatra J, Boothroyd JC, Margolis TP (2001): Unusual abundance of atypical strains associated with human ocular toxoplasmosis. J Infect Dis 184, 5: 633-639.

Hohlfeld P, Daffos F, Costa JM, Thulliez P, Forestier F, Vidaud M (1994): Prenatal diagnosis of congenital toxoplasmosis with a polymerase-chain-reaction test on amniotic fluid. N Engl J Med 331, 11: 695-699.

Homan WL, Vercammen M, De Braekeleer J, Verschueren H (2000): Identification of a 200- to 300-fold repetitive 529 bp DNA fragment in *Toxoplasma gondii*, and its use for diagnostic and quantitative PCR. Int J Parasitol 30, 1: 69-75.

Honore S, Couvelard A, Garin YJ, Bedel C, Henin D, Darde ML, Derouin F (2000): [Genotyping of *Toxoplasma gondii* strains from immunocompromised patients]. Pathol Biol (Paris) 48, 6: 541-547.

Howe DK, Sibley LD (1995): *Toxoplasma gondii* comprises three clonal lineages: correlation of parasite genotype with human disease. J Infect Dis 172, 6: 1561-1566.

Howe DK, Honore S, Derouin F, Sibley LD (1997): Determination of genotypes of *Toxoplasma gondii* strains isolated from patients with toxoplasmosis. J Clin Microbiol 35, 6: 1411-1414.

Hurtado A, Aduriz G, Moreno B, Barandika J, Garcia-Perez AL (2001): Single tube nested PCR for the detection of *Toxoplasma gondii* in fetal tissues from naturally aborted ewes. Vet Parasitol 102, 1-2: 17-27.

Jalal S, Nord CE, Lappalainen M, Evengard B (2004) Rapid and sensitive diagnosis of *Toxoplasma gondi*i infections by PCR. Clin Microbiol Infect 10, 10: 937-939.

Jauregui LH, Higgins J, Zarlenga D, Dubey JP, Lunney JK (2001): Development of a real-time PCR assay for detection of *Toxoplasma gondii* in pig and mouse tissues. J Clin Microbiol 39, 6: 2065-2071.

Jones CD, Okhravi N, Adamson P, Tasker S, Lightman S (2000): Comparison of PCR detection methods for B1, P30, and 18S rDNA genes of *T. gondii* in aqueous humor. *Invest Ophthalmol Vis Sci* 41, 3: 634-644.

Kasper DC, Sadeghi K, Prusa AR, Reischer GH, Kratochwill K, Forster-Waldl E, Gerstl N, Hayde M, Pollak A, Herkner KR (2009): Quantitative real-time polymerase chain reaction for the accurate detection of *Toxoplasma gondii* in amniotic fluid. Diagn Microbiol Infect Dis 63, 1: 10-15.

Khan A, Su C, German M, Storch GA, Clifford DB, Sibley LD (2005): Genotyping of *Toxoplasma gondii* strains from immunocompromised patients reveals high prevalence of type I strains. J Clin Microbiol 43, 12: 5881-5887.

Kompalic-Cristo A, Frotta C, Suarez-Mutis M, Fernandes O, Britto C (2007): Evaluation of a real-time PCR assay based on the repetitive B1 gene for the detection of *Toxoplasma gondii* in human peripheral blood. Parasitol Res 101, 3: 619-625.

Lavrard I, Chouaid C, Roux P, Poirot JL, Marteau M, Lemarchand B, Meyohas MC, Olivier JL (1995): Pulmonary toxoplasmosis in HIV-infected patients: usefulness of polymerase chain reaction and cell culture. Eur Respir J 8, 5: 697-700.

Liesenfeld O, Roth A, Weinke T, Foss HD, Hahn H (1994): A case of disseminated toxoplasmosis-value of PCR for the diagnosis. J Infect 29, 2: 133-138.

Lin MH, Chen TC, Kuo TT, Tseng CC, Tseng CP (2000): Real-time PCR for quantitative detection of *Toxoplasma gondii*. J Clin Microbiol 38, 11: 4121-4125.

Lindsay DS, Dubey JP (2011): *Toxoplasma gondii*: the changing paradigm of congenital toxoplasmosis. Parasitology 138, 14: 1829-1831.

Ma YY, Mu RL, Wang LY, Jiang S (2003): [Study on prenatal diagnosis using fluorescence quantitative polymerase chain reaction for congenital toxoplasmosis]. Zhonghua Fu Chan Ke Za Zhi 38, 1: 8-10.

Menotti J, Garin YJ, Thulliez P, Serugue MC, Stanislawiak J, Ribaud P, de Castro N, Houze S, Derouin F (2010): Evaluation of a new 5'-nuclease real-time PCR assay targeting the *Toxoplasma gondii* AF146527 genomic repeat. Clin Microbiol Infect 16, 4: 363-368.

Menotti J, Vilela G, Romand S, Garin YJ, Ades L, Gluckman E, Derouin F, Ribaud P (2003): Comparison of PCR-enzyme-linked immunosorbent assay and real-time PCR assay for diagnosis of an unusual case of cerebral toxoplasmosis in a stem cell transplant recipient. J Clin Microbiol 41, 11: 5313-5316.

Mesquita RT, Ziegler AP, Hiramoto RM, Vidal JE, Pereira-Chioccola VL (2010): Real-time quantitative PCR in cerebral toxoplasmosis diagnosis of Brazilian human immunodeficiency virus-infected patients. J Med Microbiol 59, 6: 641-647.

Messaritakis I, Detsika M, Koliou M, Sifakis S, Antoniou M (2008): Prevalent genotypes of *Toxoplasma gondii* in pregnant women and patients from Crete and Cyprus. Am J Trop Med Hyg 79, 2: 205-209.

Miller MA, Grigg ME, Kreuder C, James ER, Melli AC, Crosbie PR, Jessup DA, Boothroyd JC, Brownstein D, Conrad PA (2004): An unusual genotype of *Toxoplasma gondii* is common in California sea otters (Enhydra lutris nereis) and is a cause of mortality. Int J Parasitol 34, 3: 275-284.

Nowakowska D, Colon I, Remington JS, Grigg M, Golab E, Wilczynski J, Sibley LD (2006): Genotyping of *Toxoplasma gondii* by multiplex PCR and peptide-based serological testing of samples from infants in Poland diagnosed with congenital toxoplasmosis. J Clin Microbiol 44, 4: 1382-1389.

Okay TS, Yamamoto L, Oliveira LC, Manuli ER, Andrade Junior HF, Del Negro GM (2009): Significant performance variation among PCR systems in diagnosing congenital toxoplasmosis in São Paulo, Brazil: analysis of 467 amniotic fluid samples. Clinics (Sao Paulo) 64, 3: 171-6.

Okhravi N, Jones CD, Carroll N, Adamson P, Luthert P, Lightman S (2005): Use of PCR to diagnose *Toxoplasma gondii* chorioretinitis in eyes with severe vitritis. Clin Experiment Ophthalmol 33, 2: 184-187.

Prestrud KW, Asbakk K, Mork T, Fuglei E, Tryland M, Su C (2008): Direct high-resolution genotyping of *Toxoplasma gondii* in arctic foxes (*Vulpes lagopus*) in the remote arctic Svalbard archipelago reveals widespread clonal Type II lineage. Vet Parasitol 158, 1-2: 121-128.

Reischl U, Bretagne S, Kruger D, Ernault P, Costa JM (2003): Comparison of two DNA targets for the diagnosis of Toxoplasmosis by real-time PCR using fluorescence resonance energy transfer hybridization probes. BMC Infect Dis 3, 7.

Richomme C, Aubert D, Gilot-Fromont E, Ajzenberg D, Mercier A, Ducrot C, Ferte H, Delorme D, Villena I (2009): Genetic characterization of *Toxoplasma gondii* from wild boar (*Sus scrofa*) in France. Vet Parasitol 164, 2-4: 296-300.

Romand S, Wallon M, Franck J, Thulliez P, Peyron F, Dumon H (2001): Prenatal diagnosis using polymerase chain reaction on amniotic fluid for congenital toxoplasmosis. Obstet Gynecol 97, 2: 296-300.

Sabaj V, Galindo M, Silva D, Sandoval L, Rodríguez JC (2010): Analysis of *Toxoplasma gondii* surface antigen 2 gene (SAG2). Relevance of genotype I in clinical toxoplasmosis. Mol Biol Rep 37, 6: 2927-2933.

da Silva RC, Langoni H, Su C, da Silva AV (2011): Genotypic characterization of *Toxoplasma gondii* in sheep from Brazilian slaughterhouses: new atypical genotypes and the clonal type II strain identified. Vet Parasitol 175, 1-2: 173-177.

de Sousa S, Ajzenberg D, Canada N, Freire L, de Costa J, Darde ML, Thulliez P, Dubey JP (2006): Biologic and molecular characterization of *Toxoplasma gondii* isolates from pigs from Portugal. Vet Parasitol 135, 2: 133-137.

Su C, Evans D, Cole RH, Kissinger JC, Ajioka JW, Sibley LD (2003): Recent expansion of Toxoplasma through enhanced oral transmission. *Science* 299, 5605: 414-416.

Su C, Zhang X, Dubey JP (2006): Genotyping of *Toxoplasma gondii* by multilocus PCR-RFLP markers: a high resolution and simple method for identification of parasites. Int J Parasitol 36, 7: 841-848.

Su C, Shwab EK, Zhou P, Zhu XQ, Dubey JP (2010): Moving towards an integrated approach to molecular detection and identification of *Toxoplasma gondii*. Parasitology 137, 1: 1-11.

Switaj K, Master A, Skrzypczak M, Zaborowski P (2005): Recent trends in molecular diagnostics for *Toxoplasma gondii* infections. Clin Microbiol Infect 11, 3: 170-176.

Talabani H, Asseraf M, Yera H, Delair E, Ancelle T, Thulliez P, Brezin AP, Dupouy-Camet J (2009): Contributions of immunoblotting, real-time PCR, and the Goldmann-Witmer coefficient to diagnosis of atypical toxoplasmic retinochoroiditis. J Clin Microbiol 47, 7: 2131-2135.

Truppel JH, Reifur L, Montiani-Ferreira F, Lange RR, de Castro Vilani RG, Gennari SM, Thomaz-Soccol, V (2010): *Toxoplasma gondii* in Capybara (Hydrochaeris hydrochaeris) antibodies and DNA detected by IFAT and PCR. Parasitol Res 107, 1: 141-146.

Thulliez P, Daffos F, Forestier F (1992): Diagnosis of Toxoplasma infection in the pregnant woman and the unborn child: current problems. Scand J Infect Dis Suppl 84, 18-22.

Vidal JE, Colombo FA, de Oliveira AC, Focaccia R, Pereira-Chioccola VL (2004): PCR assay using cerebrospinal fluid for diagnosis of cerebral toxoplasmosis in Brazilian AIDS patients. J Clin Microbiol 42, 10: 4765-4768.

Villard O, Filisetti D, Roch-Deries F, Garweg J, Flament J, Candolfi E (2003): Comparison of enzyme-linked immunosorbent assay, immunoblotting, and PCR for diagnosis of toxoplasmic chorioretinitis. J Clin Microbiol 41, 8: 3537-3541.

Vujanić M (2012): Molecular detection and genotyping of *Toxoplasma gondii* strains isolated in Serbia. PhD thesis. University of Belgrade, Serbia.

Vujanić M, Ivović V, Kataranovski M, Nikolić A, Bobić B, Klun I, Villena I, Kataranovski D, Djurković-Djaković O (2011): Toxoplasmosis in naturally infected rodents in Belgrade, Serbia. Vector Borne Zoonotic Dis 11, 8: 1209-1211.

Wahab T, Edvinsson B, Palm D, Lindh JJ (2010): Comparison of the AF146527 and B1 repeated elements, two real-time PCR targets used for detection of *Toxoplasma gondii*. Clin Microbiol 48, 2: 591-592.

Wallon M, Franck J, Thulliez P, Huissoud C, Peyron F, Garcia-Meric P, Kieffer F (2010): Accuracy of real-time polymerase chain reaction for *Toxoplasma gondii* in amniotic fluid. Obstet Gynecol 115, 4: 727-733.

Yera H, Filisetti D, Bastien P, Ancelle T, Thulliez P, Delhaes L (2009): Multicenter comparative evaluation of five commercial methods for toxoplasma DNA extraction from amniotic fluid. J Clin Microbiol 47, 12: 3881-3886.

Chapter 6

Endemic *Toxoplasma gondii* Genotype II Causes Fatal Infections in Animal Hosts in Europe – Lessons Learnt

Pikka Jokelainen

Additional information is available at the end of the chapter

http://dx.doi.org/10.5772/49984

1. Introduction

Toxoplasma gondii is a successful protozoan parasite of domestic animals, wildlife, and humans [1]. Despite this parasite is capable of causing disease and even killing its host, majority of infections are subclinical or asymptomatic. These latent, chronic infections are beneficial for the parasite: while the host is unaware of even ever acquiring the infection, the parasite stays dormant in the tissues of the host waiting for the host to be eaten by another host.

The latent *T. gondii* infections can be detected by measuring the antibody responses raised by the host against the parasite [1]. For most host species, the seroprevalence numbers are clearly higher than incidence of clinical and fatal cases. One exception is the European brown hare (*Lepus europaeus*), a host species that appears very susceptible to the infection [2]. It is worth emphasizing that if the infection proves fatal, it is not good for the parasite, either.

For this parasite, any nucleated cell of a warm-blooded animal will do, and the intestines of Felids are the place for sexual reproduction [1]. Humans are usually nothing but a dead-end host for *T. gondii*. Animal hosts clearly outnumber human hosts living on this planet and are more important for the spread and surviving of the parasite – Felids are shedding the oocyst reservoir, migrating animals are introducing the parasite to new areas, and prey animals are harboring the parasite in their tissues ready to infect the predators and scavengers. Investigating the infections in animal hosts can provide relevant clues needed for better understanding the parasite and its epidemiology, which has implications for public health also. The larger animal host population provides more options for epidemiologic studies.

Currently, one of the major issues in human toxoplasmosis research is evaluating the effect of some characteristics of the parasite, such as its genotype, on the outcome of the infection. Little is known of this effect in many animal hosts. Applying currently available methods to genetically characterize the parasite strains that cause clinical, and at worst fatal, toxoplasmosis in different host species can provide valuable new information to further understand the interactions of *T. gondii* and its various hosts: humans, domestic animals and wildlife.

In addition, free-ranging animal hosts and pet animals sharing the urban environment with humans can be regarded as sentinels for the *T. gondii* strains present in a specific area – the ones humans may encounter there as well. Characterization of both the *T. gondii* strains that are waiting to be eaten in the tissues of animals raised for human consumption and especially the possibly more virulent strains that had killed their animal hosts following natural infection in an area may thus provide important information for human health care professionals and public health decision making. Monitoring the situation assists in rapid detection of emergence of strains new to an area and changes in infection pressure. Molecular methods also allow tracing the infection sources and following the spread of an outbreak.

Majority of the *T. gondii* strains isolated from humans and animal hosts from Europe belong to genotype II, which typically only causes chronic infections if inoculated into mice (nonvirulent in mice) [9]. This is in sharp contrast to what appears to be the case in other areas, especially South America, where high level of genetic diversity is seen in T. gondii [9]. Fatal toxoplasmosis has been reported sporadically among individuals of both domestic and wild animal species examined postmortem [1,9], but published genotyping results of the parasites causing the severe, fatal infections are scarce. Data on the genotypes causing the fatal infections is particularly interesting from an area where the predominant genotype is considered to be of low virulence, such as Europe where type II is endemic.

This chapter describes recently published results from genetic characterization of T. gondii strains that proved fatal to their animal hosts following naturally acquired infection in Europe, and discusses the lessons learnt from them.

2. Summary of recent results

The special interest or our group has been genotyping the *T. gondii* strains causing fatal infections in various host species, thus far in Finland [2-4]. Recently, our group has retrospectively searched the records of European brown hares (*Lepus europaeus*), mountain hares (*Lepus timidus*) [2], and Eurasian red squirrels (*Sciurus vulgaris*) [3] examined postmortem in 2006-2009 at the only wildlife pathology laboratory in Finland, Evira, for cases of fatal toxoplasmosis. In addition, diagnosed cases of fatal toxoplasmosis in pet cats (*Felis catus*) that were necropsied at the University of Helsinki, Finland, in 2008-2010 have been thoroughly investigated [4]. The cases were confirmed with immunohistochemical staining of sections of formalin-fixed, paraffin-embedded tissue samples; the automated IHC staining protocol is described in [2]. In these studies of ours, naturally acquired toxoplasmosis was the confirmed cause of death of 14 (8.1%) of 173 European brown hares, 4 (2.7%) of 148 mountain hares [2], 3 (15.8%) of 19 Eurasian red squirrels [3], and 6 (3.1%) of

193 cats [4]. It is, indeed, not a particularly rare cause of death in these host species. However, it is important to bear in mind that this is not a good measure of disease incidence because these numbers are strongly affected by the material submitted for examination. The material available for investigations like these studies cannot be regarded as truly representative of the host animal populations of the area. This is especially the case in wild animals submitted for post-examination: only the dead animals found by active citizens before scavengers reach the wildlife pathology laboratory. The animals that had died near human settlements are very likely overrepresented.

For the genotyping of the *T. gondii* strains, we have extracted DNA from various tissue samples of the animals that had died from the infection: both formalin-fixed paraffin embedded samples, and fresh or frozen samples if available. Although most tissues have been rich in parasites in these cases, liver has become our tissue of choice. We use direct genetic characterization of the parasites in the tissues, without a bioassay step that could have a selective effect especially in case of mixed infections with several strains. Thus far two strains have been successfully isolated directly into cell cultures and cryopreserved, and from those, the genotyping analysis has been repeated from cell culture harvested parasites. The genotyping method we use is a multilocus method based on length polymorphism of seven microsatellite markers [2, 5, 6]. Six of the markers (B18, TUB2, TgM-A, W35, B17, and M33) are used for genotyping, and one additional marker (M48) for further characterization [5, 6].

As shown in Table 1, the genotyping results of the*T. gondii s*trains causing the death of the animal hosts have been consistent with type II in all the 27 fatal cases examined from Finland thus far. Very similar results have been reported from other areas in Europe:

In Switzerland, a cat died from toxoplasmosis and the causative strain was genotyped using polymerase chain reaction-restriction fragment length polymorphism method with nine genetic markers (SAG2, SAG3, BTUB, GRA6, c22-8, c29-2, L358, PK1, and Apico) [7]. The analysis revealed type II alleles at all loci except one, Apico, which displayed a type I allele. This result is identical to the results one would obtain with this method from, for example, the reference strain PRU [1]. This commonly used genotype II reference strain was originally isolated from human fetal tissues in France and gives results that are fully consistent with genotype II with the method our group uses.

T. gondii parasites that had killed four arctic foxes (*Vulpes lagopus*) in the remote arctic archipelago Svalbard – this is very interesting from the geographical point of view - were genotyped at ten loci (SAG1 and the nine markers used in [7]) also using the polymerase chain reaction-restriction fragment length polymorphism method [8]. Three of the samples from the fatal cases had type I allele at Apico, whereas one had type II allele at all markers, and all four were interpreted as type II.

The strain that killed the cat in Switzerland was isolated by inoculation in mice and later maintained in cell cultures, but the genotyping was also performed directly from frozen tissues of the cat [7]. The genotyping of the strains that caused the deaths of the arctic foxes was done directly from the brain tissue of the foxes [8].

Species	Country of origin	Number of cases	Genotyping method used	Reference
Arctic fox (*Vulpes lagopus)*	Norway	4	PCR-RFLP	[8]
Cat (*Felis catus*)	Finland Switzerland	6 1	MS PCR-RFLP	[4] [7]
Eurasian red squirrel (*Sciurus vulgaris*)	Finland	3	MS	[3]
European brown hare (*Lepus europaeus*)	Finland	14	MS	[2]
Mountain hare (*Lepus timidus)*	Finland	4	MS	[2]

Table 1. Recent genotyping results of cases of fatal toxoplasmosis in different animal host species in Europe.

Taken together, *T. gondii* parasites belonging to the endemic genotype II that are typically nonvirulent in mice caused these altogether 32 fatal infections in altogether five different animal host species (Table 1). Genotype II was the only genotype detected from these fatal cases. Surprisingly, none of these animals had appeared to have any clear immunodeficiency or other predisposing factor. By contrast, the hares that had died from toxoplasmosis were actually heavier, in better bodily condition, than the hares that had died of other causes [2]. Interestingly, some host species, such as the European brown hares [2] and possibly also Eurasian red squirrels [3], appear extremely susceptible to the acquired *T. gondii* infection. They have relatively high proportional mortality rates from toxoplasmosis: the proportion of animals examined post-mortem that had died from toxoplasmosis is substantial.

3. Conclusions

Two conclusions and one question arise from these results summarized above:

1. These infections were naturally acquired, which supports the endemic status and dominance of *T. gondii* genotype II in Europe. These results also show its spread north, and that the parasite appears unstopped by the harsh winters and remote locations. Not on-

ly animals, but undoubtedly also humans can encounter *T. gondii* even in the northernmost parts of Europe.

2. These results further affirm that no especially virulent *T. gondii* strain is required for the infection to kill a host. Moreover, these were naturally acquired infections, implying the infection doses have been within limits of what may be encountered in the nature and the infection routes probably the ones these hosts should be most adapted to.

The question remaining unanswered is the prevalence, role, and importance of *T. gondii* strains belonging to other genotypesthan type II in Europe. More investigations in this field are ongoing, and needed. Strains belonging to other genotypes, possibly more virulent ones, could be found by characterizing more strains that cause severe or fatal infections.

Author details

Pikka Jokelainen
Veterinary Pathology and Parasitology, Department of Veterinary Biosciences, Faculty of Veterinary Medicine, University of Helsinki, Helsinki, Finland

4. References

[1] Dubey JP (2010) Toxoplasmosis of Animals and Humans.CRC Press.

[2] Jokelainen P, Isomursu M, Näreaho A, Oksanen A (2011) Natural *Toxoplasma gondii* infections in European Brown Hares and Mountain Hares in Finland: Proportional Mortality Rate, Antibody Prevalence, and Genetic Characterization. Journal of Wildlife Diseases 47: 154–163.

[3] Jokelainen P, Nylund M (2012) Acute Fatal Toxoplasmosis in Three Eurasian Red Squirrels (*Sciurus vulgaris*) Caused by Genotype II of *Toxoplasma gondii*. Journal of Wildlife Diseases, 48: 454–457.

[4] Jokelainen P, Simola O, Rantanen E, Näreaho A, Lohi H, Sukura A. Feline toxoplasmosis in Finland: Cross-sectionalepidemiological study and case series study. Journal of Veterinary Diagnostic Investigation

[5] Ajzenberg D, Dumètre A, Dardé M-L (2005) Multiplex PCR for Typing Strains of *Toxoplasma gondii*. Journal of Clinical Microbiology 43: 1940–1943.

[6] Blackston CR, Dubey JP, Dotson E, Su C, Thulliez P, Sibley D, Lehmann T (2001) High-resolution Typing of *Toxoplasma gondii* Using Microsatellite Loci. Journal of Parasitology 87: 1472–1475.

[7] Spycher A, Geigy C, Howard J, Posthaus H, Gendron K, Gottstein B, Debache K, Herrmann DC, Schares G, Frey CF (2011) Isolation and Genotyping of *Toxoplasma gondii* Causing Fatal Systemic Toxoplasmosis in an Immunocompetent 10-year-old Cat. J Vet Diagn Invest 23:104–108.

[8] Prestrud KW, Åsbakk K, Mørk T, Fuglei E, Tryland M, Su C (2008) Direct High-resolution Genotyping of *Toxoplasma gondii* in Arctic Foxes (*Vulpes lagopus*) in the

Remote Arctic Svalbard Archipelago Reveals Widespread Clonal Type II Lineage. Veterinary Parasitology 158: 121–128.
[9] Wendte JM, Gibson AK, Grigg ME (2011) Population Genetics of *Toxoplasma gondii*: New Perspectives from Parasite Genotypes in Wildlife. Veterinary Parasitology 182: 96-111.

Section 3

Clinical Issues

Chapter 7

Risk Factors, Pathogenesis and Diagnosis of Ocular Toxoplasmosis

Jean Dupouy-Camet, Hana Talabani, Emmanuelle Delair, Florence Leslé, HélèneYera and Antoine P. Brézin

Additional information is available at the end of the chapter

http://dx.doi.org/10.5772/50267

1. Introduction

Ocular toxoplasmosis (OT) is a major cause of posterior uveitis worldwide but its incidence and prevalence are difficult to establish precisely. In 1993, a survey in a French Hospital Service of Ophthalmology showed that OT was seen in less than 1 per thousand outpatients [1]. In a study performed in Germany, toxoplasmosis accounted for 4.2 % of all cases of uveitis at a referral centre [2]. Around 5000 people develop symptomatic OT each year in the United States [3]. OT is a complication of both acute acquired and reactivated congenital in immunocompetent but particularly in immunocompromissed individuals and its severity can be influenced by variation in parasite isolates, parasitic load, route of infection and host-related factors such as immune function, age and pregnancy. Diagnosis is usually based on ophthalmological examination and is confirmed by the response to specific treatment, but also by biological assays including local antibody production, PCR and western blot. All these points will be detailed below.

2. A complication of acquired and congenital infections

Classically, retinochoroiditis secondary to acquired toxoplasmosis was considered an exceptional event in immunocompetent individuals, and was usually defined as a periodic reactivation of latent cysts associated with undiagnosed congenital infections. But recent data, based on ophthalmological examination, seem to establish that acquired infection might be responsible for most cases. This fact was particularly demonstrated by outbreaks reported in Canada, Brazil and India. In Canada, amongst 100 individuals infected during a water-borne outbreak, 19 had OT [4]. In southern Brazil 17.7% of 1,042 individuals examined had OT with lesions in 0.9% of 1- to 8-year-olds and in 21.3% of all individuals older than 13, suggesting that in this population, the disease was a sequel of postnatal rather than congenital infection [5]. In India, Balasundaram et al. [6] described ocular involvement due to toxoplasmosis in 248 patients who had active retinochoroiditis and toxoplasmic serology suggesting recently acquired disease. Delair et al. [7] analysed 425 cases of OT, 100 (23.5%) were acquired, 62 (14.6%) were congenital, and 263 (61.9%) were of unknown origin. At the time of the study, the mean age of the patients with congenital OT was 9.1 +/- 8.8 years, and 21.7 +/- 12.6 years in the patients with the acquired disease ($p < 0.001$). Bilateral OT was only found in 4% of acquired cases and in 43.5% of congenital cases ($p < 0.001$) and in acquired infections, visual acuity was significantly less impaired than in congenital infections. In the United Kingdom, 50% of OT in children was acquired after birth and no clear clinical distinction could be made between acquired and congenital toxoplasmosis (CT) [8]. However, other authors have identified clinical presentations specific to each group. Montoya et al. (1996) observed that patients with post-natal acquired toxoplasmic retinochoroiditis had mostly unilateral lesions without old scars or involvement of the macula [9]. In case of congenital origin, the risk of ocular disease depends on the trimester of pregnancy when infection occurred, and on whether or not treatment was administered to the mother during pregnancy. In one study, a period exceeding 8 weeks between maternal infection and the beginning of treatment, female gender, and especially cerebral calcifications were risk factors for retinochoroiditis [10]. No significant association was found in other cohort studies between gestational age at maternal infection, prenatal treatment and the risk of developing OT [11, 12].

3. Occurrence depends on host genetic background and immune status

In mice, the severity of ocular damage is linked to many factors related to either host immunity or the parasite, such as inoculum size, infective stage (oocysts versus cysts), route of infection and the genotype of the infecting strain. However, these data are not well documented in humans. The acquired immune deficiency syndrome (AIDS) epidemic has dramatically reminded that effective host immunity was essential to limit the severity of ocular lesions. AIDS patients without highly active antiretroviral therapy can develop extensive and recurring lesions [13]. Similar lesions may also be encountered during the use of immunosuppressive drugs [9, 14]. Many studies have focused on elderly patients [15-17]. These patients can have large and multiple ocular lesions with severe vitritis and prolonged disease, in some instances similar to lesions encountered in immunocompromissed individuals, although they are otherwise healthy. Indeed, both cellular and humoral immune responses are modified with advancing age and probably contribute to the higher severity of OT in older patients [16]. A cross-sectional household study involving 499 individuals was undertaken in Minas Gerais state of Brazil, where infection with *T. gondii* is endemic. The frequency of OT increased significantly with age as approximately 50% of individuals above 60 years of age had lesions and older patients had a higher risk of OT following recently acquired infection compared to younger patients [18]. The factors responsible for recurrences are unknown, but trauma, hormonal changes and cellular or humoral immunosuppression appear to contribute to the release of parasites from tissue cysts. Bosch-Driessen et al. reported an increased incidence of recurrences after cataract surgery and during pregnancy [19]. The hormonal and immunological changes in pregnant women can cause recurrences and these authors described four women having such recurrences in every pregnancy [19]. Garweg et al. [20] reported that recurrence occurred in approximately in 4 out of 5 patients and that the risk was higher two years after the first episode. Holland et al. [21] confirmed that the risk of recurrence was the highest immediately after an episode of active disease and that recurrence had a tendency to occur in clusters. Mice with different genetic backgrounds will have different susceptibilities to the parasite [22]. In humans, an increased frequency of the HLA-Bw62 antigen was observed in patients with severe OT [23]. In mother-child pairs from Europe and North America, ocular disease in CT was associated with polymorphisms in ABCA4 encoding the ATP-binding cassette transporter and in COL2A1 encoding type II collagen [24]. Evidence will be shown below that polymorphism in cytokine genes is also an important factor triggering OT occurrence.

4. Specific parasitic genotypes could be involved

Currently, it is assumed that the population of *T. gondii* consists of 3 3 predominant clonal lineages, which differ at the DNA sequence level by 1% or less [25] but microsatellite analysis has shown the high diversity of that genus [26]. In Europe and the United States, type II is the most common cause of systemic *Toxoplasma* infection [27]. As early as 2001 Grigg et al. [28] suggested a possible correlation between severe retinal disease and atypical genotypes in immunocompetent patients as, in acquired OT, an unusual abundance of type I, or recombinant genotypes I/III were found. In Brazil, genetic studies have shown that genotypes of *T. gondii* involved in acquired OT were atypical, belonging to genotypes different from genotype II [29]. The differences in the frequency, size and multiplicity of retinochoroidal lesions may be explained by more virulent parasite genotypes that predominate in Brazil, but are rarely found in Europe. Khan et al. [30] compared 25 clinical and animal isolates of *T. gondii* from Brazil to previously characterised clonal lineages from North America and Europe. Genotypes of *T. gondii* strains isolated from Brazil were highly divergent when compared (by multilocus nested PCR analysis combined with sequencing of a polymorphic intron) to the previously described clonal lineages found in Europe. These atypical genotypes may also explain the high frequency (20% of 97 cases) of ocular involvement in the above mentioned Canadian outbreak where an atypical cougar isolate was suspected, and the 100-fold higher incidence of OT in patients born in Africa compared to patients born in Britain [31,32]. The distribution of genotypes was different in immunocompromised patients who reactivate a type II strain (if acquired in Europe), or a non–type II strain (if acquired in Africa or South America). However, direct genotyping of strains from aqueous or vitreous fluids of 20 French patients showed a predominance of the type II genotype in OT [33] so the possible link of OT with some specific genotypes is not yet clear.

5. Immune privileged status and cytokine responses are key factors in toxoplasmic retinochoroiditis

The pathogenesis of OT is directly linked to the anatomical characteristics of the eye resulting in an immune privileged status. The presence of the hemato-retinal barrier and the absence of lymphatic vessels limits the passage of inflammatory cells and lymphocytes and of antibodies and complement components [34]. In addition, the ocular characteristics of the distribution and the functions of antigen presenting cells are also of importance. For example, corneal epithelium is deprived of Langerhans cells and the dendritic cells of the ciliary epithelium are not activated by GM-CSF and do not stimulate T lymphocytes [35, 36]. There is a low expression of classical MHC class IA molecules which reduce the lytic activity of CD8+ lymphocytes usually stimulated by the MHC I molecules. MHC II molecules are not expressed in the eye, which limits CD4+ lymphocyte activation. Increased expression of surface molecules like CD46, CD55 and CD59 will also inhibit complement activation [37]. A local production of immunosuppressive cytokines, such as TGF-β, limits B and Th1 lymphocyte activation but activates Th2 lymphocytes [34, 38, 39]. Finally, retinal cells express surface molecules involved in apoptosis such as TNF- Related Apoptosis Inducing Ligand (TRAIL) and Fas ligand (FasL). FasL interacts with FasR (Fas receptor) carried by the inflammatory cells, inducing their apoptosis. This would control the entry of Fas-expressing lymphoid cells and limit the alteration of ocular cells by these cells [40, 41]. Whereas the mechanisms that underlie retinal damage in OT are yet not fully understood, the immune response might directly affect the pathogenesis of toxoplasmic retinochoroiditis and some cytokines have been shown to be fundamental to either control or block a protective response against *T. gondii* in experimental models. As early as 1998, Gazzinelli & Denkers [42] stated that initiating a strong T-cell-mediated immunity was crucial in the immune defense against *T. gondii*. High levels of gamma interferon (IFNγ) were induced by the parasite during initial infection as a result of early T-cell as well as natural killer (NK) cell activation. Induction of interleukin-12 by macrophages is a major mechanism driving early IFNγ synthesis. They also stated that "while part of the clinical manifestations of toxoplasmosis results from direct tissue destruction by the parasite, inflammatory cytokine-mediated immunopathologic changes may also contribute to disease progression". In animal experiments, many authors have described that IFNγ and TNFα, which enhance macrophage activation and induce production of other cytokines such as IL-12, give rise to a type Th1 immune response that plays a crucial role in parasite control [43]. These two cytokines could play a major role in immunological responses that control parasite proliferation by induction of indoleamine 2,3-dioxygenase production in retinal pigment epithelial cells [44]. Moreover, Gazzinelli et al. [45] observed that compared to control animals, mice treated with IFNγ or TNFα antagonists or antibodies against T cells (CD4 and CD8), showed more severe lesions characterized by exacerbated ocular damage and increased parasite detection in the eye. Conversely, a shift to a Th2 immune response with production of anti-inflammatory cytokines including IL-10, TGF-β and IL-4 promoted parasite survival, and was required to maintain immune privilege in the eye and prevent immune tissue destruction [46]. IFNγ and TNFα are also inhibitors of parasite replication in retinal pigment epithelial cells [47]. In humans, the participation of inflammatory mediators in physiopathology of OT is not yet clear. Nevertheless, a study by Yamamoto et al. [48] showed that asymptomatic patients secreted significantly more IL-12 and IFNγ in response to *T. gondii* antigens than patients with ocular damage. Conversely, acquired OT was associated with high levels of IL-1 and TNFα. They also observed that in comparison with non-infected subjects, IL-2 and IFNγ production by peripheral blood mononuclear cells in response to *T. gondii* was decreased in subjects with congenital infection, suggesting a status of parasite tolerance. Ongkosuwito et al. [49] measured the levels of six chemokines directly in aqueous humor samples from patients presenting with viral or toxoplasmic uveitis. Interestingly, IL-6 titers in patients with OT correlated with the degree of activity of toxoplasmic chorioretinitis. This cytokine is now described as essential in Th17 differentiation and Th17 cells are involved in inflammatory and autoimmune uveitis, supporting the hypothesis that the host immune response takes part in ocular damage [50]. The expansion of IL-17 producing cells in human OT has been demonstrated by Lahmar et al [51] who monitored cytokine patterns in serum and aqueous humor of subjects suffering from OT, infectious or non-infectious uveitis and cataract. High levels of IL-17 were reported in aqueous humor samples from 70 % patients presenting OT. Similar findings were also reported in patients suffering from other ocular inflammatory diseases showing that inflammatory processes could play a major role in the establishment of ocular damage in the chronic stage of OT. Due to large inter-individual variations of cytokine levels within each group of patients, no correlation was found between cytokine titers and clinical presentation. In addition, increased levels of pro-inflammatory mediators MCP-1, IL-8 and IL-6 were found in intraocular fluid samples from OT, but these variations were not specific for toxoplasmic uveitis [51]. IL-12 enhances TNF production and synthesis was higher in OT than in other ocular diseases in accordance with the importance of the Th1 response in mouse models. The Th2 cytokines (Il-4, IL-5, IL-10), which counterbalance inflammatory processes, were up-regulated and consequently the authors were unable to define the respective roles of Th1 and Th2 responses in the pathogenesis of human OT. As observed in experimental autoimmune uveitis, it is now proposed that eye damage may be induced by pathogenic responses mediated by Th-17 cells producing TNFα [52]. Conversely, host hypersensitivity pathways in the eye might be counterbalanced by IL-27 secretion up-regulated by IFNγ from Th1 cells [52]. A possible association between polymorphisms in cytokine genes and OT was searched for in patients. Specific IL1, IL10 and IFNγ alleles were preferentially found in patients with OT. No such association was found with TNFα gene polymorphisms [53-56]. A putative summary of the role of the different cytokines and T cells in defense against the parasite but also in the occurrence of tissue lesions is summarized in figure 1.

6. Diagnosis is based on clinical signs and some selected biological assays

The diagnosis is usually based on ophthalmological examination showing unilateral, whitish, fuzzy-edged, round, focal lesions surrounded by retinal edema (figure 2). Cells are found in the vitreous, particularly overlying the active lesion. In the area surrounding the active retinitis, one may see hemorrhage, as well as sheathing of the retinal blood vessels. Fluorescein angiography of the active lesion demonstrates early blockage with subsequent leakage of the lesion. Cells in the anterior chamber may also be noted and may appear to be either a granulomatous or non granulomatous uveitis. The discovery of healed pigmented

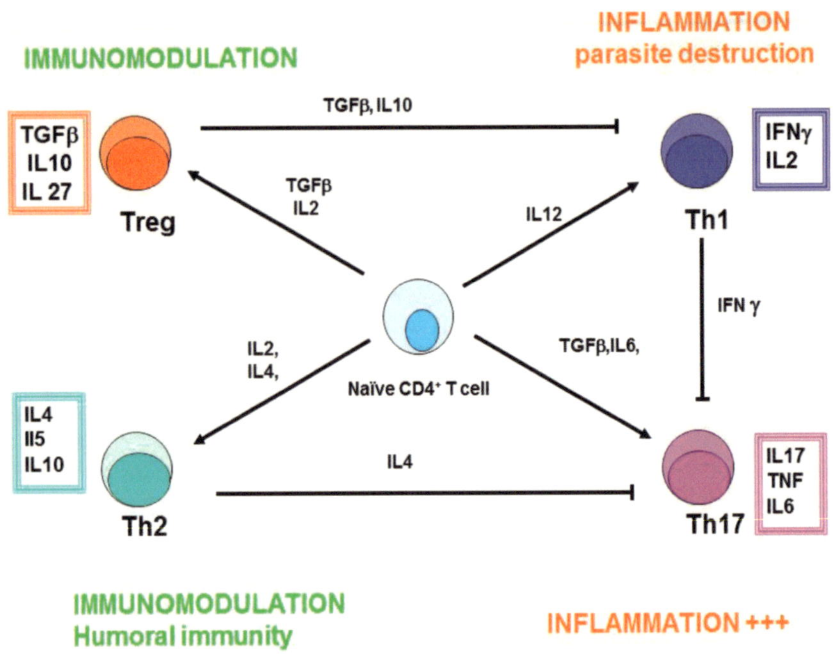

Figure 1. T cells and cytokines involved in ocular toxoplasmosis and parasite destruction

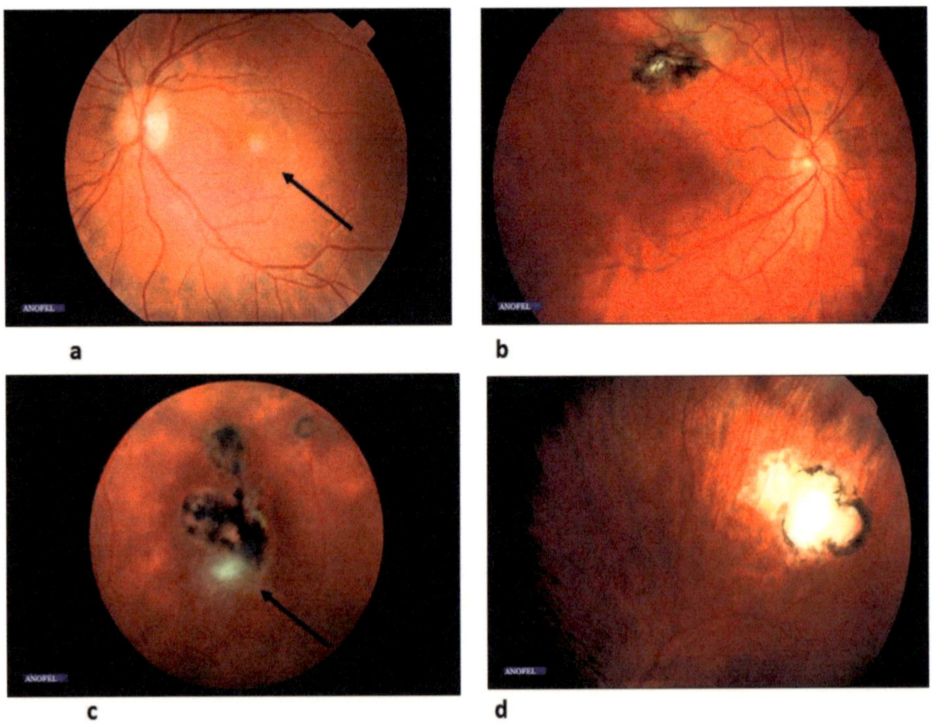

Figure 2. Eye fundus aspects of ocular toxoplasmosis. a: active lesion; b, d: scar; c: active lesion and scars (source A.P. Brézin and Anofel)

retinochoroidal scars facilitates the diagnosis [57, 58]. OT is also confirmed by a favorable clinical response to specific therapy. However, diagnosis and treatment can be delayed in patients with atypical lesions (unusual and complicated forms) or patients showing an inadequate response to antimicrobial therapy as particularly observed in elderly or immunocompromised patients [13, 17]. In such cases, rapid identification of the causative agent requires aqueous humor sampling by anterior chamber paracentesis [59]. Laboratory diagnosis is based on the comparison of antibody profiles in ocular fluid and serum samples in order to detect intraocular specific antibody synthesis, based on the Goldmann-Witmer coefficient (GWC) or on the observation of qualitative differences between eye fluid and serum by immunoblotting (IB) [60]. The GWC is based on the comparison of the levels of specific antibodies to total immunoglobulin in both aqueous humor and serum. Recent studies have shown the usefulness of PCR applied to aqueous humor, in combination with serologic tests, for the diagnosis of OT [61-68]. However, although this combined approach improves diagnostic sensitivity, the volume of the ocular fluid sample may not be adequate for PCR, IB, and GWC. We showed [68] that a combination of all three methods had a 85% sensitivity and a 93% specificity for the diagnosis of atypical or extensive toxoplasmic retinochoroiditis. The sensitivity of GWC alone for atypical uveitis (based mainly on aqueous humor samples) ranges from 39% to 93% [60, 63, 65, 67, 69-71]. Discrepancies could be explained by differences in (i) the interval between symptom onset and paracentesis, (ii) the characteristics of the uveitis (typical or atypical), (iii) underlying immunological status, and (iv), the chosen GWC positivity threshold, which ranges from 2 to 8 in the literature. The specificity of the GWC is usually high if the retinal barrier has not been impaired. IB on aqueous humor has sensitivities ranging from 50 to 81% for the diagnosis of atypical [60, 65] and typical [66, 68, 69] OT. Apparently the sensitivity of IB increases with the length of the interval between onset of symptoms and paracentesis. The sensitivity of real-time PCR ranges from 36 % to 55% [63, 67, 68]. The sensitivity was higher with a real-time PCR assay targeting the *T. gondii* repeat element of 529 base pairs [68] than with real-time PCR targeting the B1 gene (40% and 36% respectively). Real-time PCR has been shown to be more sensitive on a variety of samples when the 529-bp repeat element rather than the B1 gene was used as a target [71]. In contrast to the IB and GWC results, the results of PCR are not influenced by the interval between symptom onset and paracentesis. The total size of acute retinal foci is larger in PCR-positive patients [64, 67, 68]. PCR seems more informative than the GWC and IB for immunocompromised patients [62, 64]. The rate of detection of specific intraocular antibodies seems related to the interval between symptom onset and paracentesis. Early sampling is often associated with negative GWC results and with low IB sensitivity. The sensitivity of the GWC increases when sampling is performed at least 10 days after symptom onset, and IB was positive for 72% of cases 30 days after symptom onset [68]. Several studies have examined the influence of this interval on GWC results. Fardeau et al. [64] reported that the GWC was useless during the first 2 weeks but that its sensitivity increased sharply when anterior chamber puncture was performed between the 3rd and 8th week after symptom onset. Garweg et al. [69] showed that GWC sensitivity increased from 57% to 70% when puncture was performed at 6 weeks instead of 3 weeks. As stated above, PCR sensitivity was not influenced by this interval. Combining the three biological techniques increases the sensitivity and the specificity but sometimes the volume size of the sample is so small that it is not possible to perform all three. On the basis of the presented results, we propose an algorithm for choosing the test with the best sensitivity according to ophthalmologic findings and delay after onset of the disease (figure 3). When paracentesis is performed during the 10 days following symptom onset, real-time PCR is most suitable, especially if the patient is immunocompromised or if the total size of the foci is large (> 2 optic disc diameters). Beyond 10 days, the best choice is the GWC if old scars are present and/or if the reaction in the anterior chamber is mild to severe, or PCR if the total size of foci is large (>2 optic disc diameters); IB should be preferred when paracentesis is performed more than 30 days after symptom onset.

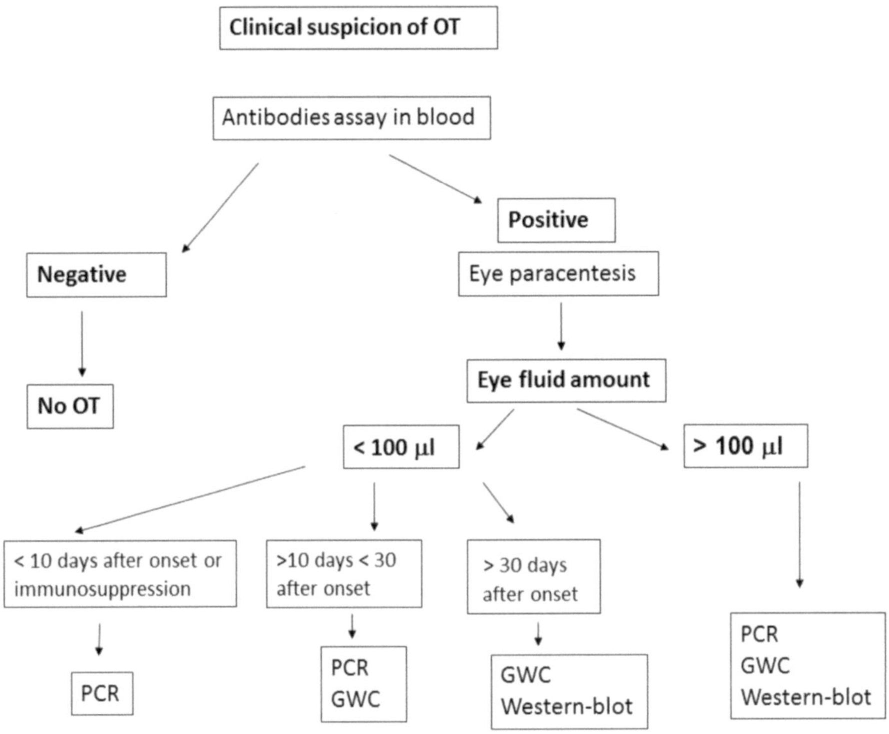

Figure 3. Algorithm for the biological diagnosis of ocular toxoplasmosis (in severely immunosuppressed patients a negative serology does not exclude OT which can be then confirmed by PCR)

7. Efficient treatments are available but there is no real mean of prevention

There is no real consensus on the treatment of retinochoroiditis [72-75]. Some experts will treat only patients in which the lesions are near the macula or the optic nerve and when there is an important hyalitis with an impairment of the optical acuity. The non-treated patient will be regularly checked. Other experts will treat all the lesions whatever their localizations and this is now possible because the recommended association pyrimethamine/azythromycine is better tolerated and has a better compliance than pyrimethamine associated to sulfadiazine [76, 77]. Corticosteroids (prednisone at 0.5 to 1mg/kg/d) are constantly administered for several weeks, except for immunocompromised patients [73, 78]. Pyrimethamine in adults is used at 100mg/d for several days then decreased at 50mg/d. It should be associated with sulfadiazine at 75mg/kg/d divided in 4 doses or better with azythromycine 250 mg/d. The total length of the treatment will be of 3 to 6 weeks, sometimes more, depending on the initial size of the lesion. In patients intolerant to treatment, clindamycine at 450-600 mg/d should be associated [79]. The treatment of congenital retinochoroiditis in newborns is based on sulfadiazine (50mg/kg/d in 2 doses) associated with pyrimethamine at 1mg/kg/d for 6 to 12 months. Fifteen mg folinic acid is given every 3 days. The prophylaxis of congenitally acquired OT is based on national programs of prevention of CT (e.g. France, Austria) but their efficiency is discussed [80-82] and depends on the local epidemiology and virulence of strains [83]. Peyron et al. [84] stated that "treating CT has little effect on the quality of life and visual function of the affected individuals". However, Kieffer et al. [10] showed that a period exceeding 8 weeks between maternal infection and the beginning of treatment was a risk factor for retinochoroiditis; therefore emphasizing the need to prevent and treat CT. Evidence for the effectiveness of prenatal or postnatal treatment for CT is still needed. Randomised controlled trials and cohort studies are in progress to provide information on prognosis, especially disability [85]. There is no radical prevention of acquired toxoplasmosis besides hygienic rules in preparing meals. Eating well done or deeply frozen meat should be particularly recommended in regions where highly pathogenic isolates are prevalent. In HIV patients, drug prevention of toxoplasmosis has been successfully used for years and is now less needed since the use of efficient HAART.

8. Conclusions

Acquired or CT can be complicated by OT. The diagnosis relies on clinical aspects, responses to specific treatment and results of biological assays. The incidence and the prevalence of this complication are both difficult to establish precisely and depend on the parasite prevalence in the general population, and are affected by different factors such as type of exposure to the parasite, genetic background of the different parasites and the host, and the type of immune response elicited by the parasite. Prevention of CT (though still discussed), and a rapid specific treatment of acquired cases could be the key measures to avoid severe visual impairment but evaluation of these procedures is urgently needed.

Author details

Jean Dupouy-Camet*, Hana Talabani, Florence Leslé and Hélène Yera
Service de Parasitologie-Mycologie, Hôpital Cochin, Assistance Publique-Hôpitaux de Paris, Université Paris Descartes, Paris, France

* Corresponding Author

Emmanuelle Delair and Antoine P. Brézin
Service d'Ophtalmologie, Hôpital Cochin, Assistance Publique-Hôpitaux de Paris, Université Paris Descartes, Paris, France

Acknowledgement

Parts of this chapter were already published in Factors of occurrence of ocular toxoplasmosis. A review. Talabani H, Mergey T, Yera H, Delair E, Brézin AP, Langsley G, Dupouy-Camet J. Parasite. 2010 Sep;17(3):177-82. This chapter is published with the help of ADERMEPT.

9. References

[1] Dupouy-Camet J, Lahmi T., Vidal-Trecan G, Ancelle T, Mondon H. Prévalence des choriorétinites toxoplasmiques chez 4019 consultants d'un service d'ophtalmologie. Bulletin Epidémiologique Hebdomadaire 1995; 95(2):7 http://archives.invs.sante.fr/beh/1995/02/beh_02_1995.pdf

[2] Jakob E, Reuland MS, Mackensen F, Harsch N, Fleckenstein M, Lorenz HM, Max R, Becker MD. Uveitis subtypes in a german interdisciplinary uveitis center-analysis of 1916 patients. J Rheumatol 2009; 36: 127-36.

[3] Jones JL, Holland GN. Annual burden of ocular toxoplasmosis in the US. Am J Trop Med Hyg 2010; 82: 464-5.

[4] Bowie WR, King AS, Werker DH, Isaac-Renton JL, Bell A, Eng SB, Marion SA. Outbreak of toxoplasmosis associated with municipal drinking water. Lancet 1997; 350:173-7.

[5] Glasner PD, Silveira C, Kruszon-Moran D, Martins MC, Burnier Júnior M, Silveira S, Camargo ME, Nussenblatt RB, Kaslow RA, Belfort Júnior R. An unusually high prevalence of ocular toxoplasmosis in southern Brazil. Am J Ophthalmol 1992; 114: 136-44.

[6] Balasundaram MB, Andavar R, Palaniswamy M, Venkatapathy N. Outbreak of acquired ocular toxoplasmosis involving 248 patients. Arch Ophthalmol 2010; 128: 28-32.

[7] Delair E, Monnet D, Grabar S, Dupouy-Camet J, Yera H, Brezin AP. Respective roles of acquired and congenital infections in presumed ocular toxoplasmosis. Am J Ophthalmol 2008;146:851–855.

[8] Stanford MR, Tan HK, Gilbert RE. Toxoplasmic retinochoroiditis presenting in childhood: clinical findings in a UK survey. Br J Ophthalmol 2006; 90: 1464-7.

[9] Montoya JG, Remington JS. Toxoplasmic chorioretinitis in the setting of acute acquired toxoplasmosis. Clin Infect Dis1996; 23: 277-82.

[10] Kieffer F, Wallon M., Garcia P, Thulliez P, Peyron F, Franck J. Risk factors for retinochoroiditis during the first 2 years of life in infants with treated congenital toxoplasmosis. Pediatr Infect Dis J 2008; 27: 27-32.

[11] Binquet C, Wallon M, Quantin C, Kodjikian L, Garweg J, Fleury J, Peyron F, Abrahamowicz M. Prognostic factors for the long-term development of ocular lesions in 327 children with congenital toxoplasmosis. Epidemiol Infect 2003; 131: 1157-68.

[12] Freeman K, Tan HK, Prusa A, Petersen E, Buffolano W, Malm G, Cortina-Borja M, Gilbert R; European Multicentre Study on Congenital Toxoplasmosis. Predictors of retinochoroiditis in children with congenital toxoplasmosis: European, prospective cohort study. Pediatrics 2008; 121, 1215-22.
[13] Holland GN, Engstrom RE Jr, Glasgow BJ, Berger BB, Daniels SA, Sidikaro Y, Harmon JA, Fischer DH, Boyer DS, Rao NA, et al. Ocular toxoplasmosis in patients with the acquired immunodeficiency syndrome. Am J Ophthalmol 1988; 106: 653-67.
[14] Ronday MJ, Ongkosuwito JV, Rothova A, Kijlstra A. Intraocular anti-*Toxoplasma gondii* IgA antibody production in patients with ocular toxoplasmosis. Am J Ophthalmol 1999; 127: 294-300.
[15] Holland G. Ocular toxoplasmosis: the influence of patient age. Mem Inst Oswaldo Cruz 2009; 104: 351-7.
[16] Johnson MW, Greven GM, Jaffe GJ, Sudhalkar H, Vine AK. Atypical, severe toxoplasmic retinochoroiditis in elderly patients. Ophthalmology1997; 104: 48-57.
[17] Labalette P, Delhaes L, Margaron F, Fortier B, Rouland JF. Ocular toxoplasmosis after the fifth decade. Am J Ophthalmol 2002; 133: 506-15.
[18] Portela RW, Bethony J, Costa MI, Gazzinelli A, Vitor RW, Hermeto FM, Correa-Oliveira R, Gazzinelli RT. A multihousehold study reveals a positive correlation between age, severity of ocular toxoplasmosis, and levels of glycoinositolphospholipid-specific immunoglobulin A. J Infect Dis 2004; 190: 175-83.
[19] Bosch-Driessen LH, Berendscho TT, Ongkosuwito JV, Rothova A. Ocular toxoplasmosis: clinical features and prognosis of 154 patients. Ophthalmology 2002; 109, 869-78.
[20] Garweg JG, Scherrer JN, Halberstadt M. Recurrence Characteristics in European Patients with Ocular Toxoplasmosis. Br J Ophthalmol. 2008;92:1253-6.
[21] Holland GN, Crespi CM, ten Dam-van Loon N, Charonis AC, Yu F, Bosch-Driessen LH, Rothova A. Analysis of recurrence patterns associated with toxoplasmic retinochoroiditis. Am J Ophthalmol, 2008;145:1007-1013.
[22] Norose K, Mun HS, Aosai F, Chen M, Piao LX, Kobayashi M, Iwakura Y, Yano A. IFN-gamma-regulated Toxoplasma gondii distribution and load in the murine eye. Invest Ophthalmol Vis Sci 2003; 44: 4375-81.
[23] Meenken C, Rothova A, de Waal LP, van der Horst AR, Mesman BJ, Kijlstra A. HLA typing in congenital toxoplasmosis. Br J Ophthalmol1995; 79: 494-7.
[24] Jamieson SE, Cordell H, Petersen E, McLeod R, Gilbert RE, Blackwell JM. Host genetic and epigenetic factors in toxoplasmosis. Mem Inst Oswaldo Cruz 2009;104:162-9.
[25] Saeij J., Boyle JP, Boothroyd JC. Differences among the three major strains of *Toxoplasma gondii* and their specific interactions with the infected host. Trends Parasitol 2005; 21: 476-81.
[26] Su C, Khan A, Zhou P, Majumdar D, Ajzenberg D, Dardé ML, Zhu XQ, Ajioka JW, Rosenthal BM, Dubey JP, Sibley LD. Globally diverse *Toxoplasma gondii* isolates comprise six major clades originating from a small number of distinct ancestral lineages. Proc Natl Acad Sci U S A. 2012;109:5844-9.

[27] Howe DK, Honoré S, Derouin F, Sibley LD. Determination of genotypes of *Toxoplasma gondii* strains isolated from patients with toxoplasmosis. J Clin Microbiol 1997; 35:1411-4.

[28] Grigg ME, Ganatra J, Boothroyd JC, Margolis TP. Unusual abundance of atypical strains associated with human ocular toxoplasmosis. J Infect Dis 2001; 184: 633-9.

[29] Vallochi AL, Muccioli C, Martins MC, Silveira C, Belfort Jr R, Rizzo LV. The genotype of *Toxoplasma gondii* strains causing ocular toxoplasmosis in humans in Brazil. Am J Ophthalmol 2005; 139: 350-1.

[30] Khan A, Jordan C, Muccioli C, Vallochi AL, Rizzo LV, Belfort R Jr, Vitor RW, Silveira C, Sibley LD. Genetic divergence of *Toxoplasma gondii* strains associated with ocular toxoplasmosis, Brazil. Emerg Infect Dis 2006; 12: 942-9.

[31] Gilbert RE, Stanford MR, Jackson H, Holliman RE, Sanders MD. Incidence of acute symptomatic toxoplasma retinochoroiditis in south London according to country of birth. BMJ 1995; 310: 1037-40.

[32] Burnett AJ, Shortt SG, Isaac-Renton J, King A, Werker D, Bowie WR. Multiple cases of acquired toxoplasmosis retinitis presenting in an outbreak. Ophthalmology 1998; 105: 1032-7.

[33] Fekkar A, Ajzenberg D, Bodaghi B, Touafek F, Le Hoang P, Delmas J, Robert PY, Dardé ML, Mazier D, Paris L. Direct genotyping of *Toxoplasma gondii* in ocular fluid samples from 20 patients with ocular toxoplasmosis: predominance of type II in France. J Clin Microbiol. 2011;49:1513-7

[34] Hori J, Vega JL, Masli S. Review of ocular immune privilege in the year 2010: modifying the immune privilege of the eye. Ocul Immunol Inflamm 2010;18: 325-333.

[35] Streilein JW. Tissue barriers, immunosuppressive microenvironments, and privileged sites: the eye's point of view. Reg Immunol 1993; 5: 253-268.

[36] Forrester JV. Privilege revisited: an evaluation of the eye's defence mechanisms. Eye (Lond) 2009; 23: 756-766.

[37] Bora NS, Gobleman CL, Atkinson JP, Pepose JS and Kaplan HJ. Differential expression of the complement regulatory proteins in the human eye. Invest Ophthalmol Vis Sci 1993; 34(13): 3579-3584.

[38] Denniston AK, Kottoor SH, Khan I, Oswal K, Williams GP, Abbott J, Wallace GR, Salmon M, Rauz S, Murray PI, Curnow SJ. Endogenous cortisol and TGF-beta in human aqueous humor contribute to ocular immune privilege by regulating dendritic cell function. J Immunol 2011;186: 305-311.

[39] Zhou R, Horai R, Mattapallil MJ,Caspi RR. A new look at immune privilege of the eye: dual role for the vision-related molecule retinoic acid. J Immunol 2011;187: 4170-4177.

[40] Ferguson TA , Griffith TS. The role of Fas ligand and TNF-related apoptosis-inducing ligand (TRAIL) in the ocular immune response. Chem Immunol Allergy, 2007; 92: 140-154.

[41] Roychoudhury J, Herndon JM, Yin J, Apte RS and Ferguson TA. Targeting immune privilege to prevent pathogenic neovascularization. Invest Ophthalmol Vis Sci 2010; 51: 3560-3566.

[42] Denkers EY, Gazzinelli RT. Regulation and function of T-cell-mediated immunity during *Toxoplasma gondii* infection. Clin Microbiol Rev 1998 ;11: 569-588.
[43] Jones LA, Alexander J, Roberts CW. Ocular toxoplasmosis: in the storm of the eye. Parasite Immunol 2006; 28: 635-42.
[44] Nagineni CN, Pardhasaradhi K, Martins MC, Detrick B, Hooks JJ. Mechanisms of interferon-induced inhibition of *Toxoplasma gondii* replication in human retinal pigment epithelial cells. Infect Immun 1996; 64: 4188-96.
[45] Gazzinelli RT, Brezin A, Li Q, Nussenblatt RB, Chan CC. *Toxoplasma gondii*: acquired ocular toxoplasmosis in the murine model, protective role of TNF-alpha and IFN-gamma. Exp Parasitol, 1994; 78: 217-29.
[46] Gaddi PJ, Yap GS. Cytokine regulation of immunopathology in toxoplasmosis. Immunol Cell Biol 2007; 85:155-9.
[47] Delair E, Creuzet C, Dupouy-Camet J, Roisin MP. In vitro effect of TNF-alpha and IFN-gamma in retinal cell infection with *Toxoplasma gondii*. Invest Ophthalmol Vis Sci. 2009;50:1754-60.
[48] Yamamoto JH, Vallochi AL, Silveira C, Filho JK, Nussenblatt RB, Cunha-Neto E, Gazzinelli RT, Belfort R Jr, Rizzo LV. Discrimination between patients with acquired toxoplasmosis and congenital toxoplasmosis on the basis of the immune response to parasite antigens. J Infect Dis 2000; 181: 2018-22.
[49] Ongkosuwito JV, Feron EJ, van Doornik CE, Van der Lelij A, Hoyng CB, La Heij EC, Kijlstra A. Analysis of immunoregulatory cytokines in ocular fluid samples from patients with uveitis. Invest Ophthalmol Vis Sci 1998; 39: 2659-65.
[50] Yoshimura T, Sonoda KH, Ohguro N, Ohsugi Y, Ishibashi T, Cua DJ, Kobayashi T, Yoshida H, Yoshimura A.. Involvement of Th17 cells and the effect of anti-IL-6 therapy in autoimmune uveitis. Rheumatology (Oxford) 2009; 48:347-54.
[51] Lahmar I, Abou-Bacar A, Abdelrahman T, Guinard M, Babba H, Ben Yahia S, Kairallah M, Speeg-Schatz C, Bourcier T, Sauer A, Villard O, Pfaff AW, Mousli M, Garweg JG, Candolfi E. Cytokine profiles in toxoplasmic and viral uveitis. J Infect Dis 2009; 199: 1239-49.
[52] Garweg JG , Candolfi E. Immunopathology in ocular toxoplasmosis: facts and clues. Mem Inst Oswaldo Cruz 2009; 104: 211-20.
[53] Cordeiro CA, Moreira PR, Costa GC, Dutra WO, Campos WR, Oréfice F, Teixeira AL Interleukin-1 gene polymorphisms and toxoplasmic retinochoroiditis. Mol Vis 2008; 14: 1845-9.
[54] Cordeiro CA, Moreira PR, Costa GC, Dutra WO, Campos WR, Oréfice F, Teixeira AL.. TNF-alpha gene polymorphism (-308G/A) and toxoplasmic retinochoroiditis. Br J Ophthalmol 2008; 92: 986-8.
[55] Cordeiro CA, Moreira PR, Andrade MS, Dutra WO, Campos WR, Oréfice F, Teixeira AL. Interleukin-10 gene polymorphism (-1082G/A) is associated with toxoplasmic retinochoroiditis. Invest Ophthalmol Vis Sci 2008; 49: 1979-82.
[56] Albuquerque MC, Aleixo AL, Benchimol EI, Leandro AC, das Neves LB, Vicente RT, Bonecini-Almeida Mda G, Amendoeira MR. The IFN-gamma +874T/A gene

polymorphism is associated with retinochoroiditis toxoplasmosis susceptibility. Mem Inst Oswaldo Cruz, 2009, 104, 451-5.
[57] Delair E, Latkany P, Noble AG, Rabiah P, McLeod R and Brezin AP. Clinical manifestations of ocular toxoplasmosis. Ocul Immunol Inflamm 2011; 19: 91-102.
[58] Kovačević-Pavićević D, Radosavljević A, Ilić A, Kovačević I, Djurković-Djaković O. Clinical pattern of ocular toxoplasmosis treated in a referral centre in Serbia. Eye (Lond) 2012;26:723-8
[59] Garweg JG, de Groot-Mijnes JD and Montoya JG. Diagnostic approach to ocular toxoplasmosis. Ocul Immunol Inflamm 2011; 19: 255-261.
[60] Robert-Gangneux F, Binisti P, Antonetti D, Brezin A, Yera H, Dupouy-Camet J. Usefulness of immunoblotting and Goldmann-Witmer coefficient for biological diagnosis of toxoplasmic retinochoroiditis. Eur J Clin Microbiol Infect Dis 2004; 23:34–38.
[61] Brezin AP, Eqwuagu CE, Silveira C, Thulliez P, Martins MC, Mahdi RM, Belfort Jr R, Nussenblatt RB. Analysis of aqueous humor in ocular toxoplasmosis. N Engl J Med 1991; 324:699.
[62] de Boer JH, Verhagen C, Bruinenberg M, Rothova A, de Jong PT, Baarsma GS, Van der Lelij A, Ooyman FM, Bollemeijer JG, Derhaag PJ, Kijlstra A. Serologic and polymerase chain reaction analysis of intraocular fluids in the diagnosis of infectious uveitis. Am J Ophthalmol 1996; 121:650–658.
[63] De Groot-Mijnes JD, Rothova A, Van Loon AM, Schuller M, Ten Dam-Van Loon NH, De Boer JH, Schuurman R, Weersink AJ. Polymerase chain reaction and Goldmann-Witmer coefficient analysis are complimentary for the diagnosis of infectious uveitis. Am J Ophthalmol 2006;141:313–318.
[64] Fardeau C, Romand S, Rao NA, Cassoux N, Bettembourg O, Thulliez P, Lehoang P.Diagnosis of toxoplasmic retinochoroiditis with atypical clinical features. Am J Ophthalmol 2002;134:196–203.
[65] Fekkar A , Bodaghi B, Touafek F, Le Hoang P, Mazier D, Paris L. Comparison of immunoblotting, calculation of the Goldmann-Witmer coefficient, and real-time PCR using aqueous humor samples for diagnosis of ocular toxoplasmosis. J Clin Microbiol 2008; 46:1965–1967.
[66] Villard, O., D. Filisetti, F. Roch-Deries, J. Garweg, J. Flament, and E. Candolfi. Comparison of enzyme-linked immunosorbent assay, immunoblotting, and PCR for diagnosis of toxoplasmic chorioretinitis. J Clin Microbiol 2003; 41:3537–3541.
[67] Westeneng AC, Rothova A, de Boer JH, de Groot-Mijnes J. Infectious uveitis in immunocompromised patients and the diagnostic value of polymerase chain reaction and Goldmann-Witmer coefficient in aqueous analysis. Am J Ophthalmol 2007;144:781–785.
[68] Talabani H, Asseraf M, Yera H, Delair E, Ancelle T, Thulliez P, Brézin AP, Dupouy-Camet J.Contributions of immunoblotting, real-time PCR, and the Goldmann-Witmer coefficient to diagnosis of atypical toxoplasmic retinochoroiditis. J Clin Microbiol 2009; 47: 2131-5.

[69] Garweg JG, Jacquier P, Boehnke M. Early aqueous humor analysis in patients with human ocular toxoplasmosis. J Clin Microbiol 2000, 38:996–1001
[70] Garweg JG, Garweg SD, Flueckiger F, Jacquier P, Boehnke M. Aqueous humor and serum immunoblotting for immunoglobulin types G, A, M, and E in cases of human ocular toxoplasmosis. J Clin Microbiol 2004; 42:4593–4598.
[71] Cassaing S, Bessieres MH, Berry A, Berrebi A, Fabre R, Magnaval JF. Comparison between two amplification sets for molecular diagnosis of toxoplasmosis by real-time PCR. J. Clin. Microbiol 2006; 44:720–724.
[72] Rothova A, de Boer JH, Ten Dam-van Loon NH, Postma G, de Visser L, Zuurveen SJ, Schuller M, Weersink AJ,. M. van Loon A, de Groot-Mijnes JD. Usefulness of aqueous humor analysis for the diagnosis of posterior uveitis. Ophthalmology 2008;115:306–311.
[73] Stanford MR, Gilbert RE. Treating ocular toxoplasmosis: current evidence. Mem Inst Oswaldo Cruz 2009;104: 312-315.
[74] de-la-Torre A, Stanford M, Curi A, Jaffe GJ and Gomez-Marin JE. Therapy for ocular toxoplasmosis. Ocul Immunol Inflamm 2011; 19: 314-320
[75] Vance SK, Freund KB, Wenick AS, Nguyen QD, Holland GN and Kreiger AE. Diagnostic and therapeutic challenges. Retina 2011;31: 1224-1230.
[76] Wakefield D, Cunningham ET Jr., Pavesio C, Garweg JG, Zierhut M. Controversies in ocular toxoplasmosis. Ocul Immunol Inflamm 2011;19: 2-9.
[77] Bosch-Driessen LH, Verbraak FD, Suttorp-Schulten MS, van Ruyven RL, Klok AM, Hoyng CB and Rothova A. A prospective, randomized trial of pyrimethamine and azithromycin vs pyrimethamine and sulfadiazine for the treatment of ocular toxoplasmosis. Am J Ophthalmol 2002; 134(1): 34-40.
[78] Yazici A, Ozdal PC, Taskintuna I, Kavuncu S and Koklu G. Trimethoprim/Sulfamethoxazole and azithromycin combination therapy for ocular toxoplasmosis. Ocul Immunol Inflamm 2009;17: 289-291.
[79] Bosch-Driessen LH and Rothova A. Sense and nonsense of corticosteroid administration in the treatment of ocular toxoplasmosis. Br J Ophthalmol 1998; 82(8): 858-860.
[80] Djurkovic-Djakovic O, Stanojevic-Paovic A, Bobic B, Bergam J, Nikolic A, Paovic J, Vukovic D. Short-term effects of the clindamycin-steroid regimen in the treatment of ocular toxoplasmosis. J Chemother. 1995 Nov;7 Suppl 4:199-201
[81] McLeod R, Kieffer F, Sautter M, Hosten T, Pelloux H. Why prevent, diagnose and treat congenital toxoplasmosis? Mem Inst Oswaldo Cruz. 2009;104:320-44.
[82] Gilbert R. Treatment for congenital toxoplasmosis: finding out what works. Mem Inst Oswaldo Cruz 2009; 104: 305-311.
[83] Faucher B, Garcia-Meric P, Franck J, Minodier P, Francois P, Gonnet S, L'Ollivier C and Piarroux R. Long-term ocular outcome in congenital toxoplasmosis: A prospective cohort of treated children. J Infect 2012; 64: 104-109.
[84] Sauer A, de la Torre A, Gomez-Marin J, Bourcier T, Garweg J, Speeg-Schatz C, Candolfi E. Prevention of retinochoroiditis in congenital toxoplasmosis: Europe versus South America. Pediatr Infect Dis J. 2011; 30:601-3.

[85] Peyron F, Garweg JG, Wallon M, Descloux E, Rolland M, Barth J. Long-term impact of treated congenital toxoplasmosis on quality of life and visual performance. Pediatr Infect Dis J 2011; 30:597-600.

[86] Wallon M, Kieffer F, Binquet C, Thulliez P, Garcia-Méric P, Dureau P, Franck J, Peyron F, Bonnin A, Villena I, Bonithon-Kopp C, Gouyon JB, Masson S, Félin A, Cornu C. Congenital toxoplasmosis: randomised comparison of strategies for retinochoroiditis prevention. Therapie 2011; 66:473-80. French.

Chapter 8

Immunological and Immunogenetic Parameters on the Diversity of Ocular Toxoplasmosis: Evidence to Support Morphological Criteria to Classify Retinal/Retinochoroidal Scar Lesions in Epidemiologic Surveys

Lílian M.G. Bahia-Oliveira, Alba L.P. Rangel, Marcela S.B. Boechat, Bianca M. Mangiavacchi, Livia M. Martins, Francielle B. Ferraz, Maycon B. Almeida, Elisa M. Waked Peixoto, Flavia P. Vieira and Ricardo G. Peixe

Additional information is available at the end of the chapter

http://dx.doi.org/10.5772/50086

1. Introduction

Toxoplasmosis is highly prevalent in Brazil, where its prevalence ranks among the highest in the world. However, the prevalence of ocular toxoplasmosis may vary from one region to another within the country, even in the face of seroprevalence of the same magnitude. For over a decade we have been studying toxoplasmosis in Campos dos Goytacazes, which has amongst the highest prevalence of the condition already reported. Local social and environmental peculiarities influence the risk factors and impact the seroprevalence when analyses are performed in local populations stratified by socioeconomic status [1]. Campos dos Goytacazes, usually referred to as Campos, is located in the northern state of Rio de Janeiro in the most important oil-producing region of Brazil. The city is composed of an area equivalent to 4,027 km^2, and with 463.731 inhabitants, it is the third most economically important city in the state of Rio de Janeiro. Some aspects related to the natural history of toxoplasmosis in Campos are connected to its historic past with respect to economic agricultural and rural activities that were linked to the Sugar Cane economy. Sugar production prevailed as the most important economic activity until the mid-80s, at which point it began gradually giving way to activities related to oil. The city still preserves its spatial organization and cultural points, which are characteristics of a city with strong rural features.

In areas with a high prevalence of infectious and parasitic diseases, such as toxoplasmosis in Campos, several challenges are posed to the health authorities with regard to diagnoses, accurate assessment of incidence and prevalence, and clinical management of disease symptoms. Our studies in toxoplasmosis have focused on the natural history, epidemiology, immune response and immunogenetics of infected individuals in order to better understand the clinical presentation of the disease. In this chapter, we present in four sections, data related to 1) the diversity of presumable toxoplasmic retinal/retinochoroidal scar lesion presentations in comparison to other population-based studies of the same nature in Brazil; 2) the profile of the *in vitro* immune response of patients in the context of the clinical presentation of ocular toxoplasmosis; 3) evidence for candidate genes that are associated with susceptibility for or protection against the development of toxoplasmic retinal lesions; and 4) the association of ocular toxoplasmosis with other infectious diseases.

2. The diversity of retinal/retinochoroidal scar lesions in *T. gondii* hyperendemic areas of Brazil

In the past, most *T. gondii* retinochoroiditis was thought to be of congenital infection origin. However, it is currently accepted that ocular disease is most likely the most common potentially severe symptomatic manifestation in acute, postnatally acquired toxoplasmosis [2, 3]. The epidemiologic studies in Brazil have contributed to changing that traditional belief. In the country, toxoplasmosis is the most frequent cause of infectious uveitis, as in many other nations [4-9,56,57]. The prevalence of ocular toxoplasmosis in areas highly endemic for *T. gondii* in Brazil has an important public health impact and differs among areas of similar seroprevalence. Population-based studies involving people of ages ranging from 10 years to older than 50 years from different regions of the country have shown that the prevalence of retinochoroiditis varies from 2.6% to 17.7% [4-8].

The population-based studies that are used to estimate ocular disease caused by *T. gondii* infection depend on the observation of retinal/retinochoroidal lesion scars via fundoscopic examinations, and as in epidemiologic surveys, it is not common to find patients with active toxoplasmic lesions. The observed difference in ocular prevalence, even in face of similar seroprevalence has oriented studies to better understand and identify the risk factors for infection and for the development of toxoplasmic ocular disease.

Holland and associates in 1996 [3] report the three types of retinochoroidal lesions in otherwise healthy patients, described in 1969 by Friedmann and Knox, which are based on the localization in the retina, size, vitreous inflammatory reaction and probable prognosis in terms of complications or decreased vision. However, for epidemiologic surveys, the lack of a classification system or a consensual proposal to describe scar lesions presumably caused by *T. gondii* infections certainly impacts the final prevalence that is determined in various studies and, perhaps more importantly, fails to describe asymptomatic, less severe scar lesions confined to the retinal pigment epithelium (RPE) that are not commonly seen by ophthalmologists in clinical settings. Such lesions might be important not only from an epidemiological point of view itself, but, if well studied, they could perhaps aid in the development of new therapeutic approaches that may benefit patients who have more severe forms of disease, especially recurrent forms of ocular toxoplasmosis.

In light of these considerations, subjective criteria certainly influence the clinical diagnosis of ocular toxoplasmosis in population-based studies, which are based on the appearance of inactive retinal/retinochoroidal scar lesions left by presumed toxoplasmic lesions that were previously active. In addition, the ophthalmologists' clinical experience on the resolution of active lesions is important for the recognition of retinal/retinochoroidal toxoplasmic scar lesions.

An important epidemiological study conducted in Brazil by Glasner and associates in 1992 reported a ranking of probability for the classification of retinal scar lesions that are presumably caused by *T. gondii* infection [4]. The system was established by the authors to try to estimate the actual prevalence of ocular toxoplasmosis in a highly endemic area for *T. gondii* infection located in a small village in southern Brazil called Erechim. According to the authors, on the basis of a conservative assessment of ophthalmic findings, 17.7% of the patients (184 out of 1042 examined) were considered to have ocular toxoplasmosis. They categorized the different types of lesions that were identified during the examination of 1042 individuals and organized them into five groups numbered 1 through 5 according to the probability that the lesion was caused by *T. gondii* infection. Those classified from grade one to grade three were considered to be definitively caused by *T. gondii* infection [4]. We found the authors' initiative very important, and with the same objective, we have proposed some descriptive criteria to classify the most commonly found retinal/retinochoroidal lesions from our population-based work in Campos dos Goytacazes [7, 10, 11]. However, as mentioned earlier, the nature of the toxoplasmic retinal/retinochoroidal scar lesions, or even active lesions described during the fundoscopic examination, is subjective. Thus, the decision as to whether a scar lesion was caused by *T. gondii* infection depends, to some extent, on subjective criteria. To minimize the intrinsic characteristic of this decisional process, in population-based studies, a group of ophthalmologists consensually decide which scar lesions have the greatest probability of being caused by toxoplasmic infection. During this process, the ophthalmologists are usually uninformed as to whether the patient serology is positive or negative for *T. gondii*.

There is a type of retinal/retinochoroidal scar lesion that is universally accepted as being healed from active retinal/retinochoroidal inflammation caused by *T. gondii* infection. These scars usually result from the active typically visible yellow-white focus with fluffy borders, which may or may not be accompanied by vitreous inflammation that limits the visualization of the posterior pole [12]. However, there exist other lesions that are equally recognized by specialists as toxoplasmic lesions, termed as "atypical" toxoplasmic lesions, and their active forms have been reviewed [3, 12]. The frequency of scar lesions healed from "atypical" active toxoplasmic lesions in population-based studies is not well known because in previous studies, with the intent of avoiding an over estimation of ocular toxoplasmosis, only scars healed from typical lesions, which are most likely equally typical in terms of toxoplasmic retinochoroidal scar lesion representativeness, have been usually used to infer the ocular prevalence of *T. gondii* infection in epidemiologic surveys. As a consequence, identifying the actual prevalence of ocular toxoplasmosis in areas highly endemic for *T. gondii* in Brazil constitutes a challenge in practice and may be underestimated. In fact, the existence of retinal/retinochoroidal scars most likely healed from non-typical toxoplasmic retinal/retinochoroidal lesions have been reported in endemic areas [4, 7, 9-11, 13] as discussed later in this section.

Two groups working independently in Rio de Janeiro state, one from the State University of North Fluminense (UENF) at Campos dos Goytacazes and another from the Oswaldo Cruz Foundation, have conducted epidemiological and human immunogenetic studies that can be directly compared because the same criteria for ocular scar lesions classification was adopted for both [9, 11]. The criteria for characterizing scar lesions that were presumably caused by *T. gondii* infection adopted by both groups were based on the morphological aspects of the scars, primarily the pigmentation and the degree of retinal tissue damage. The lesions were termed as type A, type B or type C by the Campos dos Goytacazes group [7, 11] and as type 1, type 2 or type 3, respectively, by the Oswaldo Cruz Foundation group [9]. The Oswaldo Cruz group investigated the retinochoroiditis caused by *T. gondii* infection in a rural area (Santa Rita) of Barra Mansa, located at southern part of the Rio de Janeiro state [9]. Campos dos Goytacazes and Santa Rita are both supplied by the Paraíba do Sul River, which supplies water to approximately 4.8 million persons in Brazil. The cities are located approximately 390 km from each other; Campos at north of the state and Barra Mansa in the south.

In 2005, the Campos group published a proposal (in Portuguese) to categorize/classify the diverse foci of retinochoroiditis scars found in a survey conducted from 1997-1999 on the prevalence and risk factors for *T. gondii* infection. In the proposal, the group termed the toxoplasmic scar lesion foci as type I, type II or type III [10]. In a previous publication of 2001 [7], the Campos group had termed such lesions as type A, type B and type C, respectively. However, because of the possibility of confusion and some relation with the three archetypal *T. gondii* lineages, which are termed type I, II or III based on the genomic sequence associated with their virulence in mice [14, 15], we returned to the original classification nomenclature of type A, type B and type C [7, 11]. The following descriptions in quotes are related to the three classes of retinal/retinochoroidal foci scars found in *T. gondii* seropositive individuals in endemic areas to toxoplasmosis published by both the Campos and Oswaldo Cruz Foundation groups: "class A lesions present well-marked boundaries, usually surrounded by a pigmented halo and extensive destruction of the retina and choroid. Class B lesions are characterized by a surrounding hypopigmented halo and a smaller degree of tissue destruction in comparison to class A. Class C lesions are basically areas of retinal pigment epithelium hyperplasia or atrophy with a smaller degree of tissue destruction compared to class A and B" [11] and "type 1 lesions boundaries are well marked with a halo of hyperpigmentation and central area of retinochoroidal atrophy, type 2 lesions with hypopigmented halo and central hyperpigmented area and type 3 lesions hyperpigmented or hypopigmented consistent with hyperplasia or atrophy of the retinal pigment epithelium" [1] [9].

---

[1] Translated from the original publication in Portuguese (ref.9)

Figure 1 shows representative type A, B and C scar lesions that appear isolated in one or both eyes as well as multiple lesions of different types (AB, ABC, AC and BC) in one or both eyes. Type A and B scar lesions have a higher probability of being recognized by ophthalmologists as being caused by *T. gondii* infection. Certainly, out of the context of epidemiological surveys to estimate ocular toxoplasmosis, type C scar lesions would, with very low probability, be considered as retinal scars healed from ocular toxoplasmosis. Some aspects intrinsic to this type of scar lesion led us to believe they are caused by *T. gondii* infection; these are i) their high frequency in patients who are seropositive for *T. gondii*; ii) their common association with the more typical type A and B scar lesions; and iii) their differentiated profile of the specific *in vitro* cellular immune response of patients presenting this type of lesion compared to *T. gondii* seropositive patients who present no ocular lesions. We have evidence that the profile of their specific *in vitro* cellular immune response is most likely a result of a very efficient mild to minimal inflammatory intraocular reaction against *T. gondii* that causes only superficial injury to RPE, which can result in pigmented or apigmented scars, as we shall see later in this chapter.

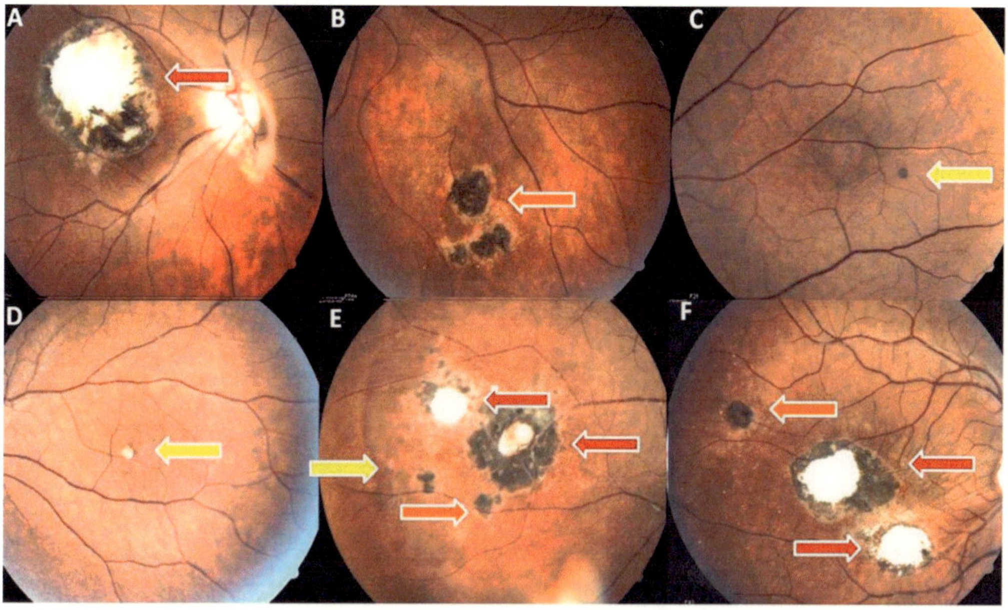

Figure 1. Fundus photograph of representative retinal/retinochoroidal non-active scar lesions. Panel A and panel B represent single type A and B scar lesions, respectively. Panels C and D represent single type C scar lesions that are hyper- and hypopigmented, respectively. The scar lesions by type are indicated by colored arrows: red represents type A scar lesions, orange represents type B scar lesions and yellow indicates type C scar lesions. The two pictures at the bottom (panels E and F) show multiple scar lesions of type ABC (with arrows red, orange and yellow) and a multiple scar lesion of type AB (with arrows red and orange).

In a survey conducted in 1997-1999 to investigate the seroprevalence of toxoplasmosis in Campos [1], during which 1436 persons were investigated and the local waterborne nature of *T. gondii* infection was shown, the study population was divided into three socio-economic strata. In addition to other factors, the geographic localization of the selected people was important for differential *T. gondii* seroprevalence levels. Then, for the groups living in slums and rural areas from Campos who shared the same lower socio-economic strata termed as population 1 (P1), the *T. gondii* age adjusted serumprevalence was 84% [1]. For the middle and upper socioeconomic groups, termed as population 2 (P2) and population 3 (P3), 62% and 23% of *T. gondii* age adjusted seroprevalence was identified, respectively. However, the lower age adjusted seroprevalence of toxoplasmosis observed for P3 (23%) and P2 (62%) in comparison with P1 (84%) [1] contrasted with the similar overall ocular prevalence found for the three populations namely, P3 (12%), P2 (10%) and P1 (12%) [7]. It is important to mention that for the estimation of ocular disease prevalence caused by *T. gondii* infection in Campos, which was published in 2001, a more conservative basis for diagnose was adopted. The diagnosis considered only the typical appearance of retinochoroidal scar lesions for the prevalence calculation [7]. For the Santa Rita study, which will be compared to the Campos study, only the population living in rural areas was evaluated, and the *T. gondii* seroprevalence was found to be 65.9%; however, no risk factor was reported [7]. For the Campos study, we observed that despite the same seroprevalence among those living in rural areas and those living in slums (both from P1 strata), the prevalence of ocular disease was different. Namely, when the lower socio-economic strata were sub-stratified according to people living in rural areas and those living in slums, we found that the prevalence of ocular disease was 14% for those living in rural areas and 8% for those living in slums [7]. For the Santa Rita study, which involved only the rural community, ocular disease prevalence was reported as 5.8%.

For the past six years, we have conducted randomized samplings of individuals older than 10 years belonging to P1 and P2 (lower and middle socio-economic strata, respectively, from the total Campos population). We have collected peripheral venal blood for *T. gondii* serologic evaluation and patients have been examined by indirect ophthalmoscopy . Some patients who may have participated from the previous survey [1] were re-evaluated clinically and serologically by collecting new blood samples for the immunological and immunogenetic studies. The results of the serologic prevalence and the prevalence of ocular disease from 411 patients that were examined over the past six years are reported in Table 1 to compare our results with the Santa Rita study population.

The frequencies of types of scar lesions, considering the total number of patients who presented scar lesions in each study, are shown in the Table 1. There were 41 persons with scar lesions out of 706 *T. gondii* seropositive individuals from Santa Rita and 94 subjects with scar lesions out 314 *T. gondii* seropositive individuals from Campos. We observed that the frequency of type A (type 1) lesions was much higher in Santa Rita (41.5%) than in Campos (19.1,%) and that the most frequent type of scar lesion per patient from Campos was type C (28.7%); in Santa Rita, the frequency of the type C (Type 3) scar lesion was 12.2%. Curiously, the frequency of type B (type 2) lesions was very similar in both areas: 24.4% in Santa Rita and 24.5% in Campos. The sum of multiple lesions types in both areas was also similar. Namely, the sum of the frequency of individuals who presented AB + ABC + AC + BC as well as 1 and 2 + 1 and 2 and 3 + 1 and 3 + 2 and 3 scar lesions was 27.7% and 22% for Campos and Santa Rita, respectively.

	Santa Rita (Barra Mansa)			Campos dos Goytacazes	
	n	%		n	%
Study population	1071			411	
T. gondii seropositivity	706	65.9		314	76.6
Type of scar lesions	n	%	Type of scar lesions	n	%
1	17	41.5	A	18	19.1
2	10	24.4	B	23	24.5
3	5	12.2	C	27	28.7
1 and 2	2	4.9	AB	9	9.6
1 and 3	4	9.8	AC	2	2.1
2 and3	2	4.9	BC	7	7.4
1, 2 and 3	1	2.4	ABC	8	8.5
Total	41	5.8%	Total	94	11.7 %*

* The total prevalence of ocular disease in Campos can be expressed in three levels.
1- Considering only the persons who present type A scar lesions, which are those universally recognized as being healed from the typical toxoplasmic retinochoroidal active lesions. This value is calculated as the sum of single type A scar lesions (n=18) plus the multiple type lesions that contain the type A scar lesion,(AB n=9) + (AC n=2) + (ABC n=8), totaling 37 individuals. This gives the prevalence of ocular disease of 11.7%.
2- Considering the individuals who present type A single and multiple type scar lesions plus the individuals presenting type B single (n=23) plus multiple type lesions (BC n=7), which adds up to a total of 67 individuals and gives a prevalence of 21.33%.
3- Considering all the people who present type A and type B single and multiple type lesions and persons who present with type C scar lesions, which totals 94 individuals and gives a prevalence of 29.9%.

Table 1. Comparison Between the *T. gondii* Seroprevalence and Retinal/Retinochoroidal Scar Lesions Prevalence from Campos dos Goytacazes (RJ) and Santa Rita (Barra Mansa-RJ)

Considering that out of 411 clinically and serologically examined patients 314 were seropositive for *T. gondii*, the seroprevalence was estimated at 76.6%. This prevalence represents the intermediate value between the prevalence observed for P1 (84%) and P2 (62%) reported in 2003 [1] and calculated by P1(84%) + P2(62%)/2 = 73%. The same was observed for the expected and found toxoplasmic ocular prevalence; i.e., adopting the same highly conservative criteria of 2001 to compute toxoplasmic scar lesions and considering only the individuals who presented typical lesions (type A scar single or multiple lesions, i.e., the sum of type A scar lesions plus scar lesions of type AB, ABC and AC), we found a toxoplasmic ocular prevalence of 11.7% (37 out of 314 individuals). Once again, the prevalence corresponded to that would be expected from that observed in 2001: 10% for P1 and 12% for P2 [7], as P1(10 %) + P2(12%)/2 = 11%. However, if we consider type B and type BC scar lesions together with type A and type AB, ABC, and AC scar lesions to calculate the toxoplasmic ocular prevalence in Campos, we find 21.33% (67 out of 314). Furthermore, if we additionally consider type C scar lesions to calculate the frequency, the prevalence of toxoplasmic ocular lesions in Campos increases to 29.9% (94 out of 314). It is important to keep in mind that the prevalence values are related to the population extract P1 plus P2 older than 10 years and that it is after the age of 10 that we observe a substantial increase in

T. gondii seroprevalence for P1 and P2, based on previous studies in Campos [1]. Furthermore, it is only after 10 years of age that we observe the elevation of ocular toxoplasmosis prevalence in population-based studies in general [2].

In the context of the diversity of retinal/retinochoroidal scar lesions found in epidemiologic surveys in Brazil, another important report from the Erechim area was conducted by Silveira and associates in 1999 [13], seven years after the study conducted by Glasner and associates in 1992 [4]. A group of patients that were previously examined in 1992 presented a type of hyperpigmented scar lesion presumably caused by *T. gondii* infection and termed as "atypical" in comparison with those were termed as "typical" lesions. Some of those patients had "atypical" scar lesions that evolved to "typical" toxoplasmic retinal lesions in the time frame of 7 years. The description of the hyperpigmented "atypical" lesions from patients of Erechim fulfills all but one of the criteria we have used to classify type B toxoplasmic scar lesions in Campos [13]. The difference between Silveira's description and our description is that we do not consider size to define the type of scar in any of our classification criteria. Instead, we consider the type of pigment distribution in the scar and the degree of the retinal tissue damage, namely the degree of tissue damage that can be inferred by indirect opththalmoscopy, considering the natural limitations for this type of examination in terms of tissue evaluation damage. In the referred study from Erechim, Silveira and associates showed that at 7-year follow-up, 3 persons of 13 subjects presented "atypical" scar lesions that evolved to "typical" toxoplasmic retinochoroidal scars. They concluded that the typical new lesions arose from or adjacent to the pre-existing atypical lesions in two of the three patients based on photographs and drawing of atypical scar lesion location seven years prior [13].

As stated earlier, the criteria used to classify scar lesions as type A, B or C are morphological based on the pigment appearance and the degree of retinal damage. However, we believe that information regarding their size and localization could be useful for future comparative studies in other endemic areas of Brazil and abroad. We present the frequency of localization and sizes of 85 scar lesions from 49 patients, some of which were involved in immunological and immunogenetic studies conducted in Campos [16-18]. In Figure 2, a fundoscopy picture from a normal (presenting no retinal damage) individual is shown. The numbers indicate four retinal region (code/index) that are used to compute the scar lesion localization for frequency calculation purposes, as shown in Table 2. Each retinal region shown in Figure 2 is assigned an arbitrary number (index/code) as follows: equatorial (1), macula (2), posterior pole / macula (3), posterior pole (4); the periphery (5) shown in Table 2 does not appear in Figure 2 because it is not usually visible in fundoscopic pictures. Each scar lesion was computed independently if an individual exhibited more than one type of scar lesion in one or both eyes, such as A, B or C or a combination of types, such as AB, AC, ABC, or BC, irrespective of their locations. Thus, from the 49 individuals who presented scar lesions, a total of 15 type A scar lesions, 34 type B scar lesions and 36 type C scar lesions were considered for analysis, totaling 85 scar lesions.The median value of scar from the most severe lesions (type A) that was 2, presentes a numeric value (index/code) arbitrarily attributed to denote location on the retina, that was lower compared to values observed for the locations of type B (median value= 4) and C (median value =5) scar lesions. This fact illustrates that the median locations of type A scar lesions (median value =2) are preferably in regions closer to the macula (see Figure 2), whereas type C lesions are preferentially located in peripheral regions of retina. The statistical comparison among the different types of toxoplasmic scar lesion locations was tested using a Kruskal-Wallis test followed by a Dunns test. A significant difference ($p \leq 0.01$) was found between the localization of type A scars and type C scars. No significant difference between the locations of type A and B scar lesions was found. Between type B and type C scar lesions, a significant difference ($p < 0.01$) was also found.

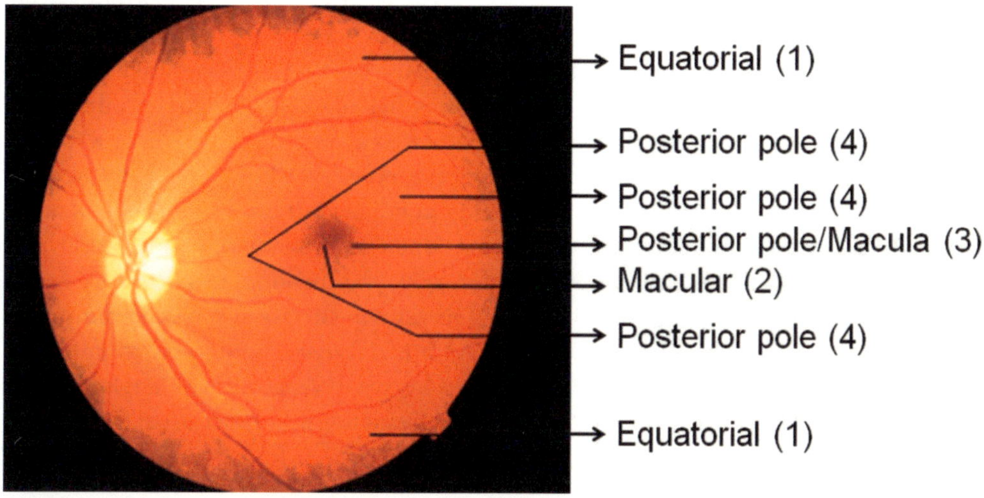

Figure 2. Fundoscopic photograph of a normal retina indicating the regions: equatorial (1) macular (2), posterior pole/macula (3) and posterior pole (4). Region 5, which corresponds to the periphery, is not shown (see text and Table 2).

Lesion localization region	Location Code (Index) of lesion in retina	Frequency of occurrence (n) of each scar type lesion
Equatorial	1	A(6) B (15) C (9)
Macular	2	A(5) B (1) C (0)
Posterior pole/Macula	3	A(1) B (0) C (0)
Posterior pole	4	A(1) B (5) C (2)
Periphery	5	A(2) B (13) C (25)

Table 2. Frequency of the Topographic Location of Retinal/Retinochoroidal Scar Lesions of type A, type B and type C in the retina

The sizes of the same 85 scar lesions were also measured in terms of optic disc size (disc diameter, dd) at the slit lamp with a 78 D lens in a normal clinical ophthalmoscopic examination.. Table 3 shows the scar lesion types sizes that were categorized in 4 size ranges: 0 to 0.5 dd, 0.6 to 1 dd, 1.1 to 1.5 dd, and 1.6 to 2.0 dd. The four size ranges corresponded to a code/index number from 1 to 4, respectively, for the statistical analysis objective. The diameter of the optical disc of each subject was used as a parameter for determining the size of the scar lesions of the same person. There is no proportional relationship defined between the disc diameter and the arbitrary attributed code/index number. The frequency of occurrence by size of each of the 15 type A scar lesions, 34 type B and 36 type C scar lesions is shown in Table 3, where the three scar type sizes were compared in terms of the relationship between the type and the size range measured for the disc diameter (dd), as explained above. The type A scar lesions (healed from the most severe lesions) exhibited sizes significantly larger (median value = 2.2) $p \leq 0.001$ than the type C scar lesions (median value = 1.0) but not significantly larger than type B scar lesions (median value =1.8), which are of middle severity in terms of retinal damage. A significant difference ($p \leq 0.001$) relative to the size of the type B ocular scar lesions was also observed in comparison with type C scar lesions, which were on average smaller than type B lesions. It is important to mention that the age of the patient can influence the size of the optical nerve (diameter) [19], which can interfere with these types of measurements. However, the average age between groups did not differ statistically, and therefore this factor likely did not affect our evaluation. Nonetheless, the size measurement was not considered in our proposed criteria to classify scar type lesions, and it is discussed here solely to provide a better representation of the diversity of the scar lesions we have found with a reference for the measurement, which can be useful for comparative studies in other areas from Brazil and abroad.

Size of lesion in diameter disk (dd)	Size code (index) of retinal lesion	Frequency of occurrence (n) of each lesion type
0 – 0.5	1	A(3) B (17) C (35)
0.6 – 1	2	A(7) B (9) C (1)
1.1 – 1.5	3	A(2) B (6) C (0)
1.6 – 2.0	4	A(3) B (2) C (0)

Table 3. Frequency of the Size of Retinal/Retinochoroidal Scar Lesions of type A, type B and type C in the Retina

The average age between groups did not differ statistically. The average age of patients presenting scar lesions of type A was 44 yrs and AC 52 yrs which are higher in comparison with the other types of lesions (type B, BC and ABC 29 yrs, type AB 32 yrs and type C 36 yrs) and consistent with previous findings that have shown that age is an important factor for the severity of ocular toxoplasmosis [20]. Nevertheless, if we assume that the "atypical" hypermigmented scar lesions that were described to occur in *T. gondii* seropositive patients from Erechim [13] are the same type of type B scar lesion we describe for patients from

Campos, the data are similar regarding the age of the patients presenting those lesions, which were more common among younger patients (under 17 years of age) compared to older individuals [13]. This fact might indicate that type B scar lesions would be related to more recent infections. Unfortunately, age as a function of the type of scar lesion was not reported in the Santa Rita study [9]. We can conclude from the set of data presented and reported from other studies that the lack of a set of consensual criteria for scar lesions presumably caused by *T. gondii* infection may account, at least partially, for the differences in the reports of categorization/classification of toxoplasmic ocular prevalence observed in Brazil.

3. Immunological parameters in the context of the diversity of retinal/retinochoroidal scar lesions from *T. gondii* seropositive patients

T. gondii infection in both mice and humans is characterized by a host response with high levels of pro-inflammatory cytokines, such as interleukin 12 (IL-12), tumor necrosis factor (TNF)-α and interferon gamma (IFN- γ), all of which have been implicated in both the regulation of parasitic replication in the host as well as in the ocular pathology [11, 16, 21-24]. The importance of the immune response of patients infected with *T. gondii* against the parasite has been recognized, together with other variables comprising the multifactorial nature of ocular toxoplasmosis. In this section, we present results from the *in vitro* parameters of the cellular immune response of *T. gondii* seropositive patients with and without ocular retinal/retinochoroidal scars and control groups of seronegative patients exposed to the same risk of infection, which involved the consumption of untreated water from wells or other natural water sources [1], against soluble antigens from *T. gondii* tachyzoite forms (STAg). Cytokines, chemokines, and isotypes of immunoglobulins have been evaluated in an effort to identify potential predictive factors for the development or prevention of ocular disease. All of the immunological parameters have been analyzed considering different groups of patients arranged according to the similarity in the retinal/retinochoroidal scar lesion group.

A pro-inflammatory specific T helper 1 (Th-1) oriented response is observed mainly in groups of patients presenting retinochoroidal scar healed from severe lesions, which suggests that the exacerbation of the immune response can be related to tissue damage, and its attenuation/regulation may be related to the development of minor retinal damages. The central role of IFN-γ seems to be important in both cases, namely, in exacerbated and in the regulated context of in vitro cellular immune response, suggesting that the cellular immune responses against *T. gondii* in the eye should be suitably tailored [11, 16, 21-23], as we shall see later. Other molecules and cells related to the regulation of secretion of IFN-γ include IL-13, chemokines, isotypes of immunoglobulins, NK cells and T CD8 lymphocytes in relation to the development or prevention of development of toxoplasmic ocular pathology have also been investigated [11, 16, 21, 22]. The immunological parameters studied have also made way for the election of candidate genes to be investigated in studies of genetic association with ocular toxoplasmosis, as we shall see in the next section.

However, we have evaluated many immunological parameters we have chosen three to better illustrate the profile of the cellular immune response as a function of the type of scar lesion presented by patients. The first is IFN-γ, the prototype of Th-1 response that has been shown to be of vital importance for inducing anti-*T. gondii* effectors mechanisms to control the parasite replication in the host [25]. The second, IL-13, is a Th-2 cytokine whose functions overlap considerably with those of IL-4, and it is important for the control of the Th-1 response but that has not been well studied in toxoplasmosis. The third chemokine, CXCL 10 (interferon gamma-induced protein 10- IP-10), is secreted in response to IFN-γ stimulation. Recently, it was demonstrated in a murine model that treatment of chronically infected mice with anti-CXCL10 antibodies led to decreases in the numbers of CD3+, CD4+, and CD8+ T cells and the amount of IFN-γ mRNA expression in the retina and an increase in replicating parasites and ocular pathology, which provides evidence that the maintenance of the T-cell response and the control of *T. gondii* in the eye during chronic infection is dependent on CXCL10 [26]. Cytokines and chemokine measurements were carried out using supernatants collected from PBMC cultures stimulated with *T. gondii* antigens. The concentrations were determined by using the BD Cytometric Bead Array (CBA) human chemokine kit and Th1/Th2 cytokine kits and Human IL-13 Flex Set, according to the manufacturer's protocol (BD Pharmingen).

Table 4 summarizes the individuals for which the specific immune response against *T. gondii* has been evaluated. The *T. gondii* serology and age range is provided. All the seronegative (SN) individuals, seropositive (SP) without ocular scar lesions (NL) and individuals with retinal or retinochoroidal scar lesions categorized as type A, type B or type C, as explained above, were sex- and age-matched among the groups. We observed that there was a similarity in terms of the profile of the *in vitro* immune response between patients who presented multiple scar type lesions and patients who presented single type A or B scar lesions, depending on which cytokine had been considered among the groups for comparison. Then immunological analysis, presented in Figure 3 and Figure 4, show the patients presenting multiple type scar lesions (AB, ABC, AC or BC) grouped in two different ways. This optional arrangement of patients, considering the multiple types of scar lesions, has helped us to propose three settings of immune responses that match the clinical presentation of ocular toxoplasmosis, which has been inferred in our studies by the morphological appearance of the retinal/retinochoroidal lesions. The reasoning behind the optional arrangements is related to the common presence of type B and type A scar lesions in two (AB and ABC) out of the four (AB, ABC, AC and BC) multiple type scar lesions. In Figure 3, they were grouped as follows: patients with AB, ABC and AC scar lesions are all included in the type A scar lesion group, which we considered the highest categorization in terms of tissue damage severity of scar lesion, and the patients presenting scar lesions of type BC were included in the group of type B scar lesions. The type C scar lesion group is composed of individuals presenting only type C scar lesions.

Concerning to the cytokine and chemokine production, we observed two levels of production that are termed as high or low levels. As a consequence, individuals producing low or high levels of cytokines or chemokines are termed high or low cytokine/chemokine producers. To calculate the frequency of high and low levels of production, an arbitrary cutoff value was established for each cytokine and chemokine based on the visual dispersion graphics, where it was possible to determine a dividing line that separated the secretion levels into two scattered clusters, one high and another low. The capability of producing low and high levels of IFN-γ is a phenotypic characteristic that is genetically associated with a single nucleotide polymorphism in the first intron of the human IFN-γ gene, as determined by Pravica and colleagues in 2000 [27]. The capability of producing low and high levels of IFN-γ can be observed in other infectious disease [28, 29]. The levels secreted by each patient that fell above the cutoff values were considered high values, and the levels that fell below the cutoff values were considered low values. The median value of the two cytokines IFN-γ and IL-13 and the chemokine CXCL10 secretion was utilized to help to establish the exact numeric cutoff values to be used for each cytokine and chemokine: 29.58ng./mL, 194.12 pg/mL, and 113.72 ng/mL for IFN-γ, IL-13 and CXCL10, respectively. Those median values refer to patients who presented type C scar lesions. This group was chosen because it exhibited the best spreading profile, producing two very clearly separated clusters corresponding to levels of high and low producers of the two cytokines and the chemokine that were evaluated.

Groups	Toxoplasmosis serology and scar lesion type	n	Mean Age (SE)[1]
1	SN[2]	9	29.6 (5.2)
2	SP[3]/NL[4]	21	28.8 (4.7)
3	SP/type A[5-6]	18	35.5 (6.0)
4	SP/type B[5-6]	21	27.5 (4.4)
5	SP/type C[5]	20	31.7 (5.1)

[1] (SE) = standard error
[2] *T. gondii*-seronegative individuals (SN)
[3] *T. gondii*-seropositive individuals (SP) without ocular lesions [4](NL)
[5] *T. gondii*-seropositive individuals (SP) with retinochoroidal/retinal scars lesions categorized as class type A, type B or type C.
[6] In the group of type A scar lesions, individuals with single type A scar lesions (N=4) and multiple scars lesions type AB (N=5), ABC (N=7) and AC (N=2) were also included, totaling the 18 individuals shown in the table. In the group of type B scar lesions, individuals with single type B lesions (N=14) and individuals with multiple scars lesions type BC (N=7) were included, totaling the 21 individuals shown in the table.

Table 4. Groups of Individuals Involved in Immunological Studies According to *Toxoplasma gondii* Serology, Age and the Presence or Absence of Retinal/Retinochoroidal Scar Lesions.

Figure 3 shows the frequency of IFN-γ, IL-13 and the chemokine CXCL 10 secretion, considering only patients who produced high levels of each cytokine, i.e., the high producers. The lowest frequency of high IFN-γ producers (43%) was observed in the group of patients with type B scar lesions even compared with patients presenting no lesions (SL) (52%), and the highest (61%) was observed in the group that presented type A scar lesions; 50% of the patients with type C lesions presented high levels of IFN-γ production. However, for IL-13 production, we observed that the lowest frequency of high producers was observed among patients with type A (28%) scar lesions, in comparison with patients who presented no lesions (SL) (29%). The highest production levels were observed among patients who presented type C scar lesions (50%); 30% of the patients with type B scar lesions presented high levels of IL-13 production. Curiously, for the CXCL 10 chemokine, which is inducible in response to IFN-γ, the highest frequency of high producers was observed among patients with type C scar lesions (53%), and the lowest frequency of high producers was observed among patients with type B scar lesions (21%), which is comparable to the frequency of high production observed in patients without ocular lesions (SL) (23%); 38% of patients with type A scar lesions were high producers of CXCL10. These data suggest that CXCL10 in humans can have the same role regarding *T. gondii* infection that it plays in mice: to control the numbers of CD3+, CD4+, and CD8+ T cells and the amount of IFN-γ mRNA expression in the retina and, in consequence, the replication of parasites in the eye during the chronic phase of *T. gondii* infection [26]. In addition, it is evident that patients who present type C scar lesions secrete high levels of IL-13, a cytokine that can control the levels of pro-inflammatory cytokines without affecting IFN-γ secretion within the eye, as shown in experimental models. The role of IL-13 was shown to inhibit pro-inflammatory cytokines, with the exception of IFN-γ, within the eye in a model of endotoxin-induced uveitis (EIU) in the Lewis rats. Intraocular injection of IL-13 significantly inhibited the production of pro-inflammatory cytokines and resulted in less intense ocular inflammation without down-regulating the levels of local IFN-γ [30]. In addition, the induced auto-immune uveitis with human retinal S-antigen in monkeys was treated with human recombinant IL-13 [31]. The injection of IL-13 significantly inhibited the inflammation in the eyes where the disease was present when the treatment was initiated. The beneficial effect of IL-13 extended into the 4-week follow-up period; however, after cessation of therapy, there was a progressive increase of inflammation in the IL-13 treated group. Nevertheless, the authors concluded that attention should be paid to the promising modality of treatment for severe uveitis with IL-13 [31]. The profile of the immune response against *T. gondii* exhibited by patients who presented type C scar lesions is suggestive of a favorable inflammatory environment within the eye for the maintenance of a controlled response to prevent both parasite growth and tissue damage, which could be caused by the parasite growth itself and/or may be a consequence of an exacerbated immune response against the parasite. In this context, it is important to highlight the fundamental importance that has been demonstrated for the role of IFN-γ in toxoplasmosis [25].

IFN-γ can induce tryptophan degradation, which is critical to the parasite's survival [32]. The effects of interferon on multiplication of *T. gondii* in *in vitro* systems seem to be dependent on cell type, and a diversity of molecular mechanisms is evident depending on the cell type or system. It has been shown in neuronal tissues and cells that nitric oxide (NO) production is an important factor for parasite growth inhibition [33]. However, parasite growth inhibition was found to be independent of a nitric oxide-mediated or tryptophan starvation mechanism [34]. The control of parasite interconversion between tachyzoites and bradyzoites in the eye is also fundamentally dependent on IFN-γ [35]. Furthermore, in primary cultures of human retinal pigment cells (HRPE), *T. gondii* replication was inhibited by the induction of indoleamine 2,3-dioxygenase (IDO), which degrades tryptophan to kynurenine. However, nitric oxide production was not detected in this system [36].

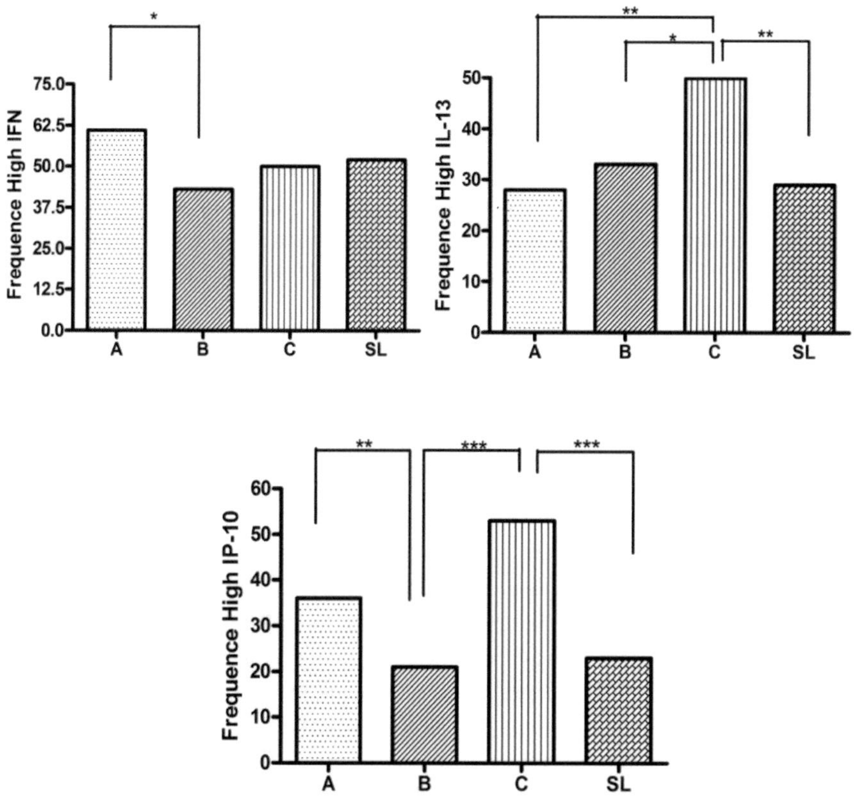

Figure 3. Frequency of high IFN-γ IL-13 and CXCL10 (IP-10) producers, which were grouped according to the type of scar lesion, as shown in Table 4. The frequency of non-infected seronegative individuals (SN) is not shown because in none of them PBMC produced high levels of IFN-gamma, IL-13 and or CXCL10 (IP-10) under stimulation with soluble *T. gondii* antigens (STAg). The exact Fisher's test was used to compare the groups in terms of the differences in the frequencies of high cytokines/chemokine producers. Significances were found at the levels of * $p < 0.05$, ** $p < 0.01$ and *** $p < 0.001$. Significant differences were found between type A and type B scar lesions for IFN-γ production (* $p < 0.05$), between type C and all the other types of scars lesions regarding IL-13 secretion, and between type C and all the other types of scars lesions groups for CXCL10 (IP-10). The data regarding PBMC IFN-γ, IL-13 and CXCL10 from non-infected (SN) individuals in response to *T. gondii* soluble antigens is not shown because none of those patients produced high levels of those cytokines or chemokine.

Based on fundoscopic examinations, type C scar lesions seem to be areas of RPE hyperplasia or atrophy. However, they must to be better characterized by new high-resolution cross-sectional imaging of the retinal tissues (such as using spectral domain optical coherence tomography) in order to better clarify their structural changes in the retinal layers. As mentioned earlier some aspects showed here led us to accept the relationship between type C scar lesions and *T. gondii* infection one of them is the profile of cellular specific immune response of patients who present only type C scar lesions, which is concomitantly abundant for IFN-γ, IL-13 and CXCL10. The reproduction of this type of scar lesion in experimental models would be of value to better understand their meaning in ocular toxoplasmosis. Because we have been working in a highly endemic area to toxoplasmosis and the majority of the population is *T. gondii* seropositive, we cannot rule out the possibility of an association between the type C scar lesions and other infectious or non-infectious conditions whose natures could be genetically predisposed and prevalent in the Campos population.

As stated previously, patients were grouped in an optional way. Those presenting only type A scar lesions comprised a distinct group, taking into account the possibility that in patients presenting only type A scar lesions, the course of the immune response could be different from that which occurred in patients who presented multiple type scar lesions. There are rational and intuitive aspects to this arrangement that are related to various factors, like the tendency for the production of higher IFN-γ levels of in PBMC cultures of patients who present only type A scar lesions in response to parasitic antigens and the clinical observation that some patients can present type A scar lesions soon after an episode of acute ocular toxoplasmosis without a previous history of ocular toxoplasmosis. However, some patients present a slower evolution, from mild to severe scar lesions, as described by Silveira and associates in a well documented report [13]. As previously stated in this chapter, this observation concerns the evolution of hyperpigmented "atypical" toxoplasmic retinal scar lesions (similar in appearance to the type B toxoplasmic scar lesions that we have described) evolving to "typical" toxoplasmic retinochoroidal lesions (similar in appearance to the type A toxoplasmic scar lesions that we have described). Then for the analysis of the immune response as a function of the clinical presentation of ocular toxoplasmosis inferred by the morphological appearance of the retinal/retinochoroidal scar lesions, the patients were optionally arranged into three groups as follows: i) patients presenting only type A scar lesions; ii) patients presenting only type B scar lesions plus patients presenting all the multiple type scar lesions (AB + ABC + AC + BC); and iii) patients presenting only type C scar lesions. Figure 4 summarizes the *in vitro* parameters of the cellular immune response against *T. gondii* antigens by PBMC of patients in the context of the retinal/retinochoroidal lesions considering the three groups of type A, type C and type B plus the multiple type scar lesions. Similarly, as shown in Figure 3, considering the profiles of the frequency of high IFN-γ, IL-13 and CXCL10 production by PBMC of patients stimulated with *T. gondii* soluble antigens (STAg), we identified three possible settings of the immune response that can be associated with the type of scar lesion. As shown in Figure 4 the Platonic solid octahedron is suitable for representing the diversity of scar lesions as a function of the three settings of immune responses. On the two edges are the polar scar lesions, type A and type C. In the top is the type A scar, which is caused by the most severe type of lesion, and in the bottom is the type C scar that likely resulted from a less severe lesions type. Both types of scar lesions respectively correlate with the setting of an exacerbated and an adequately regulated Th-1 response. In the four central vertices are type B scar lesions and the multiple type scar lesions AB, AC and BC, and in the center of the octahedron is the multiple type scar lesion ABC, all of which correlate with the setting of an immune response characterized by lower levels of Th-1 (IFN-γ and CXCL10) and Th-2 (IL-13) compared with type A and C scar lesions. Taking into account this fact, it is possible that other T cells subtypes, such as Th-17, for instance, can be important in this setting. Reinforcing this supposition is the fact that we have observed recent associations of ocular toxoplasmosis and polymorphisms in the *NOD2* (nucleotide-binding oligomerization domain-containing protein 2) gene and increased IL-

17A production by PBMC under *T. gondii* antigenic stimulation in patients with chronic or active ocular toxoplasmosis [37]. This fact could explain the lower levels of IL-13, IFN-γ and CXCL10 observed for patients who present type B and multiple type scar lesions. However, we have not analyzed patients considering their type of scar lesion groups for the mentioned genetic association study due to sample size restrictions, and the genetic association found for *NOD2* refers to the presence of ocular scar lesions without precisely identifying what type of scar lesion it could be.

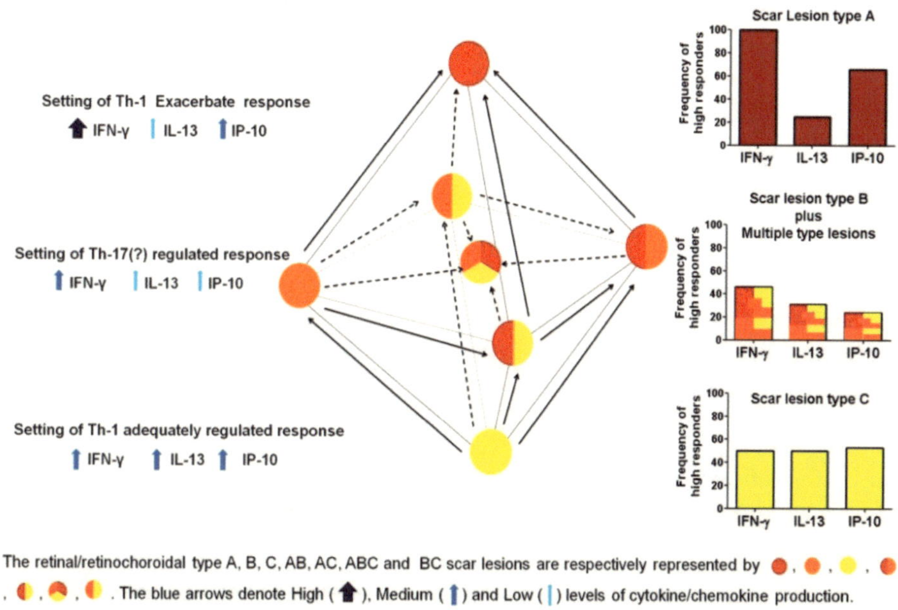

Figure 4. A Diagram representing retinal/retinochoroidal toxoplasmic scar lesions, as a function of three different settings of cellular immune response. The platonic solid octahedron in the center is suitable for representing the diversity of scar lesions as a function of the three settings of immune response. On the two edges are the type A (at the top) and type C (at the bottom) scar lesions. In the four central vertices of octahedron are represented the type B scar lesion and the multiple type scar lesions AB, AC and BC, and in the center is a multiple type scar lesion of type ABC. The dotted and solid arrows denote the possible evolution of one type of scar lesion toward another type of lesion of greater severity. Not all possibilities of evolution are shown in the picture. The frequencies of IFN-γ, IL-13 and CXCL10 (IP-10) high-responders that are shown in the graphics at right define the three settings of the immune response shown at left. Each of the three settings correlates with each of the three groups: with the scar lesions of the type A at the edge, with the scar lesion of type C at the bottom, or with the type B scar lesion plus all the multiple type lesions. The blue arrows shown in the settings denote the levels of cytokines and chemokine, as shown in the figure. The scar lesion types are represented by colored circles, as explained in the figure.

The data regarding PBMC IFN-γ, IL-13 and CXCL10 from non-infected (SN) individuals in response to *T. gondii* soluble antigens is not shown in Figure 3 and Figure 4 because none of those patients produced high levels of the cytokines or chemokine in question. In conclusion, elements from the cellular immune response, evaluated in PBMC cultures of population-based studies evidence that the morphological aspects of retinal/retinochoroidal scar lesions can be associated with three settings of immune response in areas of high prevalence of ocular toxoplasmosis. The three settings are i) a Th-1 prominent response with high levels of IFN-γ, moderate to low levels of CXCL10 and low levels of IL-13, which relate to single type A scar lesions that are healed from the most severe toxoplasmic ocular lesions; ii) a cellular response with moderate to low levels of IFN-γ and IL-13 and low levels of CXCL10, which relate to multiple type and type B scar lesions; and iii) a sharply regulated Th-1 response with moderate to high levels of CXCL 10 and IL-13 and moderate levels of IFN-γ, which relate to type C scar lesions and could protect against tissue damage due to parasite replication within the eye.

4. Ocular toxoplasmosis in association with other infectious diseases: Could this impact the clinical presentations of toxoplasmic scar lesions in population-based surveys?

The interaction with other pathogens co-infecting *T. gondii* seropositive patients will depend on their exposure to such eventually co-prevalent parasites in the same area and on the type of immune response driven against them. The disease manifestation of *T. gondii* infected patients who become infected with HIV exemplify well this type of interaction and modification on the clinical presentation of ocular toxoplasmosis in the face of concomitant infections [3].

The scar lesions left by healed uveitis caused by *T. gondii* infections result from the previous process of uveal inflammation, which they have in common with other infectious and non-infectious agents that also cause uveitis, the possibility to compromise the iris, the cilliary body, the choroid adjacent structures of the eye including the vitreous, the retina and the optic disc. In this context, the thesis dedicated to this specific issue entitled "Infectious uveitis new developments in etiology and pathogenesis" from De Visser [38] underlines the necessity in clinical practice to have the support of laboratory data for the confirmation of a suspected diagnosis, as similar clinical features may be caused by different pathogens. The prompt identification of infectious uveitis entities is of vital importance for treatment regimens and visual prognoses of intraocular infections, and differ completely from non-infectious disorders treatments.

The thesis also reports on the similarity between retinal/retinochoroidal scar lesions left by Rubella eye infection and those left by ocular toxoplasmosis in a well-documented retrospective study. The clinical presentations of the focal retinal scars in 11 patients with intraocular proof of Rubella virus and in 17 patients with intraocular proof of *T. gondii* infection are compared. Photographic and angiographic records of the 28 patients were masked for identification and for infectious agent and were evaluated by four specialists in the field of ocular toxoplasmosis. It is reported that no differences were observed between the retinochoroidal scar lesions in Rubella virus-positive and *T. gondii*-positive patients. Retinochoroidal scar lesions were considered consistent with the diagnosis of ocular toxoplasmosis in 55% of Rubella virus-positive patients and in 88% of *T. gondii*-positive patients by at least three out of the four experts. According to the author of the thesis, two experts considered the retinal lesions in *T. gondii*-positive patients more frequently "consistent with the diagnosis of ocular toxoplasmosis" (P = .010 and P = 0.011). There was a substantial agreement between the four experts (Fleiss' Kappa = 0.623) [38].

We cannot rule out the fact that none of the patients have been considered as cases of ocular toxoplasmosis in the Campos dos Goytacazes surveys or in surveys from other parts of Brazil, as scar lesions left from Rubella virus infection as opposed to *T. gondii* ocular infection were present in their eyes. However, we have to take into account that Rubella was a highly prevalent virus worldwide, including in Brazil, and it is probable that if ocular lesions left by Rubella infection were as frequent as in toxoplasmosis, such lesions would already have been described as a causative entity of uveitis with epidemiologic importance. Rubella virus-caused lesions currently no longer occur due to the vaccination program against Rubella virus that was undertaken in many countries, including in Brazil where it was introduced 15 years ago. Hence, despite the clinical relevance of the similarity between the Rubella virus- caused lesions and toxoplasma retinal/retinochoroidal scar lesions, we believe that from an epidemiologic perspective, this similarity is not relevant. However, these data reinforce that the search for parameters, other than the morphological and serological, for classifying retinal/retinochoroidal scar lesions presumably caused by *T. gondii* infections should be pursued. Parameters of cellular specific immune response or the genotyping of candidate genes with the potential to differentiate between infectious agents that produce similar ocular lesions could be of help for disease management.

We have reported recently in Campos that the host immune response to *T. gondii* and *Ascaris lumbricoides* evidence co-immune modulation properties that can influence the outcome of both infections. One of the most impressive aspect of the immune response of co-infected individuals is the prominent specific secretion of IL-13 against *Ascaris* and *T. gondii* antigens by PBMC of patients who present type C scar lesions in addition to middle to high secretion levels of IFN-γ [11]. This aspect of the immune response seems to be important for the control of the parasite retinal replication and most likely for the maintenance of an equilibrated *T. gondii* load and the interconversion of tachyzoites and bradyzoites in the eye tissues. *T. gondii* and *A. lumbricoides* are both parasites that infect hosts orally; however, they elicit polar type I or type II host responses, respectively. Because both parasites are endemic in tropical areas, it is likely that co-infections with these organisms have been common throughout human evolution. If this is the case, then the host immune response mounted against both parasites may have adapted to permit such co-parasitism. The possibility of *A. lumbricoides* to produce some type of ocular scar lesion in humans seems not to be of epidemiologic importance, as we have not detected ocular scar lesions in patients seronegative to *T. gondii* and positive to *A. lumbricoides* in our surveys.

The recent adoption of massive anti-helminthic treatments for people living in poor communities as a measure of public health policy has made difficult the research on individuals co-infected with *A. lumbricoides* and *T. gondii* in Campos dos Goytacazes as well as in other parts of Brazil. For this reason, we have begun to work with an experimental model of co-infection with *T. gondii* and *Heligmosomoides polygyrus*, which has been shown as valid model for studying parasites that evoke polar Th-1 and Th-2 in mice. *H. polygyrus* is a gastrointestinal worm, a natural parasite to mice, which evokes a polarized Th2 response in the host and blocks the type 1 immune response [39, 40]. It has been shown that a previous infection with the helminth can inhibit the development of CD8 T-cell immune response against *T. gondii,* thus compromising long-term protection against a protozoan parasite [41], which illustrates the adequacy of the model for studying the interaction between helminthic and *T. gondii* infections.

5. Immunogenetic studies: Candidate genes on ocular toxoplasmosis

Studies on genetic association in human toxoplasmosis in the past have provided evidence of associations between human leukocyte antigen (HLA) genes with the susceptibility to toxoplasmic encephalitis in AIDS patients (42) and with the outcome of congenital toxoplasmosis [43]. However, no causal relationships have been proven so far. We have conducted genetic association studies of candidate genes which potentially influence the profile of the inflammatory response against *T. gondii* (17, 18, 37) in patients with ocular toxoplasmosis by means of single nucleotide polymorphisms (SNPs) analysis. Significant associations between genetic polymorphisms and ocular disease in family-based studies have been found for Toll-like receptor-9, (*TLR-9*) [17], $P2X_7$ purinoceptor 7 (*P2RX7*) [18] and nucleotide-binding oligomerization domain-containing protein 2 (*NOD2*) [37] genes. These studies are currently being expanded to be replicated into population n-based investigational projects. All of these genes are related to innate immunity and have been described in processes of inflammasome assembly, which plays an important role in processing IL-1 beta and other IL-1 beta cytokine family member (IL-18, IL-33) precursors in active cytokines, promoting a pro-inflammatory response [44].The SNPs rs352140 at *TLR-9* and rs3135499 at *NOD2* were statistically significantly associated with the manifestation of ocular toxoplasmosis [17, 37] while the absence of the SNP rs1718119 at *P2RX7* was strongly associated with protection to ocular disease manifestation [18] as we shall see in detail.

The product of the *P2RX7* belongs to the family of purinoceptors for ATP, 595 amino acids in length and highly polymorphic. The relative amount of $P2X_7$ function varies between human individuals because of the numerous single nucleotide polymorphisms; combinations of these polymorphisms give rise to various haplotypes that can modify $P2X_7$ function and result in either loss or gain of function [45]. Splice isoforms that can alter receptor expression and function and modify the signaling properties downstream of receptor have also been described [45].

The receptor functions as a ligand-gated ion channel and is responsible for ATP-dependent lysis of macrophages by means of the formation of membrane pores that are permeable to large molecules. The receptor $P2X_7$ functions as a pro-inflammatory receptor in cells of the monocyte/macrophage lineage and is activated by extracellular ATP released from a variety of cellular sources including platelets and damaged cells [46] Its expression is up-regulated by IFN-γ and can lead directly to the killing of intracellular pathogens including *T. gondii* [46, 47]. $P2X_7$ stimulates inflammasome activation and secretion of IL-1β [48].

Polymorphisms at the *P2RX7* have been investigated in a cooperative immunogenetic study involving patients from United State and Campos dos Goytacazes in Brazil. The studies comprised 149 child in 149 child/parent trios from North America and 60 families with 68 affected with postnatal ocular toxoplasmosis offspring in Brazil [18]. For the United states casuistic, an association between the derived C(+)G(−) allele and a second synonymous variant rs1621388 in linkage disequilibrium with it; and clinical signs of disease *per se.* were observed . Analysis of clinical sub-groups showed associations with retinal disease and brain calcifications (OR=3.0 to 4.25; 0.004<P<0.009). The association with toxoplasmic retinochoroiditis was replicated in a family-based study from Campos dos Goytacazes (60 families; 68 affected offspring), where the ancestral T(+) allele (f= 0.296) at SNP rs1718119 which contains the Ala-348 to Thr polymorphism was strongly protective (OR= 0.27; 95% CI: 0.09–0.80) [18]. This last association at SNP rs1718119 was recently replicated in a case-control study with 361 non-related individuals. The study confirmed the protective association of the T(+) allele (f= 0.296) (OR =0,3; 95% CI: 0,15-0,59 chi-square value = 13,53 *p* corrected for multiple comparisons = 0.0132) for patients with type B scar lesions [49]

The SNPs at the *P2RX7* may be associated with a gain or loss of function of the receptor. Data from Stokes and colleagues [50] showed the gain of function for $P2X_7$ haplotypes carrying rs1718119 SNP, which matches our recent case-control data that confirmed a strong protection due to the ancestral allele T(+) for the *P2RX7* associated with the development of ocular disease. Therefore, it is reasonable to speculate that the ancestral allele (that do not carry the rs1718119 SNP and do not contain the Ala-348 to Thr polymorphism) would help to protect against an exacerbated immune response as a consequence of the gain of function conferred by the rs1718119 SNP, which would lead to an immune response with high levels of pro-inflammatory cytokines, such as IL-1 β and IFN-γ, and could contribute to retinal tissue damage. Our data provides evidence that the Th-1 specific immune response is centered in the IFN-γ secretion by PBMC of patients with the different types of retinal/retinochoroidal scar lesions, which also reinforces the supposition that an exacerbated immune response in an environment with prolonged inflammatory mediators can contribute to retinal/retinochoroidal damage.

Albuquerque and colleagues described an association between the IFN-γ +874T/A gene polymorphism with toxoplasmic retinochoroiditis susceptibility [51]. This study is related to the Santa Rita (Barra Mansa) casuistic, as described previously in this chapter. The authors found that AA homozygous individuals showed a 1.62-fold higher risk than other genotypes (AT and TT) for developing toxoplasmic retinochoroiditis [51]. Regarding the IFN-γ +874T/A gene polymorphism, it was demonstrated that the polymorphism is linked to high and low producer phenotypes [27, 28] and the genotype AA is associated with the phenotype for low IFN-γ capacity of production in contrast to the AT or TT genotypes that are linked with a phenotype for a middle and high IFN-γ capacity of production respectively [29]. The T to A polymorphism coincides with a putative NF-kappa B binding site that may have functional consequences for the transcription of the human IFN-γ gene [27]. In the Santa Rita study, the IFN-γ production by PMBC of the patients was not reported. However, considering that this cytokine is a very important to parasite control replication, the patients presenting the AA genotype for the IFN-γ +874 T/A polymorphism likely have a similar profile of specific cellular immune response with that observed for the group that presented lesions of types B and BC, as shown in Figure 3, and multiple type scar lesions, as shown in Figure 4. Namely, they would tend to produce moderate to low levels of IFN-γ and IL-13 and low levels of CXCL 10, which most likely causes an immune response that is not sufficient to efficiently prevent/control parasite proliferation; as a consequence, retinal/retinochoroidal tissues damage occurs. It is important to note that to determine the frequency of the genotype AA among individuals grouped by the type of scar lesions, in association with phenotypic parameters of the immune response, like cytokines and chemokines, would be of value to improve our understanding of the possible pathological mechanisms that occur in the different types of scar lesions in ocular toxoplasmosis.

Other reports in the literature have described genetic association studies of cytokines with toxoplasmic ocular diseases in Brazil. However, they describe small casuistic related to patients from ophthalmologic reference centers and do not find significant associations [52-54], although one suggests the association of polymorphism at IL-1 alfa gene and the recurrence of ocular toxoplasmosis [54].

6. Conclusion

We have presented data related to a decade of research on a hyperendemic area to *T. gondii* infection, considering aspects linked to the clinical presentation of ocular disease in a population exposed to high risk of waterborne toxoplasmosis, the profile of *in vitro* specific immune response in the function of the disease's clinical presentation, and genetic association studies with candidate genes in ocular toxoplasmosis.

It is important to consider the conclusions and advances that can be derived based on the study of PBMC from patients who exhibit different clinical presentations of ocular toxoplasmosis, stimulated *in vitro* with parasite antigens. One can argue that the study of the specific responses of PBMC *in vitro* does not reflect the eye's immune-privileged environment, for instance. However, the study of PBMC represents is a non-invasive approach that is adequate for population-based studies such that in the genomic medicine era, it will improve our understanding of relevant gene response, i.e., their activation and regulation in inflammatory process within the eye. The associations between phenotype and genotype data from cohorts accelerate our understanding of the molecular mechanisms involved in the disease's pathology. Our data on $P2X_7$ genotyping genes together with the PBMC immune profile illustrate this aspect. Namely, our initial hypothesis on an exacerbation of the inflammatory response with high levels of pro-inflammatory cytokines, especially IFN-γ secretion, concomitant with relatively low levels of anti-inflammatory cytokines like IL-13 secretion in response to parasite antigens, which was identified by *in vitro* PBMC stimulation experiments and could contribute to the development of ocular disease, is reinforced by the findings on *P2RX7* genotypingat the SNP rs1718119. This data showed that the ancestral allele is highly protective for the development of ocular disease. The SNP rs1718119 has been demonstrated to confer a gain of function to the receptor $P2X_7$, imbuing it with a more vigorous pro-inflammatory response. Therefore, the presence of the ancestral allele would protect the eye tissues from harmful exacerbations of immune responses, which corroborates our previous interpretations from PBMC experiments, as described above. Furthermore, the similarity of immunologic parameters between the mouse model and human infection, such as that observed for IFN-γ and CXCL10, motivates the development of innovative protocols using PBMC to access the gene response at the patient level. This approach is both feasible and suitable. For instance, in a given patient, it is possible to study PBMC to access the expression of the $P2X_7$ protein, the product of the same *P2RX7* that is expressed in retinal epithelial cells. Concerning the relevance of this approach, it is worth mentioning that primary cultures of human retinal epithelial cells that express $P2X_7$ protein [55] are responsive to IFN-γ stimulation leading to *T. gondi*i elimination in a pathway independent of nitric oxide (NO) [36].

The interpretations of our data on PBMC *in vitro* stimulation with *T. gondii* antigens together with the candidate genes genotyping relevant to the innate immune response, targeting the parasite, contribute to a better understanding of the immunological pathogenesis of infectious diseases that has been recently achieved. However, many issues remain to be addressed before the clinical exploitation of these findings can be realized. The function of these elements and their interplay with one another and with other components in the immune system are complex, and it is crucial to determine the balance between their beneficial and pathological roles in ocular toxoplasmosis.

Finally, the immune responses of patients from population-based studies who exhibit diverse scar lesions that are likely caused by *T. gondii* infection illustrate the multifactorial nature of ocular toxoplasmosis. Beyond host genetics and interactions with other pathogens that we have mentioned in this chapter, there are many other factors, such as environmental questions, the age at which individuals are infected, the parasitic load in the host, and the parasite genetic background that are equally important for disease manifestation. Therefore, all of these aspects, in addition to those not mentioned here or unknown, that characterize the multifactorial nature of ocular toxoplasmosis cannot be considered separately, and their interaction in and with the host will be expressed by one single feature that represents the profile of the immune response mounted by the host. The immune response will be subject to influences by every factor and will ultimately impact the different clinical presentation of ocular toxoplasmosis.

Author details

Lílian M.G. Bahia-Oliveira*, Alba L.P. Rangel, Marcela S.B. Boechat,
Bianca M. Mangiavacchi**, Livia M. Martins**, Francielle B. Ferraz**,
Maycon B. Almeida and Flavia P. Vieira

Laboratório de Biologia do Reconhecer (LBR) Centro de Biociências e Biotecnologia (CBB) Universidade Estadual do Norte Fluminense Darcy Ribeiro (UENF), Campos dos Goytacazes, RJ, Brazil

* Corresponding Author

** Equal Contribution

Elisa M. Waked Peixoto and Ricardo G. Peixe
Laboratório de Biologia do Reconhecer (LBR) Centro de Biociências e Biotecnologia (CBB) Universidade Estadual do Norte Fluminense Darcy Ribeiro (UENF),Campos dos Goytacazes, RJ, Brazil
Faculdade de Medicina de Campos, Campos dos Goytacazes, RJ, Brazil

Acknowledgement

The following grants supported this work: FAPERJ E-26/112.045/2008; E-26/110.869/2009; E26/111.131/2010; E-26/111.305/2010

We thank Jennifer Blackwell, Ricardo Gazzinelli and Miriam Dutra for their partnership on genetic studies and JP Dubey for research support. We are thank to Fernando Orefice and Wesley Campos for their participation on the fundoscopic examinations of patients in Campos dos Goytacazes and Liliani Souza Elias, Fernando Cesar Lopes and Flavia Rangel for their technical support. We thank Dr. Daíse Malheiros Meira, for her brilliant and original suggestion to propose a classification of the retinal/retinochoroidal scars in terms of the degree of retinal tissues destruction.

7. References

[1] Bahia-Oliveira LM, Jones JL, Azevedo-Silva J, Alves CC, Orefice F, Addiss DG. Highly endemic, waterborne toxoplasmosis in north Rio de Janeiro state, Brazil. Emerg Infect Dis. 2003;9(1):55-62. Epub 2003/01/21.

[2] Gilbert RE, Stanford MR. Is ocular toxoplasmosis caused by prenatal or postnatal infection? The British journal of ophthalmology. 2000;84(2):224-6. Epub 2000/02/03.

[3] Holland GN, O'Connor GR, Belfort Junior R, al. E. Toxoplasmosis. St. Louis: Mosby; 1996.

[4] Glasner PD, Silveira C, Kruszon-Moran D, Martins MC, Burnier Junior M, Silveira S, et al. An unusually high prevalence of ocular toxoplasmosis in southern Brazil. American journal of ophthalmology. 1992;114(2):136-44. Epub 1992/08/15.

[5] de Abreu MT, Boni D, Belfort Junior R, Passos A, Garcia AR, Muccioli C, et al. Toxoplasmose ocular em Venda Nova do Imigrante, ES, Brasil. Arquivos Brasileiros de Oftalmologia. 1998;61:540-5.

[6] Garcia JL, Navarro IT, Ogawa L, de Oliveira RC, Kobilka E. [Seroprevalence, epidemiology and ocular evaluation of human toxoplasmosis in the rural zone Jauguapita (Parana) Brazil]. Revista panamericana de salud publica = Pan American journal of public health. 1999;6(3):157-63. Epub 1999/10/12. Soroprevalencia, epidemiologia e avaliacao ocular da toxoplasmose humana na zona rural de Jaguapita (Parana), Brasil.

[7] Bahia Oliveira LM, Wilken de Abreu AM, Azevedo-Silva J, Orefice F. Toxoplamosis in southeastern Brazil: an alarming situation of highly endemic acquired and congennital

infection. Recent trends in research on congennital toxoplasmosis: International Journal for Parasitology; 2001. p. 133-6.

[8] Portela RW, Bethony J, Costa MI, Gazzinelli A, Vitor RW, Hermeto FM, et al. A multihousehold study reveals a positive correlation between age, severity of ocular toxoplasmosis, and levels of glycoinositolphospholipid-specific immunoglobulin A. J Infect Dis. 2004;190(1):175-83. Epub 2004/06/15.

[9] Aleixo AL, Benchimol EI, Neves Ede S, Silva CS, Coura LC, Amendoeira MR. [Frequency of lesions suggestive of ocular toxoplasmosis among a rural population in the State of Rio de Janeiro]. Revista da Sociedade Brasileira de Medicina Tropical. 2009;42(2):165-9. Epub 2009/05/19. Frequencia de lesoes sugestivas de toxoplasmose ocular em uma populacao rural do Estado do Rio de Janeiro.

[10] Orefice F, Bahia Oliveira LM. Toxoplasmose. In: Médica C, editor. Uveíte Clínica e cirúrgica. 2 ed. Rio de Janeiro2005.

[11] Bahia-Oliveira LM, Silva JA, Peixoto-Rangel AL, Boechat MS, Oliveira AM, Massara CL, et al. Host immune response to Toxoplasma gondii and Ascaris lumbricoides in a highly endemic area: evidence of parasite co-immunomodulation properties influencing the outcome of both infections. Mem Inst Oswaldo Cruz. 2009;104(2):273-80. Epub 2009/05/12.

[12] Smith JR, Cunningham ET, Jr. Atypical presentations of ocular toxoplasmosis. Current opinion in ophthalmology. 2002;13(6):387-92. Epub 2002/11/21.

[13] Silveira C, Belfort R, Jr., Muccioli C, Abreu MT, Martins MC, Victora C, et al. A follow-up study of Toxoplasma gondii infection in southern Brazil. American journal of ophthalmology. 2001;131(3):351-4. Epub 2001/03/10.

[14] Sibley LD, Boothroyd JC. Virulent strains of Toxoplasma gondii comprise a single clonal lineage. Nature. 1992;359(6390):82-5. Epub 1992/09/03.

[15] Khan A, Taylor S, Su C, Mackey AJ, Boyle J, Cole R, et al. Composite genome map and recombination parameters derived from three archetypal lineages of Toxoplasma gondii. Nucleic acids research. 2005;33(9):2980-92. Epub 2005/05/25.

[16] Peixoto-Rangel AL. Investigação de Fatores Imunogenéticos Associados à Manifestação de Retinocoroidites Toxoplásmicas em Área Altamente Endêmica para Toxoplasmose. [Tese de Doutorado] Campos dos Goytacazes: Universidade Estadual do Norte Fluminense Darcy Ribeiro; 2008.

[17] Peixoto-Rangel AL, Miller EN, Castellucci L, Jamieson SE, Peixe RG, Elias LD, et al. Candidate gene analysis of ocular toxoplasmosis in Brazil: evidence for a role for toll-like receptor 9 (TLR9). Mem I Oswaldo Cruz. 2009;104(8):1187-90.

[18] Jamieson SE, Peixoto-Rangel AL, Hargrave AC, de Roubaix LA, Mui EJ, Boulter NR, et al. Evidence for associations between the purinergic receptor P2X(7) (P2RX7) and toxoplasmosis. Genes Immun. 2010;11(5):374-83.

[19] Kee C, Koo H, Ji Y, Kim S. Effect of optic disc size or age on evaluation of optic disc variables. The British journal of ophthalmology. 1997;81(12):1046-9. Epub 1998/03/14.

[20] Holland GN. Ocular toxoplasmosis: the influence of patient age. Mem Inst Oswaldo Cruz. 2009;104(2):351-7. Epub 2009/05/12.

[21] Azevedo-Silva J. Avaliação da Resposta Imunológica contra Antígenos de Toxoplasma gondii e Ascaris lumbricoides em Pacientes Residentes em Áreas Co-endêmicas para Ambos os Parasitas em Campos dos Goytacazes/RJ. [Dissertação de Mestrado] Campos dos Goytacazes: Universidade Estadual do Norte Fluminense Darcy Ribeiro; 2001.

[22] Boechat MSB. Perfil de Quimiocinas em Indivíduos Portadores de Lesão Ocular Decorrente da Infecção pelo Toxoplasma gondii. [Dissertação de Mestrado] Campos dos Goytacazes: Universidade Estadual do Norte Fluminense Darcy Ribeiro; 2008.

[23] Garweg JG, Candolfi E. Immunopathology in ocular toxoplasmosis: facts and clues. Mem Inst Oswaldo Cruz. 2009;104(2):211-20. Epub 2009/05/12.

[24] Lahmar I, Abou-Bacar A, Abdelrahman T, Guinard M, Babba H, Ben Yahia S, et al. Cytokine profiles in toxoplasmic and viral uveitis. J Infect Dis. 2009;199(8):1239-49. Epub 2009/03/24.

[25] Suzuki Y, Orellana MA, Schreiber RD, Remington JS. Interferon-gamma: the major mediator of resistance against Toxoplasma gondii. Science. 1988;240(4851):516-8. Epub 1988/04/22.

[26] Norose K, Kikumura A, Luster AD, Hunter CA, Harris TH. CXCL10 is required to maintain T-cell populations and to control parasite replication during chronic ocular toxoplasmosis. Investigative ophthalmology & visual science. 2011;52(1):389-98. Epub 2010/09/03.

[27] Pravica V, Perrey C, Stevens A, Lee JH, Hutchinson IV. A single nucleotide polymorphism in the first intron of the human IFN-gamma gene: absolute correlation with a polymorphic CA microsatellite marker of high IFN-gamma production. Human immunology. 2000;61(9):863-6. Epub 2000/10/29.

[28] Gomes JAS, Bahia-Oliveira LMG, Rocha MOC, Martins-Filho OA, Gazzinelli G, Correa-Oliveira R. Evidence that development of severe cardiomyopathy in human Chagas' disease is due to a thl-specific immune response. Infect Immun. 2003;71(3):1185-93.

[29] Ben Selma W, Harizi H, Bougmiza I, Hannachi N, Ben Kahla I, Zaieni R, et al. Interferon gamma +874T/A polymorphism is associated with susceptibility to active pulmonary tuberculosis development in Tunisian patients. DNA and cell biology. 2011;30(6):379-87. Epub 2011/02/22.

[30] Lemaitre C, Thillaye-Goldenberg B, Naud MC, de Kozak Y. The effects of intraocular injection of interleukin-13 on endotoxin-induced uveitis in rats. Investigative ophthalmology & visual science. 2001;42(9):2022-30. Epub 2001/08/02.

[31] Roberge FG, de Smet MD, Benichou J, Kriete MF, Raber J, Hakimi J. Treatment of uveitis with recombinant human interleukin-13. The British journal of ophthalmology. 1998;82(10):1195-8. Epub 1999/01/30.

[32] Pfefferkorn ER. Interferon gamma blocks the growth of Toxoplasma gondii in human fibroblasts by inducing the host cells to degrade tryptophan. Proceedings of the National Academy of Sciences of the United States of America. 1984;81(3):908-12. Epub 1984/02/01.

[33] Gazzinelli RT, Eltoum I, Wynn TA, Sher A. Acute cerebral toxoplasmosis is induced by in vivo neutralization of TNF-alpha and correlates with the down-regulated expression

of inducible nitric oxide synthase and other markers of macrophage activation. Journal of immunology. 1993;151(7):3672-81. Epub 1993/10/01.

[34] Halonen SK, Weiss LM. Investigation into the mechanism of gamma interferon-mediated inhibition of Toxoplasma gondii in murine astrocytes. Infect Immun. 2000;68(6):3426-30. Epub 2000/05/19.

[35] Norose K, Mun HS, Aosai F, Chen M, Piao LX, Kobayashi M, et al. IFN-gamma-regulated Toxoplasma gondii distribution and load in the murine eye. Investigative ophthalmology & visual science. 2003;44(10):4375-81. Epub 2003/09/26.

[36] Nagineni CN, Pardhasaradhi K, Martins MC, Detrick B, Hooks JJ. Mechanisms of interferon-induced inhibition of Toxoplasma gondii replication in human retinal pigment epithelial cells. Infect Immun. 1996;64(10):4188-96. Epub 1996/10/01.

[37] Dutra MS, Béla SR, Peixoto-Rangel AL, Fakiola M, Gazzinelli A, Quites HF, et al. Association of a NOD2 gene polymorphism and responsiveness of Th17 lymphocytes with ocular toxoplasmosis. The Journal of Infectious Diseases (accepted for publication).

[38] de Visser L. Infectious uveitis: New developments in etiology and pathogenesis. [PhD Thesis] Netherlands: Utrecht University 2009.

[39] Svetic A, Madden KB, Zhou XD, Lu P, Katona IM, Finkelman FD, et al. A primary intestinal helminthic infection rapidly induces a gut-associated elevation of Th2-associated cytokines and IL-3. Journal of immunology. 1993;150(8 Pt 1):3434-41. Epub 1993/04/15.

[40] Setiawan T, Metwali A, Blum AM, Ince MN, Urban JF, Jr., Elliott DE, et al. Heligmosomoides polygyrus promotes regulatory T-cell cytokine production in the murine normal distal intestine. Infect Immun. 2007;75(9):4655-63. Epub 2007/07/04.

[41] Khan IA, Hakak R, Eberle K, Sayles P, Weiss LM, Urban JF, Jr. Coinfection with Heligmosomoides polygyrus fails to establish CD8+ T-cell immunity against Toxoplasma gondii. Infect Immun. 2008;76(3):1305-13. Epub 2008/01/16.

[42] Suzuki Y, Wong SY, Grumet FC, Fessel J, Montoya JG, Zolopa AR, et al. Evidence for genetic regulation of susceptibility to toxoplasmic encephalitis in AIDS patients. J Infect Dis. 1996;173(1):265-8. Epub 1996/01/01.

[43] Mack DG, Johnson JJ, Roberts F, Roberts CW, Estes RG, David C, et al. HLA-class II genes modify outcome of Toxoplasma gondii infection. International journal for parasitology. 1999;29(9):1351-8. Epub 1999/12/01.

[44] Stutz A, Golenbock DT, Latz E. Inflammasomes: too big to miss. The Journal of clinical investigation. 2009;119(12):3502-11. Epub 2009/12/04.

[45] Sluyter R, Stokes L. Significance of P2X7 receptor variants to human health and disease. Recent patents on DNA & gene sequences. 2011;5(1):41-54. Epub 2011/02/10.

[46] Correa G, Marques da Silva C, de Abreu Moreira-Souza AC, Vommaro RC, Coutinho-Silva R. Activation of the P2X(7) receptor triggers the elimination of Toxoplasma gondii tachyzoites from infected macrophages. Microbes and infection / Institut Pasteur. 2010;12(6):497-504. Epub 2010/03/20.

[47] Lees MP, Fuller SJ, McLeod R, Boulter NR, Miller CM, Zakrzewski AM, et al. P2X7 receptor-mediated killing of an intracellular parasite, Toxoplasma gondii, by human

and murine macrophages. Journal of immunology. 2010;184(12):7040-6. Epub 2010/05/22.

[48] Qu Y, Franchi L, Nunez G, Dubyak GR. Nonclassical IL-1 beta secretion stimulated by P2X7 receptors is dependent on inflammasome activation and correlated with exosome release in murine macrophages. Journal of immunology. 2007;179(3):1913-25. Epub 2007/07/21.

[49] Ferraz FB. Estudo caso-controle e frequências alélicas de SNPs de P2RX7 em coorte de indivíduos com lesão ocular toxoplásmica no norte do estado do Rio de Janeiro. [Dissertação de mestrado] Campos dos Goytacazes: Universidade Estadual do Norte Fluminense Darcy Ribeiro; 2012.

[50] Stokes L, Fuller SJ, Sluyter R, Skarratt KK, Gu BJ, Wiley JS. Two haplotypes of the P2X(7) receptor containing the Ala-348 to Thr polymorphism exhibit a gain-of-function effect and enhanced interleukin-1beta secretion. FASEB journal : official publication of the Federation of American Societies for Experimental Biology. 2010;24(8):2916-27. Epub 2010/04/03.

[51] Albuquerque MC, Aleixo AL, Benchimol EI, Leandro AC, das Neves LB, Vicente RT, et al. The IFN-gamma +874T/A gene polymorphism is associated with retinochoroiditis toxoplasmosis susceptibility. Mem Inst Oswaldo Cruz. 2009;104(3):451-5. Epub 2009/06/24.

[52] Cordeiro CA, Moreira PR, Costa GC, Dutra WO, Campos WR, Orefice F, et al. TNF-alpha gene polymorphism (-308G/A) and toxoplasmic retinochoroiditis. The British journal of ophthalmology. 2008;92(7):986-8. Epub 2008/06/26.

[53] Cordeiro CA, Moreira PR, Costa GC, Dutra WO, Campos WR, Orefice F, et al. Interleukin-1 gene polymorphisms and toxoplasmic retinochoroiditis. Molecular vision. 2008;14:1845-9. Epub 2008/10/23.

[54] Cordeiro CA, Moreira PR, Andrade MS, Dutra WO, Campos WR, Orefice F, et al. Interleukin-10 gene polymorphism (-1082G/A) is associated with toxoplasmic retinochoroiditis. Investigative ophthalmology & visual science. 2008;49(5):1979-82. Epub 2008/04/26.

[55] Yang D, Elner SG, Clark AJ, Hughes BA, Petty HR, Elner VM. Activation of P2X receptors induces apoptosis in human retinal pigment epithelium. Investigative ophthalmology & visual science. 2011;52(3):1522-30. Epub 2010/11/13.

[56] Melamed J. Contributions to the history of ocular toxoplasmosis in Southern Brazil. Memórias do Instituto Oswaldo Cruz. 2009;104(2):358-63.

[57] Dubey J, Gennari S, Lago E, Su C, Jones J. Toxoplasmosis in humans and animals in Brazil: high prevalence, high burden of disease, and epidemiology. Parasitology. 2012. doi:10.1017/S0031182012000765

Chapter 9

Pseudo Toxoplasmosis

Yoshiaki Shimada

Additional information is available at the end of the chapter

http://dx.doi.org/10.5772/50708

1. Introduction

Signs that may be included in the clinical presentation of congenital toxoplasmosis may be observed in infants without identification of *Toxoplasma gondii* or other intrauterine infection. When congenital toxoplasmosis is excluded, these case are diagnosed as having pseudo toxoplasmosis (Hervouet, 1961), pseudo-TORCH (*toxoplasma,* rubella, cytomegalovirus, and herpes simplex) syndrome (Baraitser et al., 1983; Burn et al., 1986; Cohen et al., 2012; Ishitsu et al., 1985; Knoblauch et al., 2003; Kulkarni et al., 2010; Nakamura et al., 2011; Reardon et al., 1994; Vivarelli et al., 2001; Watts et al., 2008; Wieczorek et al., 1995) or congenital infection-like syndrome (Abdel-Salam & Zaki, 2009; al-Dabbous et al., 1998; al-Gazali et al., 1999; Dale et al., 2000; Knoblauch et al., 2003; Kulkarni et al., 2010; Mishra et al., 2002; Mizuno et al., 2011; Slee et al.,1999).

These signs include microcephaly (Aalfs et al., 1995; Abdel-Salam & Zaki, 2009; Abdel-Salam et al., 1999; Abdel-Salam et al., 2000; Ahmadi & Bradfield, 2007; Aicardi & Goutières, 1984; al-Dabbous et al., 1998; al-Gazali et al., 1999; Alzial et al., 1980; Angle et al., 1994; Atchaneeyasakul et al., 1998; Baraitser et al., 1983; Bogdan, 1951; Book et al., 1953; Briggs et al., 2008; Burn et al., 1986; Cantú et al., 1977; Casteels et al., 2001; Dale et al., 2000; Eventov-Friedman et al., 2009; Feingold & Bartoshesky 1992; Fisch et al., 1973; Fryns et al., 1995; Hoyeraal et al., 1970; Hordijk et al., 1996; Hreidarsson et al., 1988; Ishitsu et al., 1985; Jarmas et al., 1981; Kloepfer et al., 1964; Knoblauch et al., 2003; Komai et al., 1955; Kozma et al., 1996; Kulkarni et al., 2010; Leung, 1985; Limwongse et al., 1999; McKusick et al., 1966; Mishra et al., 2002; Nakamura et al., 2011; Nemos et al., 2009; Ostergaard et al., 2012; Pearson et al., 2008; Reardon et al., 1994; Sadler & Robinson, 1993; Simonell et al., 2002; Slee et al., 1999; Strauss et al., 2005; Tenconi et al., 1981; Trzupek et al., 2007; van den Bosch, 1959; van Genderen et al., 1997; Vasudevan et al., 2005; Vivarelli et al., 2001; Warburg & Heuer, 1994; Wieczorek et al., 1995), intracranial calcifications (Abdel-Salam & Zaki, 2009; Aicardi & Goutières, 1984; al-Dabbous et al., 1998; al-Gazali et al., 1999; Asai et al., 2012; Baraitser et al., 1983; Bogdan, 1951; Briggs et al., 2008; Burn et al., 1986; Cohen et al., 2012; Dale et al., 2000;

Hervouet, 1961; Ishitsu et al., 1985; Knoblauch et al., 2003; Kulkarni et al., 2010; Mishra et al., 2002; Mizuno et al., 2011; Nakamura et al., 2011; Reardon et al., 1994; Revesz et al., 1992; Slee et al., 1999; Vivarelli et al., 2001; Watts et al., 2008; Wieczorek et al., 1995) and retinal changes (Abdel-Salam et al., 1999; Abdel-Salam et al., 2000; Ahmadi & Bradfield, 2007; Alzial et al., 1980; Angle et al., 1994; Asai et al., 2012; Atchaneeyasakul et al., 1998; Bogdan, 1951; Burn et al., 1986; Cantú et al., 1977; Casteels et al., 2001; Eventov-Friedman et al., 2009; Feingold & Bartoshesky 1992; Fryns et al., 1995; Hervouet, 1961; Hordijk et al., 1996; King et al., 1998; Limwongse et al., 1999; McKusick et al., 1966; Revesz et al., 1992; Sadler & Robinson, 1993; Simonell et al., 2002; Strauss et al., 2005; Tenconi et al., 1981; Trzupek et al., 2007; van Genderen et al., 1997; Vasudevan et al., 2005; Warburg & Heuer, 1994; Watts et al., 2008).

The majority of the cases have a family history (Abdel-Salam & Zaki, 2009; Aicardi & Goutières, 1984; al-Dabbous et al., 1998; al-Gazali et al., 1999; Alzial et al., 1980; Atchaneeyasakul et al., 1998; Baraitser et al., 1983; Bogdan, 1951; Book et al., 1953; Briggs et al., 2008; Burn et al., 1986; Cantú et al., 1977; Cohen et al., 2012; Dale et al., 2000; Fisch et al., 1973; Hordijk et al., 1996; Ishitsu et al., 1985; Jarmas et al., 1981; Knoblauch et al., 2003; Kozma et al., 1996; Leung, 1985; Limwongse et al., 1999; McKusick et al., 1966; Reardon et al., 1994; Sadler & Robinson, 1993; Simonell et al., 2002; Slee et al., 1999; Trzupek et al., 2007; van Genderen et al., 1997; Vivarelli et al., 2001; Warburg & Heuer, 1994), and thus a genetic basis has been proposed.

To diagnose the clinical entities described below, evidence of congenital infection including toxoplasmosis is the most important exclusion criterion. Misdiagnosis would result in erroneous counseling as to risk of recurrence (Aicardi et al., 2012).

2. Clinical entities

2.1. Aicardi syndrome

2.1.1. Overview

Aicardi syndrome (MIM: 304050) is a congenital disorder characterized by a triad of signs, including corpus callosum agenesis, severe epilepsy, and chorioretinal lacunae (Aicardi et al., 1965; Dennis & Bower, 1972).

2.1.2. History

In 1965, Aicardi et al. reported eight female infants with spasms in flexion, callosal agenesis and various ocular abnormalities. In 1972, Dennis & Bower also reported a female patient and established the Aicardi Syndrome.

2.1.3. Genetics

The Aicardi syndrome is believed to an X-linked dominant disorder lethal to males and the cases of Aicardi syndrome are female infants, and males with the XXY genotype (Hopkins et al., 1979). Mutations in the CDKL5 gene on chromosome Xp22 have been found in these patients (Nemos et al., 2009).

2.1.4. Differential diagnosis

Although the Aicardi syndrome normally has a poor prognosis, there is a heterogeneity of clinical severity. A mild case of a chorioretinal defect and a hypoplastic disc has been reported (King et al., 1998). The case was misdiagnosed as having cerebral and retinal toxoplasmosis.

The presence of corpus dysgenesis supports the diagnosis of Aicardi syndrome. In addition, the Aicardi syndrome does not cause intracranial calcifications which are likely to be present in cases of congenital toxoplasmosis (Table 1). Ocular abnormality is various, however, chorioretinal lacunae are thought to be pathognomonic.

		inheritance	microcephaly	intracranial calcification	retinal changes	
2.1	Aicardi Syndrome MIM: 304050	X-linked dominant	+	-	+ (chorioretinal lacuna)	corpus agenesis
2.2	Aicardi-Goutières Syndrome (AGS) MIM: 225750, 610181, 610329, 610333, 612952	autosomal recessive	+ (post-natal)	+ (basal ganglia)	-	CSF lymphocytosis
2.3	Hoyeraal-Hreidarsson syndrome (HHS) MIM: 300240	X-linked recessive	+	-	-	severe aplastic anemia
2.4	Microcephaly, lymphedema, chorioretinal dysplasia syndrome (MLCRD) MIM: 152950	autosomal dominant	+	-	+ (chorioretinal dysplasia)	pedal lymphedema
2.5	Microcephaly and chorioretinopathy with or without mental retardation, autosomal recessive MIM: 251270	autosomal recessive	+	-	+ (chorioretinal dysplasia)	
2.6	Pseudo-TORCH syndrome (narrowly-defined) MIM: 251290	autosomal recessive	+	+	-	overlapping with AGS (2.2)
2.7	Revesz syndrome MIM: 268130	autosomal dominant	not apparent	+	+ (exudative retinopathy)	severe aplastic anemia
	congenital toxoplasmosis	-	+	+	+	

Table 1. Clinical findings of the patients affected by congnetial toxoplasmosis and the pseudo toxoplasmosis

2.2. Aicardi-Goutières Syndrome (AGS)

2.2.1. Overview

The AGS is a rare neurodevelopmental genetic disorder associated with intracranial calcification, leukocytosis in the cerebrospinal fluid (CSF), and microcephaly. (Aicardi & Goutières, 1984; Aicardi et al., 2012)

2.2.2. History

In 1984, Aicardi & Goutières reported eight infants with spasticity, acquired microcephaly, bilateral symmetrical calcifications in the basal ganglia and chronic CSF lymphocytosis in five consanguineous families.

2.2.3. Genetics

Approximately 90% of individuals with characteristic findings of AGS have been found to have mutations in the TREX1 gene on chromosome 3p21.31 (AGS1, MIM: 225750), RNASEH2A gene on chromosome 19p13.2 (AGS4, MIM: 610333), RNASEH2B gene on chromosome 13q14.3 (AGS2, MIM: 610181), RNASEH2C gene on chromosome 11q13.1 (AGS3, MIM: 610329), and SAMHD1 gene on chromosome 20q11.23 (AGS5, MIM: 612952). (Aicardi et al., 2012)

Mutations in TREX1 have also been found in some patients with systemic lupus erythematodes (SLE). Siblings with SLE who present with congenital infection-like intracranial calcification (Dale et al., 2000), may be associated with AGS. (Aicardi et al., 2012) It has also been suggested that the narrowly-defined pseudo-TORCH syndrome (2.6) shows a phenotypic overlap and that most cases of pseudo-TORCH syndrome are in fact AGS. (Aicardi et al., 2012)

2.2.4. Differential diagnosis

In case of AGS, leukocytosis in the CSF and increased concentrations of interferon-alfa (IFN-α) in the CSF are found (Aicardi et al., 2012) and microcephaly is absent at birth (Aicardi & Goutières, 1984). The onset occurs at 3-6 months of age in many patients.

Ocular structures are almost invariably normal on examination. (Aicardi et al., 2012) (Table 1)

2.3. Hoyeraal-Hreidarsson syndrome (HHS)

2.3.1. Overview

The HHS (MIM: 300240) is a severe multisystemic disorder with pre- and postnatal growth retardation, progressive pancytopenia, microcephaly, and cerebellar hypoplasia. (Aalfs et al., 1995; Knight et al., 1999; Pearson et al., 2008)

2.3.2. *History*

In 1970, Hoyeraal et al. reported two brothers with hypoplastic thrombocytopenia, microcephaly and cerebral malformations. In 1988, Hreidarsson et al. also reported an affected boy. In 1995, Aalfs et al. reported another male patient and proposed to use the eponym HHS. The first symptoms of pancytopenia did not occur before the age of five months and continued to deteriorate for years, despite extensive therapeutic measures.

2.3.3. *Genetics*

Mutations in the DKC1 gene on chromosome Xq28 have been found in the patients including the family reported by Aalfs et al. in 1995. (Knight et al., 1999) The gene is also responsible for X-linked dyskeratosis congenita (DKC, MIM: 305000), an inherited bone-marrow-failure syndrome characterized by skin pigmentation, nail dystrophy and leucoplakia which usually develop towards the end of the first decade of life. The HHS is revealed to be a severe variant of DKC. (Knight et al., 1999; Pearson et al., 2008)

2.3.4. *Differential diagnosis*

The HHS is marked by severe aplastic anemia. While retinopathy can be induced by anemia, ocular abnormality or intracranial calcification is not usually observed in cases of HSS. (Table 1)

2.4. Microcephaly, lymphedema, chorioretinal dysplasia syndrome (MLCRD)

2.4.1. *Overview*

As its name implies, the MLCRD (MIM: 152950) is characterized by a triad of signs including microcephaly, lymphedema, and chorioretinal dysplasia. (Angle et al., 1994; Casteels et al., 2001; Eventov-Friedman et al., 2009; Feingold & Bartoshesky 1992; Fryns et al., 1995; Limwongse et al., 1999; Ostergaard et al., 2012; Strauss et al., 2005; Vasudevan et al., 2005). Mental retardation is also usually present. Different combinations of these signs inherited in an autosomal dominant pattern have been reported (Leung, 1985; Hordijk et al., 1996; Simonell et al., 2002). Cases with these signs have been assumed to belong to the same spectrum of genetic disorders.

An autosomal recessive form of microcephaly with chorioretinopathy (McKusick et al., 1966) has been reported and categorized as microcephaly and chorioretinopathy with or without mental retardation, autosomal recessive (MIM: 251270) (2.5).

2.4.2. *History*

In 1981, Tenconi et al. reported patients with microcephaly and chorioretinopathy in an autosomal dominant pattern, and Jarmas et al. reported two brothers with microcephaly and retinal folds. In 1985, Leung investigated the combination of microcephaly and lymphedema in at least 4 generations of a Chinese family. In 1992, Feingold & Bartoshesky described two unrelated boys with microcephaly, lymphedema and chorioretinal dysplasia and proposed that the combination represents a single syndrome.

2.4.3. Genetics

Mutations in the KIF11 gene on chromosome 10q23 have been identified in some patients with the MLCRD. (Ostergaard et al., 2012)

2.4.4. Differential diagnosis

Congenital lymphedema is confined to the dorsa of the feet (Angle et al., 1994; Casteels et al., 2001; Eventov-Friedman et al., 2009; Feingold & Bartoshesky 1992; Fryns et al., 1995; Leung, 1985; Limwongse et al., 1999; Strauss et al., 2005; Vasudevan et al., 2005) and this is hardly observed in cases of congenital toxoplasmosis. (Table 1)

Intracranial calcifications, which are likely to be present in cases of congenital toxoplasmosis are not observed in cases of MLCRD. (Table 1)

2.5. Microcephaly and chorioretinopathy with or without mental retardation, autosomal recessive

2.5.1. Overview

While the combination of microcephaly and chorioretinopathy with or without mental retardation can be caused by heterozygous mutation in the KIF11 gene known as MLCRD (MIM: 152950) (2.4), autosomal recessive inheritance has also been suggested in familial cases (McKusick et al., 1966). A discovery of causative homozygous mutation (Puffenberger et al., 2012) has proved the independent entity, microcephaly and chorioretinopathy with or without mental retardation, autosomal recessive (MIM: 251270).

2.5.2. History

The role of consanguinity in congenital microcephaly was repeatedly reported (Kloepfer et al., 1964; Komai et al., 1955; van den Bosch, 1959). In 1966, McKusick et al. described eight individuals of microcephaly in two sibships of an imbred group. All of them had pigmentary abnormality of the fundus with mental retardation.

2.5.3. Genetics

A homozygous mutation in the TUBGCP6 gene on chromosome 22q13.33 was found in four cases reported by McKusick et al. in 1966. (Puffenberger et al., 2012)

2.5.4. Differential diagnosis

Microcephaly and chorioretinopathy with or without mental retardation, autosomal recessive produces the symptoms similar to those of the MLCRD (MIM: 152950) spectrum

(2.4). Intracranial calcifications are not observed as in MLCRD. (Table 1) Lymphedema is considered to be pathognomonic for the MLCRD, has not been reported in cases of Microcephaly and chorioretinopathy with or without mental retardation, autosomal recessive. (Table 1)

2.6 Pseudo-TORCH syndrome (narrowly-defined)

2.6.1. Overview

Narrowly-defined pseudo-TORCH syndrome (al-Dabbous et al., 1998; Baraitser et al., 1983; Briggs et al., 2008; Burn et al., 1986; Cohen et al., 2012; Ishitsu et al., 1985; Knoblauch et al., 2003; Kulkarni et al., 2010; Nakamura et al., 2011; Reardon et al., 1994; Vivarelli et al., 2001; Watts et al., 2008; Wieczorek et al. 1995), also called Baraitser-Reardon syndrome (Vivarelli et al., 2001), or band-like calcification with simplified gyration and polymicrogyria (BLCPMG; MIM: 251290) (Abdel-Salam & Zaki, 2009; Briggs et al., 2008; O'Driscoll et al., 2010), is associated with microcephaly and intracranial calcifications mimicking congenital toxoplasmosis in the absence of infection.

2.6.2. History

In 1983, Baraitser et al. reported two brothers with microcephaly and intracranial calcifications. The bilateral symmetrical calcification was in white matter and thalamus. In 1994, Reardon et al. reported nine patients from four families with microcephaly, intracranial calcifications and CNS disease and described them as "congenital intrauterine infection-like syndrome".

In 2001, Vivarelli et al. reported five patients in three families and proposed to use the eponym, Baraitser-Reardon syndrome. In 2008, Briggs et al. also reported five patients in three families with a pattern of BLCPMG as a distinct "pseudo-TORCH" phenotype.

2.6.3. Genetics

Mutations in the OCLN gene on chromosome 5q13.2 have been found in a part of affected individuals, categorized as BLCPMG. (O'Driscoll et al., 2010) A part of the cases of the pseudo-TORCH syndrome without the OCLN mutation may in fact be cases of Aicardi-Goutières Syndrome (2.2). (Aicardi et al., 2012)

2.6.4. Differential diagnosis

As some cases of pseudo-TORCH syndrome are thought to be in fact AGS (Aicardi et al., 2012), there is a phenotype overlap between pseudo-TORCH syndrome and AGS (2.2).

Ocular changes are not reported with pseudo-TORCH syndrome / AGS. (Table 1)

2.7. Revesz syndrome

2.7.1. Overview

Revesz syndrome (MIM: 268130), also known as cerebroretinal microangiopathy with calcifications and cysts (CRMCC) is a rare and fatal disorder, characterized by intrauterine growth retardation, bilateral exudative retinopathy, intracranial calcification and cysts. (Asai et al., 2012; Revesz et al. 1992; Savage et al., 2008)

2.7.2. History

In 1992, Revesz et al. reported a 6-month old boy presenting with bilateral leucocoria. The retinal appearance resembled Coat's disease. Widespread grey and white matter calcification in the brain and severe aplastic anemia were also noted. His platelet count eventually became impossible to control and the patient died at 19 months of age. In 1994, Kajtár & Méhes reported the second case, a 2-year old girl with thrombocytopenic purpura and bilateral progressive Coats'-like retinopathy.

2.7.3. Genetics

A heterozygous mutation in the gene encoding TRF1-interacting nuclear factor-2 (TINF2) on chromosome 14q12 has been found in a case of Revesz syndrome. (Savage et al., 2008) Another heterozygous truncating mutation in the TINF2 gene has been identified in a case. (Sasa et al., 2012) TINF2 is a component of the shelterin telomere protection complex, TINF2 mutations result in very short telomeres.

An inherited bone marrow failure syndrome, dyskeratosis congenital-3 (MIM: 613990) is also caused by the mutations in the TINF2 mutations.

2.7.4. Differential diagnosis

While Revesz syndrome marked by the severe aplastic anemia is related to HHS (2.3), Revesz syndrome causes Coats'-like retinopathy and intracranial calcification. A case reported as "congenital infection-like syndrome with intracranial calcification" (Mizuno et al., 2011) may be a case of Revesz syndrome. (Asai et al., 2012)

Coats'-like retinopathy is exudative, easily distinguishable from chorioretinal lacunae or dysplasia on ophthalmoscopy. (Table 1)

3. Pseudo-pseudo toxoplasmosis

3.1. Background

Even though clinical differential diagnosis summarized in Table 1 can be helpful, there are exceptions. A case of congenital toxoplasmosis can have the look of one of pseudo toxoplasmosis entities. A serological investigation for toxoplasmosis also has its indications and limitations. (Johnson et al., 1993).

3.2. Case report

A male infant was delivered by Cesarean section at 37 weeks of gestation. (Ozeki et al., 2010) There was no family history for microcephaly, retinitis pigmentosa or consanguinity. The mother was type 1 diabetic and had once experienced an intrauterine fetal death. At 20 weeks pregnant, microcephaly had been detected by ultrasonography. Toxoplasmosis had been suspected, but the treatment was withheld because of only a slightly elevated maternal *Toxoplasma* specific immunoglobulin M (IgM) antibody, 1.4 index by enzyme linked immnosorbent assay (ELISA) and a borderline IgG avidity index, 50% at 28 weeks pregnant.

The infant weighing 2,858 g with Apgar score 9/10, respectively, had microcephaly, marked lymphoedema of dorsum of both feet and chorioretinal dysplasia in the both eyes (Figure 1). The electroretinogram was nearly nonrecordable. A computed tomography (CT) scan was negative for brain calcifications or hydrocephalus. Hepatic calcifications, splenomegaly, and ascites were not noted. *Toxoplasma* IgM (ELISA) was negative (0.1 index) while IgG was positive (70 index).

Toxoplasma gondii DNA was detected in the serum by polymerase chain reaction (PCR) (Figure 1(d)) to confirm the diagnosis of congenital toxoplasmosis.

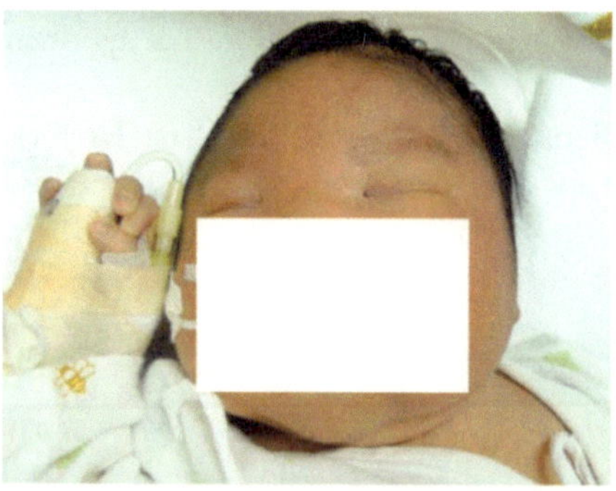

(a) microcephaly

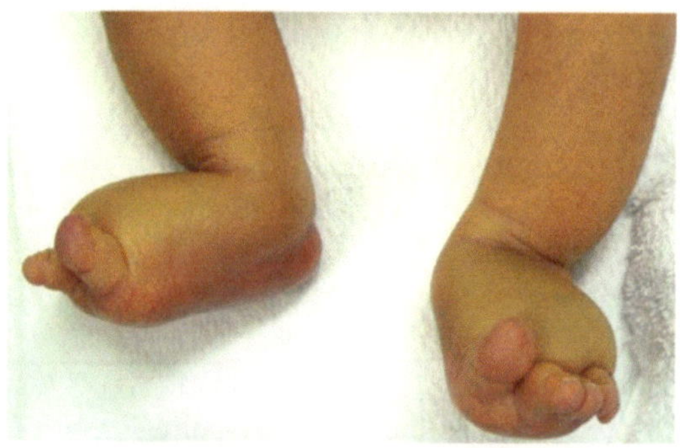

(b) lymphedema confined to the dorsum of the feet

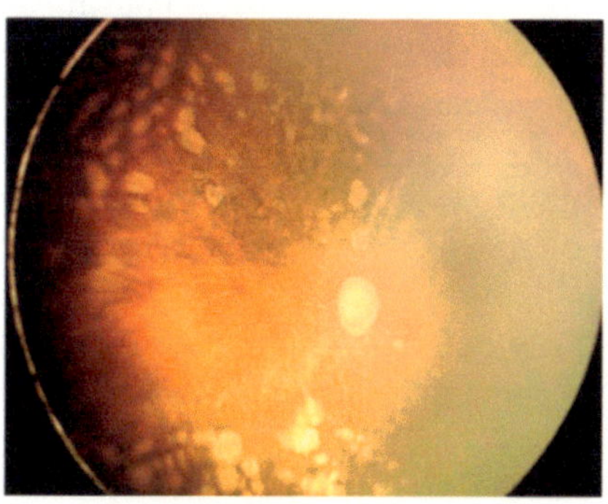

(c) chorioretinal dysplasia

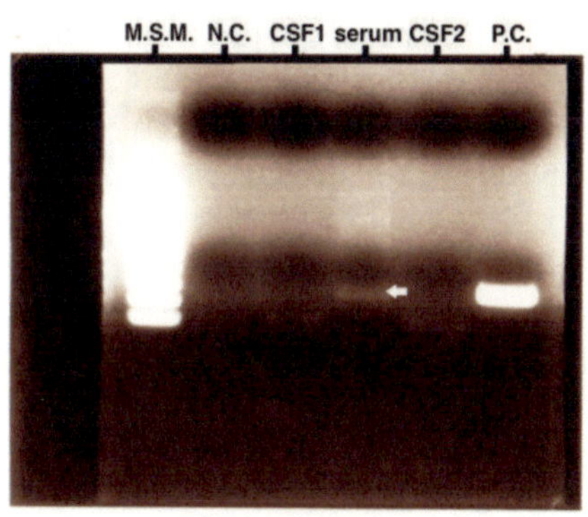

(d) PCR showing positive *Toxoplasma gondii* DNA

Figure 1.

3.3. Comment

The newborn presented with the complete triad of the MLCRD (2.4), i.e., microcephaly, lymphedema and chorioretinal dysplasia. (Table 1) He had apparent dorsal lymphedema that is hardly observed with toxoplasmosis. Brain calcifications, hydrocephalus, ascites or splenomegaly, that are more likely present in cases of congenital toxoplasmosis, could not be found. Moreover, *Toxoplasma* IgM was negative.

The present case indicates that suspected cases of congenital toxoplasmosis or pseudo toxoplasmosis should be examined for *Toxoplasma* DNA by PCR. (Ozeki et al., 2010)

Author details

Yoshiaki Shimada
Fujita Health University Banbuntane Hotokukai Hospital, Japan

4. References

Aalfs, C. M. & Hennekam, R. C. (1995). Differences between the Hoyeraal-Hreidarsson syndrome and an autosomal recessive congenital intrauterine infection-like syndrome, Am J Med Genet 58(4):385.

Aalfs, C. M., van den Berg, H., Barth, P. G. & Hennekam, R. C. (1995). The Hoyeraal-Hreidarsson syndrome: the fourth case of a separate entity with prenatal growth retardation, progressive pancytopenia and cerebellar hypoplasia, Eur J Pediatr 154(4):304-308.

Abdel-Salam, G. M., Czeizel, A. E., Vogt, G. & Imre, L. (2000). Microcephaly with chorioretinal dysplasia: characteristic facial features, Am J Med Genet 95(5):513-515.

Abdel-Salam, G. M., Vogt, G., Halász, A. & Czeizel, A. (1999). Microcephaly with normal intelligence, and chorioretinopathy, Ophthalmic Genet 20(4):259-264.

Abdel-Salam, G. M. & Zaki, M. S. (2009). Band-like intracranial calcification (BIC), microcephaly and malformation of brain development: a distinctive form of congenital infection like syndromes, Am J Med Genet A 149A(7):1565-1568.

Aicardi, J., Crow, Y. J. & Stephenson, J. B. P. (2012). Aicardi-Goutières Syndrome, in Pagon, R. A., Bird, T. D., Dolan, C. R, Stephens, K. & Adam, M. P. of Editors., SourceGeneReviews™ [Internet]. Seattle (WA): University of Washington, Seattle; 1993-. 2005 Jun 29 [updated 2012 Mar 01].

Aicardi, J. & Goutières, F. (1984). A progressive familial encephalopathy in infancy with calcifications of the basal ganglia and chronic cerebrospinal fluid lymphocytosis, Ann Neurol 5(1):49-54.

Aicardi, J., Lefebvre, J. & Lerique Koechlin, A. (1965). A new syndrome: Spasms in flexion, callosal agenesis, ocular abnormalities, Electroencephalogr Clin Neurophysiol 19(6):609-610.

Ahmadi, H. & Bradfield, Y. S. (2007). Chorioretinopathy and microcephaly with normal development, Ophthalmic Genet 28(4):210-215.

al-Dabbous, R., Sabry, M. A., Farah, S., al-Awadi, S. A., Simeonov, S. & Farag, T. I. (1998). The autosomal recessive congenital intrauterine infection-like syndrome of microcephaly, intracranial calcification, and CNS disease: report of another Bedouin family, Clin Dysmorphol 7(2):127-130.

al-Gazali, L. I., Sztriha, L., Dawodu, A., Varady, E., Bakir, M., Khdir, A. & Johansen, J. (1999). Complex consanguinity associated with short rib-polydactyly syndrome III and congenital infection-like syndrome: a diagnostic problem in dysmorphic syndromes, J Med Genet 36(6):461-466.

Alzial, C., Dufier, J. L., Aicardi, J., de Grouchy, J. & Saraux H. (1980). Ocular abnormalities of true microcephaly, Ophthalmologica 180(6):333-339.

Angle, B., Holgado, S., Burton, B. K, Miller, M. T., Shapiro, M. J. & Opitz, J. M. (1994). Microcephaly, lymphedema, and chorioretinal dysplasia: report of two additional cases, Am J Med Genet 53(2):99-101.

Asai, D., Imamura, T. & Hosoi, H. (2012). Comments on the article by Mizuno Y. et al. entitled "Congenital infection-like syndrome with intracranial calcification", Brain Dev 34(6):539.

Atchaneeyasakul, L. O., Linck, L. & Weleber, R. G. (1998). Microcephaly with chorioretinal degeneration, Ophthalmic Genet 19(1):39-48.

Baraitser, M., Brett, E. M. & Piesowicz, A. T. (1983). Microcephaly and intracranial calcification in two brothers, J Med Genet 20(3):210-212.

Bogdan, A. (1951). Microcephaly with chorioretinopathy, cerebral calcification and internal hydrocephalus, Proc R Soc Med 44(3):225-226.

Book, J. A., Schut, J. W. & Reed, S. C. (1953). A clinical and genetical study of microcephaly, Am J Ment Defic 57(4):637-660.

Briggs, T. A., Wolf, N. I., D'Arrigo, S., Ebinger, F., Harting, I., Dobyns, W. B., Livingston, J. H., Rice, G. I., Crooks, D., Rowland-Hill, C. A., Squier, W., Stoodley, N., Pilz, D. T. & Crow, Y. J. (2008). Band-like intracranial calcification with simplified gyration and polymicrogyria: a distinct "pseudo-TORCH" phenotype, Am J Med Genet A 146A(24):3173-3180.

Burn, J., Wickramasinghe, H. T., Harding, B. & Baraitser, M. (1986). A syndrome with intracranial calcification and microcephaly in two sibs, resembling intrauterine infection, Clin Genet 30(2):112-116.

Cantú, J. M., Rojas, J. A., García-Cruz, D., Hernández, A., Pagán, P., Fragoso, R. & Manzano, C. (1977). Autosomal recessive microcephaly associated with chorioretinopathy, Hum Genet 36(2):243-247.

Casteels, I., Devriendt, K., Van Cleynenbreugel, H., Demaerel, P., De Tavernier, F. & Fryns, J. P. (2001). Autosomal dominant microcephaly--lymphoedema-chorioretinal dysplasia syndrome, Br J Ophthalmol 85(4):499-500.

Cohen, M. C., Karaman, I., Squier, W., Farrel, T. & Whitby, E. H. (2011). Recurrent pseudo-torch appearences of the brain presenting as "dandy-walker" malformation, Pediatr Dev Pathol 15(1):45-49.

Dale, R. C., Tang, S. P., Heckmatt, J. Z. & Tatnall, F. M. (2000). Familial systemic lupus erythematosus and congenital infection-like syndrome, Neuropediatrics 31(3):155-158.

Dennis, J. & Bower, B. D. (1972). The Aicardi syndrome, Dev Med Child Neurol 14(3):382-390.

Eventov-Friedman, S., Singer, A. & Shinwell, E. S. (2009). Microcephaly, lymphedema, chorioretinopathy and atrial septal defect: a case report and review of the literature, Acta Paediatr 98(4):758-759.

Feingold, M. & Bartoshesky, L. (1992). Microcephaly, lymphedema, and chorioretinal dysplasia: a distinct syndrome? Am J Med Genet 43(6):1030-1031.

Fisch, R. O., Ketterling, W. C., Schacht, L. E. & Letson, R. D. (1973). Ocular abnormalities of a child associated with familial microcephaly, Am J Ophthalmol 76(2):260-264.

Fryns, J. P., Smeets, E. & Van den Berghe, H. (1995). On the nosology of the "primary true microcephaly, chorioretinal dysplasia, lymphoedema" association, Clin Genet 48(3):131-133.

Hervouet, M. F. (1961). Apropos of pseudo-toxoplasmosis, Bull Soc Ophtalmol Fr 4:223-226.

Hoyeraal, H. M., Lamvik, J. & Moe, P. J. (1970). Congenital hypoplastic thrombocytopenia and cerebral malformations in two brothers, Acta Paediatr Scand 59(2):185-191.

Hopkins, I. J., Humphrey, I., Keith, C. G., Susman, M., Webb, G. C. & Turner, E. K. (1979). The Aicardi syndrome in a 47, XXY male, Aust Paediatr J 15(4):278-280.

Hordijk, R., Van de Logt, F., Houtman, W. A. & Van Essen, A. J. (1996). Chorioretinal dysplasia-microcephaly-mental retardation syndrome: another family with autosomal dominant inheritance, Genet Couns 7(2):113-122.

Hreidarsson, S., Kristjansson, K., Johannesson, G. & Johannsson, J. H. (1988). A syndrome of progressive pancytopenia with microcephaly, cerebellar hypoplasia and growth failure, Acta Paediatr Scand 77(5):773-775.

Ishitsu, T., Chikazawa, S. & Matsuda, I. (1985). Two siblings with microcephaly associated with calcification of cerebral white matter, Jpn J Human Genet 30(3):213-217.

Jarmas, A. L., Weaver, D. D., Ellis, F. D. & Davis, A. (1981). Microcephaly, microphthalmia, falciform retinal folds, and blindness. A new syndrome, Am J Dis Child 135(10):930-933.

Johnson, J. D., Butcher, P. D., Savva, D. & Holliman, R. E. (1993). Application of the polymerase chain reaction to the diagnosis of human toxoplasmosis, J Infect 26(2):147-158.

Kajtár, P. & Méhes, K. (1994). Bilateral coats retinopathy associated with aplastic anaemia and mild dyskeratotic signs, Am J Med Genet 49(4):374-377.

King, A. M., Bowen, D.I., Goulding, P. & Doran, R. M. (1998). Aicardi syndrome, Br J Ophthalmol 82(4):457.

Kloepfer, H.W., Platou, R. V. & Hansche, W. J. (1964). Manifestations of a recessive gene for microcephaly in a population isolate, J Genet Hum 13:52-59.

Knight, S. W., Heiss, N. S., Vulliamy, T. J., Aalfs, C. M., McMahon, C., Richmond, P., Jones, A., Hennekam, R. C., Poustka, A., Mason, P. J. & Dokal, I. (1999). Unexplained aplastic anaemia, immunodeficiency, and cerebellar hypoplasia (Hoyeraal-Hreidarsson syndrome) due to mutations in the dyskeratosis congenita gene, DKC1, Br J Haematol 107(2):335-339.

Knoblauch, H., Tennstedt, C., Brueck, W., Hammer, H., Vulliamy, T., Dokal, I., Lehmann, R., Hanefeld, F. & Tinschert, S. (2003). Two brothers with findings resembling congenital intrauterine infection-like syndrome (pseudo-TORCH syndrome), Am J Med Genet A 120A(2):261-265.

Komai, T., Kishimoto, K. & Ozaki, Y. (1955). Genetic study of microcephaly based on Japanese material, Am J Hum Genet 7(1): 51–65.

Kozma, C., Scribanu, N. & Gersh, E. (1996). The microcephaly-lymphoedema syndrome: report of an additional family, Clin Dysmorphol 5(1):49-54.

Kulkarni, A.M., Baskar, S., Kulkarni, M. L., Kulkarni, A. J., Mahuli, A. V, Vittalrao, S. & Kulkarni, P. M. (2010). Fetal intracranial calcification: pseudo-TORCH phenotype and discussion of related phenotypes, Am J Med Genet A 152A(4):930-937.

Leung, A. K. (1985). Dominantly inherited syndrome of microcephaly and congenital lymphedema, Clin Genet 27(6):611-612.

Limwongse, C., Wyszynski, R. E., Dickerman, L.H. & Robin, N. H. (1999). Microcephaly-lymphedema-chorioretinal dysplasia: a unique genetic syndrome with variable expression and possible characteristic facial appearance, Am J Med Genet 86(3):215-218.

McKusick, V. A., Stauffer, M., Knox, D. L. & Clark, D. B. (1966). Chorioretinopathy with hereditary microcephaly, Arch Ophthalmol 75(5):597-600.

Mishra, D., Gupta, V. K., Nandan, D. & Behal, D. (2002). Congenital intrauterine infection like syndrome of microcephaly, intracranial calcification and CNS disease, Indian Pediatr 39(9):866-869.

Mizuno, Y., Takahashi, K., Igarashi, T., Saito, M. & Mizuguchi, M. (2011). Congenital infection-like syndrome with intracranial calcification, Brain Dev 33(6):530-533.

Nakamura, K., Kato, M., Sasaki, A., Kanai, M. & Hayasaka, K. (2011). Congenital dysplastic microcephaly and hypoplasia of the brainstem and cerebellum with diffuse intracranial calcification, J Child Neurol 27(2):218-221.

Nemos, C., Lambert, L., Giuliano, F., Doray, B., Roubertie, A., Goldenberg, A., Delobel, B., Layet, V., N'guyen, M. A., Saunier, A., Verneau, F., Jonveaux, P. & Philippe, C. (2009). Mutational spectrum of CDKL5 in early-onset encephalopathies: a study of a large collection of French patients and review of the literature, Clin Genet 76(4):357-371.

O'Driscoll, M. C., Daly, S. B., Urquhart, J. E., Black, G. C., Pilz, D. T., Brockmann, K., McEntagart, M., Abdel-Salam, G., Zaki, M., Wolf, N. I., Ladda, R. L., Sell, S., D'Arrigo, S., Squier, W., Dobyns, W. B., Livingston, J. H. & Crow, Y. J. (2010). Recessive mutations in the gene encoding the tight junction protein occludin cause band-like calcification with simplified gyration and polymicrogyria, Am J Hum Genet 87(3):354-364.

Ostergaard, P., Simpson, M. A., Mendola, A., Vasudevan, P., Connell, F. C., van Impel, A., Moore, A. T., Loeys, B. L., Ghalamkarpour, A., Onoufriadis, A., Martinez-Corral, I., Devery, S., Leroy, J. G., van Laer, L., Singer, A., Bialer, M. G., McEntagart, M., Quarrell, O., Brice, G., Trembath, R. C., Schulte-Merker, S., Makinen, T., Vikkula, M., Mortimer, P. S., Mansour, S. & Jeffery, S. (2012). Mutations in KIF11 cause autosomal-dominant microcephaly variably associated with congenital lymphedema and chorioretinopathy, Am J Hum Genet 90(2):356-362.

Ozeki, Y., Shimada, Y., Tanikawa, A., Horiguchi, M., Takeuchi, M. & Yamazaki, T. (2010). Congenital toxoplasmosis mimicing microcephaly-lymphoedema-chorioretinal dysplasia, Jpn J Ophthalmol 54(6):626-628.

Pearson, T., Curtis, F., Al-Eyadhy, A., Al-Tamemi, S., Mazer, B., Dror, Y., Abish, S., Bale, S., Compton, J., Ray, R., Scott, P. & Der Kaloustian, V. M. (2008). An intronic mutation in DKC1 in an infant with Høyeraal-Hreidarsson syndrome, Am J Med Genet A 146A(16):2159-2161.

Puffenberger, E. G., Jinks, R. N., Sougnez, C., Cibulskis, K., Willert, R. A., Achilly, N. P., Cassidy, R. P., Fiorentini, C. J., Heiken, K. F., Lawrence, J. J., Mahoney, M. H., Miller, C. J., Nair, D. T., Politi, K. A., Worcester, K. N., Setton, R. A., Dipiazza, R., Sherman, E. A., Eastman, J. T., Francklyn, C., Robey-Bond, S., Rider, N. L., Gabriel, S., Morton, D. H. & Strauss, K. A. (2012). Genetic mapping and exome sequencing identify variants associated with five novel diseases, PLoS One 7(1):e28936.

Reardon, W., Hockey, A., Silberstein, P., Kendall, B., Farag, T. I., Swash, M., Stevenson, R. & Baraitser, M. (1994). Autosomal recessive congenital intrauterine infection-like syndrome of microcephaly, intracranial calcification, and CNS disease, Am J Med Genet 52(1):58-65.

Revesz, T., Fletcher, S., al-Gazali, L.I. & DeBuse, P. (1992). Bilateral retinopathy, aplastic anaemia, and central nervous system abnormalities: a new syndrome?, J Med Genet 29(9):673-675.

Sadler, L. S. & Robinson, L. K. (1993). Chorioretinal dysplasia-microcephaly-mental retardation syndrome: report of an American family, Am J Med Genet 47(1):65-68.

Sasa, G. S., Ribes-Zamora, A., Nelson, N. D., Bertuch, A. A. (2012). Three novel truncating TINF2 mutations causing severe dyskeratosis congenita in early childhood, Clin Genet 81(5):470-478.

Savage, S. A., Giri, N., Baerlocher, G. M., Orr, N., Lansdorp, P. M. & Alter, B. P. (2008). TINF2, a component of the shelterin telomere protection complex, is mutated in dyskeratosis congenita, Am J Hum Genet 82(2):501-509.

Simonell, F., Testa, F., Nesti, A., de Crecchio, G., Bifani, M., Cavaliere, M. L., Rinaldi, E. & Rinaldi, M. M. (2002). An Italian family affected by autosomal dominant microcephaly with chorioretinal degeneration, J Pediatr Ophthalmol Strabismus 39(5):288-292.

Slee, J., Lam, G. & Walpole, I. (1999). Syndrome of microcephaly, microphthalmia, cataracts, and intracranial calcification, Am J Med Genet 84(4):330-333.

Strauss, R. M., Ferguson, A. D., Rittey, C. D. & Cork, M. J. (2005). Microcephaly-lymphoedema-chorioretinal-dysplasia syndrome with atrial septal defect, Pediatr Dermatol 22(4):373-374.

Trzupek, K. M., Falk, R. E., Demer, J. L. & Weleber, R. G. (2007). Microcephaly with chorioretinopathy in a brother-sister pair: evidence for germ line mosaicism and further delineation of the ocular phenotype, Am J Med Genet A 143A(11):1218-1222.

van den Bosch, J. (1959). Microcephaly in the Netherlands: a clinical and genetical study, Ann Hum Genet 23(2):91-116.

van Genderen, M. M., Schuil, J. & Meire, F. M. (1997). Microcephaly with chorioretinopathy. A report of two dominant families and three sporadic cases, Ophthalmic Genet 18(4):199-207.

Vasudevan, P. C., Garcia-Minaur, S., Botella, M. P., Perez-Aytes, A., Shannon, N. L. & Quarrell, O. W. (2005). Microcephaly-lymphoedema-chorioretinal dysplasia: three cases to delineate the facial phenotype and review of the literature, Clin Dysmorphol 14(3):109-116.

Vivarelli, R., Grosso, S., Cioni, M., Galluzzi, P., Monti, L., Morgese, G. & Balestri, P. (2001). Pseudo-TORCH syndrome or Baraitser-Reardon syndrome: diagnostic criteria, Brain Dev 23(1):18-23.

Tenconi, R., Clementi, M., Moschini, G. B., Casara, G. & Baccichetti, C. (1981). Chorio-retinal dysplasia, microcephaly and mental retardation. An autosomal dominant syndrome, Clin Genet 20(5):347-351.

Warburg, M. & Heuer, H. E. (1994). Chorioretinal dysplasia-microcephaly-mental retardation syndrome, Am J Med Genet 52(1):117.

Watts, P., Kumar, N., Ganesh, A., Sastry, P., Pilz, D., Levin, A. V. & Chitayat, D. (2008). Chorioretinal dysplasia, hydranencephaly, and intracranial calcifications: pseudo-TORCH or a new syndrome? Eye 22(5):730-733.

Wieczorek, D., Gillessen-Kaesbach, G. & Passarge, E. (1995). A nine-month-old boy with microcephaly, cataracts, intracerebral calcifications and dysmorphic signs: an additional observation of an autosomal recessive congenital infection-like syndrome? Genet Couns 6(4):297-302.